DSM-5®
Handbook on the Cultural Formulation Interview

DSM-5®
Handbook on the Cultural Formulation Interview

Edited by

Roberto Lewis-Fernández, M.D., M.T.S.
Neil Krishan Aggarwal, M.D., M.B.A., M.A.
Ladson Hinton, M.D.
Devon E. Hinton, M.D., Ph.D.
Laurence J. Kirmayer, M.D.

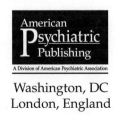

American Psychiatric Publishing
A Division of American Psychiatric Association

Washington, DC
London, England

If you would like to buy between 25 and 99 copies of this or any other American Psychiatric Publishing title, you are eligible for a 20% discount; please contact Customer Service at appi@psych.org or 800-368-5777. If you wish to buy 100 or more copies of the same title, please e-mail us at bulksales@psych.org for a price quote.

Copyright © 2016 American Psychiatric Association
ALL RIGHTS RESERVED

Manufactured in the United States of America on acid-free paper
19   18   17   16   15   5   4   3   2   1
First Edition

Typeset in Adobe's Palatino LT Std and HelveticaNeue LT Std.

American Psychiatric Publishing

A Division of American Psychiatric Association
1000 Wilson Boulevard
Arlington, VA 22209-3901
www.appi.org

Library of Congress Cataloging-in-Publication Data

DSM-5® handbook on the cultural formulation interview / edited by Roberto Lewis-Fernández, Neil Krishan Aggarwal, Ladson Hinton, Devon E. Hinton, Laurence J. Kirmayer. — First edition.
    p. ; cm.
    Handbook on the cultural formulation interview
    Includes bibliographical references and index.
    ISBN 978-1-58562-492-8 (pbk. : alk. paper)
    I. Lewis-Fernández, Roberto, 1958- , editor. II. Aggarwal, Neil Krishan, editor. III. Hinton, Ladson, 1958- , editor. IV. Hinton, Devon E., editor. V. Kirmayer, Laurence J., 1952- , editor. VI. American Psychiatric Association, issuing body. VII. Title: Handbook on the cultural formulation interview.
    [DNLM: 1. Diagnostic and statistical manual of mental disorders. 5th ed. 2. Interview, Psychological—methods. 3. Culturally Competent Care—methods. 4. Ethnopsychology—methods. 5. Mental Disorders—ethnology. WM 143]
    RC467
    616.89—dc23

2015007125

British Library Cataloguing in Publication Data
A CIP record is available from the British Library.

Contents

Contributors

Neil Krishan Aggarwal, M.D., M.B.A., M.A.
Assistant Professor of Clinical Psychiatry, Columbia University; Research Psychiatrist, New York State Psychiatric Institute, New York, New York

Iqbal Ahmed, M.D.
Faculty Psychiatrist, Tripler Army Medical Center, Honolulu, Hawaii; Clinical Professor of Psychiatry, Uniformed Services University for Health Sciences, Bethesda, Maryland; Clinical Professor of Psychiatry and Geriatric Medicine, University of Hawaii, Honolulu, Hawaii

Renato D. Alarcón, M.D., M.P.H.
Emeritus Professor of Psychiatry, Mayo Clinic College of Medicine, Rochester, Minnesota; Honorio Delgado Chair, Universidad Peruana Cayetano Heredia, Lima, Peru

Tichianaa Armah, M.D.
Assistant Clinical Professor of Psychiatry, Yale University School of Medicine, New Haven, Connecticut

Sofie Bäärnhielm, M.D., Ph.D.
Consultant Psychiatrist and Director, Transcultural Centre, Stockholm County Council, Stockholm, Sweden

Kavoos Ghane Bassiri, M.S., LMFT, LPCC, CGP
President and Chief Executive Officer, Richmond Area Multi-Services; Associate Clinical Professor, Department of Psychiatry, University of California San Francisco School of Medicine, San Francisco, California

Triptish Bhatia, Ph.D.
Chief Investigator, Global Research Initiative Program, National Institutes of Health (USA); Department of Psychiatry, Post-Graduate Institute of Medical Education and Research—Dr. Ram Manohar Lohia Hospital, New Delhi, India

James Boehnlein, M.D., M.Sc.
Professor of Psychiatry, Oregon Health & Science University, Portland, Oregon

Francisco Collazos, M.D.
Adjunct Professor of Psychiatry and Legal Medicine, Universitat Autònoma de Barcelona; Staff Psychiatrist, Servei de Psiquiatria, Hospital Universitari Vall d'Hebron, Barcelona, Spain

Lizardo Cruzado, M.D.
Instructor in Psychiatry, Universidad Peruana Cayetano Heredia; Staff Psychiatrist, Instituto Nacional de Salud Mental "Honorio Delgado-Hideyo Noguchi," Lima, Peru

Smita Neelkanth Deshpande, M.D., D.P.M.
Consultant, Professor, and Head, Department of Psychiatry and De-addiction Services, Post-Graduate Institute of Medical Education and Research—Dr. Ram Manohar Lohia Hospital, New Delhi, India

Ravi DeSilva, M.D., M.A.
Associate Director of Inpatient Psychiatry, Milstein Hospital, Columbia University Medical Center, New York, New York.

Esperanza Díaz, M.D.
Associate Professor of Psychiatry, Yale University School of Medicine, New Haven, Connecticut

Irene Falgàs, M.D.
Researcher, Vall d'Hebron Institut de Recerca; Psychiatrist, Servei de Psiquiatria, Hospital Universitari Vall d'Hebron, CIBERSAM, Barcelona, Spain

David M. Gellerman, M.D., Ph.D.
Assistant Clinical Professor of Psychiatry, University of California Davis School of Medicine, Sacramento; Staff Psychiatrist, VA Northern California Health Care System, Mather, California

Simon Groen, M.A.
Cultural Anthropologist, De Evenaar, Centre for Transcultural Psychiatry, GGZ Mental Health Care, Beilen, The Netherlands

Jaswant Guzder, M.D.
Associate Professor, Department of Psychiatry, McGill University; Head of Child Psychiatry, Jewish General Hospital Institute of Community and Family Psychiatry, Montreal, Quebec, Canada

Rita Hargrave, M.D.
Clinical Instructor, University of California Davis School of Medicine, Sacramento, California

Mark L. Hatzenbuehler, Ph.D.
Assistant Professor of Sociomedical Sciences, Mailman School of Public Health, Columbia University, New York, New York

Devon E. Hinton, M.D., Ph.D.
Associate Professor of Psychiatry, Massachusetts General Hospital, Harvard Medical School, Boston, Massachusetts

Ladson Hinton, M.D.
Professor of Psychiatry, University of California Davis School of Medicine, Sacramento, California

Sushrut Jadhav, M.B.B.S., M.D., MRCPsych, Ph.D.
Senior Lecturer in Cross-Cultural Psychiatry, University College London, London, United Kingdom

Oscar Jiménez-Solomon, M.P.H.
Research Coordinator, New York State Center of Excellence for Cultural Competence, New York State Psychiatric Institute, New York, New York

Laurence J. Kirmayer, M.D.
James McGill Professor and Director, Division of Social and Transcultural Psychiatry, McGill University, Montreal, Quebec, Canada

Arthur Kleinman, M.D.
Esther and Sidney Rabb Professor of Anthropology, Department of Anthropology, Harvard University; Professor of Medical Anthropology and Professor of Psychiatry, Department of Global Health and Social Medicine, Harvard Medical School; Victor and William Fung Director, Harvard University Asia Center, Cambridge, Massachusetts

Peter C. Lam, M.P.H.
Data Analyst, New York State Center of Excellence for Cultural Competence, New York State Psychiatric Institute, New York, New York

Martin La Roche, Ph.D.
Assistant Professor of Psychology, Department of Psychiatry, Boston Children's Hospital/Harvard Medical School, Boston, Massachusetts

Roberto Lewis-Fernández, M.D., M.T.S.
Professor of Psychiatry, Columbia University Medical Center; Director, New York State Center of Excellence for Cultural Competence and Hispanic Treatment Program, New York State Psychiatric Institute, New York, New York; Lecturer, Department of Global Health and Social Medicine, Harvard Medical School, Boston, Massachusetts

Russell F. Lim, M.D., M.Ed.
Health Sciences Clinical Professor of Psychiatry and Director of Diversity Education and Training, University of California Davis School of Medicine, Sacramento, California

Francis G. Lu, M.D.
Luke and Grace Kim Professor in Cultural Psychiatry, Emeritus, University of California Davis School of Medicine, Sacramento, California

K. Musa Misiani, B.Sc. Hons
Medical Student, University of Nairobi, and Research Associate, Africa Mental Health Foundation, Nairobi, Kenya

Abednego M. Musau, M.B.Ch.B.
Researcher, Africa Mental Health Foundation, Nairobi, Kenya

Victoria M. Mutiso, M.Sc., Ph.D.
Research Director, Africa Mental Health Foundation, Nairobi, Kenya

Rhodah Mwangi, B.A.
Communications Officer, Africa Mental Health Foundation, Nairobi, Kenya

David M. Ndetei, M.B.Ch.B., D.P.M., MRCPsych, FRCPsych, M.D., D.Sc.
Professor of Psychiatry, University of Nairobi, and Founding Director, Africa Mental Health Foundation, Nairobi, Kenya

Vishwajit Laxmikant Nimgaonkar, M.D., Ph.D.
Professor of Psychiatry and Human Genetics, Departments of Psychiatry and Human Genetics, University of Pittsburgh, Pittsburgh, Pennsylvania

John E. Pachankis, Ph.D.
Associate Professor of Epidemiology, Yale School of Public Health, New Haven, Connecticut

Adil Qureshi, Ph.D.
Psychologist, Servei de Psiquiatria, Hospital Universitari Vall d'Hebron; Adjunct Professor, Institute for the International Education of Students, Barcelona, Spain

Hans Rohlof, M.D.
Clinical Psychiatrist and Researcher, Head of the Outpatient Refugee Clinic, Centrum '45, Oegstgeest, The Netherlands

Cécile Rousseau, M.D.
Professor, Division of Social and Cultural Psychiatry, Department of Psychiatry, McGill University, Montreal, Quebec, Canada

Monica Scalco, M.D., Ph.D.
Assistant Professor of Psychiatry, University of Toronto, Toronto, Ontario, Canada

Angela Tang Soriano, M.S.S.W., LCSW
Director of Operations, Richmond Area Multi-Services, San Francisco, California

Rob van Dijk, M.Sc.
Medical Anthropologist, Parnassia Academy, Parnassia Psychiatric Institute, The Hague, The Netherlands

Hendry Ton, M.D., M.S.
Health Sciences Associate Clinical Professor, Director of Medical Student Education in Psychiatry, Director of Cultural Competency and Professionalism, and Director of Education at the Center for Reducing Health Disparities, Department of Psychiatry and Behavioral Sciences, University of California Davis School of Medicine; Medical Director, Transcultural Wellness Center, Sacramento, California

Johann Vega-Dienstmaier, M.D.
Assistant Professor of Psychiatry, Universidad Peruana Cayetano Heredia; Staff Psychiatrist, Hospital Nacional Cayetano Heredia, Lima, Peru

Mitchell G. Weiss, M.D., Ph.D.
Professor, Department of Epidemiology and Public Health, Swiss Tropical and Public Health Institute, and University of Basel, Basel, Switzerland

Joseph Westermeyer, M.D., Ph.D.
Professor of Psychiatry, University of Minnesota; Staff Physician, Minneapolis VA Health Care Center, Minneapolis, Minnesota

Disclosure of Competing Interests

The following contributors to this book have indicated a financial interest in or other affiliation with a commercial supporter, a manufacturer of a commercial product, a provider of a commercial service, a nongovernmental organization, and /or a government agency, as listed below:

Iqbal Ahmed, M.D.—Chief Editor and formerly Managing Editor for Psychiatry section for eMedicine, Medscape, an online Internet textbook of medicine, 2001 to present

Roberto Lewis-Fernández, M.D.—*Research support:* Principal Investigator of an investigator-initiated study with Eli Lilly

Russell Lim, M.D.—*Book royalties: Clinical Manual of Cultural Psychiatry,* APPI, 2014

The following contributors to this book have indicated no competing interests to disclose during the year preceding manuscript submission:

Neil Krishan Aggarwal, M.D., M.B.A., M.A.

Renato D. Alarcón, M.D., M.P.H.

Sofie Bäärnhielm, M.D., Ph.D.

Kavoos Ghane Bassiri, M.S., LMFT, LPCC, CGP

Triptish Bhatia, Ph.D.

James Boehnlein, M.D., M.Sc.

Francisco Collazos, M.D.

Lizardo Cruzado, M.D.

Smita Neelkanth Deshpande, M.D., D.P.M.

David M. Gellerman, M.D., Ph.D.

Simon Groen, M.A.

Jaswant Guzder, M.D.

Rita Hargrave, M.D.

Mark L. Hatzenbuehler, Ph.D

Devon E. Hinton, M.D., Ph.D.

Ladson Hinton, M.D.

Sushrut Jadhav, M.B.B.S., M.D., MRCPsych, Ph.D.

Oscar Jiménez-Solomon, M.P.H.

Laurence J. Kirmayer, M.D., FRCPC

Martin La Roche, Ph.D.

Francis G. Lu, M.D.

Abednego M. Musau, M.B.Ch.B.

Victoria M. Mutiso, M.Sc., Ph.D.

Rhodah Mwangi, B.A.

David M. Ndetei, M.B.Ch.B., D.P.M., MRCPsych, FRCPsych, M.D., D.Sc.

Vishwajit Laxmikant Nimgaonkar, M.D., Ph.D.

John E. Pachankis, Ph.D.

Adil Qureshi, Ph.D.

Cécile Rousseau, M.D.

Hans Rohlof, M.D.

Monica Scalco, M.D., Ph.D.

Angela Tang Soriano, M.S.S.W., LCSW

Hendry Ton, M.D., M.S.

Rob van Dijk, M.Sc.

Johann Vega-Dienstmaier, M.D.

Mitchell G. Weiss, M.D., Ph.D.

Joseph Westermeyer, M.D., Ph.D.

Foreword

In the 1970s, when I began my research and writing, cultural psychiatry as a field was principally concerned with epidemiological and clinical studies of diseases that were either common or uncommon in Europe and America (Kleinman 1978; Kleinman et al. 1978). The leading questions turned on whether the common diseases differed in symptomatology or prevalence in the non-Western world and among members of minorities in the West, and what kind of conditions the uncommon diseases were. When mental health services were considered, and often they were not because they were so thin on the ground then, the chief issues were why people from different racial, ethnic, and cultural groups failed to access psychiatric services or why those who were in treatment did not comply.

My generation of cultural psychiatrists and psychiatric anthropologists decisively shifted the central concerns in another direction. We asked research questions about the ideas that patients and family members held concerning sickness and treatment, and we compared those ideas with those held by practitioners, who also could be understood as participating in cultures (both professional and personal). My own contributions were to set out a method to elicit patient, family, and practitioner models of illness and treatment experiences (*explanatory models*) and to understand them as representative of *local moral worlds* in which culture, among other things, shaped *what was at stake* for individuals and in relationships. I also introduced the notion of the *category fallacy*, which resulted from the application of professional biomedical categories in places where those categories had no local cultural significance but instead imposed an alien ideology on indigenous illness experiences and treatment practices, thereby distorting both. I was interested in using these ideas to help understand clinical reality (what practices were at stake for clinicians in particular health care institutions) and the patient-doctor relationship as social processes shaped by cultural, political, economic, institutional, and other social forces.

I attempted to introduce these ideas into clinical practice, not only in psychiatry but also in internal medicine and family medicine, through a National Institute of Mental Health–funded clinical anthropology predoctoral and postdoctoral training program (organized with Byron Good and Mary-Jo Good), M.D.-Ph.D. and master's-level programs, clinical rounds at the University of Washington Medical Center, Seattle, and Cambridge Hospital in Cambridge, Massachusetts, and many presentations and publications. Four of the editors of this important volume (Roberto Lewis-Fernández, Neil Aggarwal, Ladson Hinton, and Devon Hinton) were my former students. Mitchell Weiss, another former trainee, developed a more systematic measure of explanatory models that facilitated matters. They, along with other contributors, have moved this field forward significantly by developing the cultural formulation approach, which I regard as the single most practically useful contribution of cultural psychiatry and medical anthropology to clinical work in psychiatry and, because this approach is also relevant, in primary care and medicine generally.

A little additional background information is needed to clarify the substantial advance that this volume represents. I cochaired the Task Force on Culture for DSM-IV. That group developed many cultural materials, of which very few were included in DSM. An earlier version of the cultural formulation was outlined in Appendix I, the ninth appendix, in DSM-IV (American Psychiatric Association 1994). It was little more than a template, the details of which were left for clinicians to fill in and develop.

Over the years, a number of clinical researchers around the world, including especially the editors of this book, developed the cultural formulation into the detailed, evidence-based, and clinically useful interview methodology detailed in this volume. The chapters on the cultural formulation before DSM-5 (American Psychiatric Association 2013) (Chapter 1), on the core and informant versions of the Cultural Formulation Interview (CFI) (Chapter 2), and on implementation (Chapter 4) disclose the very substantial research that has gone into establishing the CFI as an implementable best practices approach that can be systematically taught and applied in the field, evaluated, assembled into an implementation package, and scaled up. This is an impressive achievement, and one that holds the promise of becoming truly influential in clinical settings. Looking back over the 40 years since I introduced the explanatory model approach in the academic literature, it is shocking but also inspiring to see how far this field of clinically applied studies has come.

Although I enthusiastically applaud the achievement, I also recognize the importance of considering the cultural formulation's potential limits and also its potential, like all interventions, for unintended consequences. After I introduced the explanatory model approach, for example, I received many invitations from medical schools and hospitals to visit, deliver grand rounds or a named lecture, and meet with residents, students, and faculty. The purpose was usually to use my presence to focus on cultural issues of salience in medicine. On teaching rounds with inpatients during these visits, I was regaled with accounts of explanatory models—one patient, one model—as if they were fixed in time and materialized like other clinical "substances": electrolytes, hematocrit, and so forth. This entification of meaning produced exactly the opposite effect from the one the explanatory models approach was meant to achieve. Instead of opening conversations between patients and physicians, it stopped them. In other words, explanatory models were appropriated by powerful biomedical structures—cognitive, institutional, and cultural—in such a way as to undermine their value. I hope the same thing does not happen with the cultural formulation, but I think we should be prepared that such an unintended consequence could occur. To my mind, the greatest danger for all cultural interventions is that they will end up stereotyping patients and families with biased and superficial representations that will meet regulatory requirements, and therefore be seen as bureaucratically useful, yet only bring greater misunderstanding and stigma into the clinical relationship. How to prevent this from happening is the question that the contributors to and readers of this book will need to think hard about (Kleinman 1988, 1995). The fact that the

Explanatory Model supplementary module explicitly asks patients about changes in explanatory models throughout the illness experience is a step in a better direction (see supplementary modules in Appendix C in this handbook).

My suggestion is that the cultural formulation be taught and used with two explicit sensitivities in mind: first, a recognition that medicine itself is a particular cultural reality whose influence must be accounted for and, second, an awareness of the outcome of the CFI, assessing what, in any given case, it has accomplished and including a systematic checklist to rule out introduction of stereotypes. The exemplary chapter on the field testing of core and informant versions of the CFI (Chapter 2, "The Core and Informant Cultural Formulation Interviews in DSM-5") demonstrates that there are various measures of successful application and that, properly used, the CFI need not contribute to the problem of stereotyping, although it remains for me a concern. Applied with these two sensitivities taken into account, the CFI has great promise. Hence I see this volume as a major step forward in making the contributions of cultural psychiatry and medical anthropology available in the clinic.

Arthur Kleinman, M.D.

References

American Psychiatric Association: Diagnostic and Statistical Manual of Mental Disorders, 4th Edition. Washington, DC, American Psychiatric Association, 1994

American Psychiatric Association: Diagnostic and Statistical Manual of Mental Disorders, 5th Edition. Arlington, VA, American Psychiatric Association, 2013

Kleinman A: Concepts and a model for the comparison of medical systems as cultural systems. Soc Sci Med 12(2B):85–95, 1978 358402

Kleinman A: Rethinking Psychiatry. New York, Free Press, 1988

Kleinman A: Introduction, in Writing at the Margin. Berkeley, University of California Press, 1995, pp 1–18

Kleinman A, Eisenberg L, Good B: Culture, illness, and care: clinical lessons from anthropological and cross-cultural research. Ann Intern Med 88:251–258, 1978

Preface

This handbook on how to conduct a cultural assessment using the DSM-5 (American Psychiatric Association 2013) Cultural Formulation Interview (CFI) is directed at clinicians, administrators, policy makers, advocates, and other practitioners who work together to engage patients in the delivery of mental health care. We aim to make it easier for providers to account for the influence of culture in their work, in order to enhance patient-clinician communication in all clinical encounters—not only among participants judged to be culturally different—and improve outcomes of care. Accordingly, our primary audience is the clinician in mental health practice, of any discipline, who evaluates and negotiates treatments with patients on a regular basis. However, other stakeholders in care, including patients, will find guidance in these chapters, especially in the descriptions of the elements of culture—including the culture of mental health practice—that shape for all of us our understandings of illness, experiences of distress, and expectations and concerns about care, whether we are positioned as clinicians or as patients in any given clinical encounter.

The CFI and this book are the products of the work of many people over the last two decades, particularly since the publication of DSM-IV (American Psychiatric Association 1994). Published in DSM-5 in 2013, the CFI emerged from efforts, especially in North America and Europe, to develop questionnaires, interview protocols, and semistructured instruments to help clinicians obtain the information that the DSM-IV Outline for Cultural Formulation described as basic to cultural assessment. Many of the authors of these pre-CFI assessment tools were members of the DSM-5 Cross-Cultural Issues Subgroup, which led the CFI development process from 2007 to 2013. Many others participated in the DSM-5 international field trial that tested the feasibility, acceptability, and perceived clinical utility of one of the three CFI components, the 16-item core CFI, for use in daily mental health practice (note usage of CFI to indicate multiple components and core CFI to indicate the 16-question interview). Still others contributed their extensive clinical-cultural expertise to summarize for clinicians the elements of cultural assessment that guided the development of each CFI component and module. This handbook, and indeed the CFI itself, would not be possible without their work.

In this handbook, we describe and illustrate the use of the core CFI, the CFI–Informant Version for obtaining collateral information, and the 12 supplementary modules that expand on these basic assessments. The chapters include case vignettes, and video commentaries flesh out the use of these components. (The videos may be viewed at www.appi.org/Lewis-Fernandez. See also "Video Guide" in the handbook.) We also devote considerable attention to the issues of how to implement the CFI in contemporary practice—including its application in different clinical settings (e.g., inpatient units, emergency departments) and in diverse international contexts—and how to train clinicians at all stages of professional development in its use. Further work is ongoing, in many parts of the world, to disseminate the CFI, facilitate and test its implementation, train practitioners, and examine its effectiveness. Feedback can be provided at www.dsm5.org/Pages/Feedback-Form.aspx. An online training video developed by the New York State Office of Mental Health will also be available in the near future to encourage implementation of the CFI in public mental health systems. Information on this video will be available at the Web site of the New York State Center of Excellence for Cultural Competence at New York State Psychiatric Institute: www.nyspi.org/culturalcompetence. Our hope is that these multiple efforts will result in a maximally effective CFI that can be widely applied and can help enhance clinical care.

Roberto Lewis-Fernández, M.D., M.T.S.
September 26, 2014

References

American Psychiatric Association: Diagnostic and Statistical Manual of Mental Disorders, 4th Edition. Washington, DC, American Psychiatric Association, 1994
American Psychiatric Association: Diagnostic and Statistical Manual of Mental Disorders, 5th Edition. Arlington, VA, American Psychiatric Association, 2013

Video Guide

The Video Learning Experience

The videos can be viewed online at **www.appi.org/Lewis-Fernandez.**

To illustrate use of the Cultural Formulation Interview (CFI), the *DSM-5® Handbook on the Cultural Formulation Interview* includes access to a video with segments of a complete core CFI titled *Full CFI* in addition to 17 videos that demonstrate the application of portions of the core CFI and several supplementary modules. Pertinent videos are highlighted and described in selected, content-related chapters. Viewers may note that some of the filmed interviews are meant to demonstrate use of the semistructured questions in a short period of time; although these tend not to deviate from the recommended wording, users may choose instead to tailor the questions to their clinical situation, for example, by using only selected questions, altering the wording while adhering to the intent of the question, and interspersing more expressions of empathy or statements intended to evoke further elaboration of the interview topics. Viewers may also note that the videos feature clinicians with various degrees of experience using the CFI; some have memorized it, whereas others read questions aloud. This variation is deliberate, intended to portray clinicians in natural practice settings and to avoid the impression that all CFI questions must be memorized prior to use. The theme uniting all videos is the clinician's commitment to discovering the patient's interpretations of the illness experience.

Using the Book and the Videos Together

We recommend that readers use the boldface video prompts ▶ embedded in the text as signals for viewing the associated clips in the online viewer at www.appi.org/Lewis-Fernandez. The cues identify the vignettes by title and run time. (The videos are optimized for most current operating systems, including mobile operating systems iOS 5.1 and Android 4.1 and higher.)

Descriptions of the Videos

Video 1: Full CFI (6:57)

The relationship between the individual and her social network is on display, illustrating use of the core CFI, which includes segments of a full CFI evaluation.

Video 2: What does that have to do with my lungs? (4:26)

The consultation aims to elucidate the patient's interpretations of her illness and of her caregivers' behavior to understand her objections to recommended treatment.

Video 3: They get outta whack sometimes (2:19)

Several aspects of the patient's explanatory model are explored.

Video 4: If it's not one thing, it's another (3:46)

As the interview progresses, the patient begins to disclose the stressors associated with her condition and the role her social network plays in how she views her condition.

Video 5: DWI (3:46)

Using the CFI supplementary module on level of functioning to assess how a patient's drinking problem affects his work, earnings, life goals, and relationships is illustrated.

Video 6: The family (2:35)

The clinician conducts the core CFI with a woman with postpartum depression, exploring the important role that the patient's family members play in her social network.

Video 7: Bridging the gap (3:57)

Through use of the core CFI, the patient's preferences for care, which include reflecting on the role of his faith in treatment and asking what kinds of help would be most beneficial considering his faith and values, are ascertained.

Video 8: Crisis of faith (3:54)

The supplementary module Spirituality, Religion, and Moral Traditions is used to elicit faith-related elements of support and conflict for a young man in the emergency department who is struggling with thoughts of suicide.

Video 9: A small town, which is why I'm here (4:39)

A psychiatrist conducts an interview with a patient whose symptoms of anxiety are best understood within the framework of his migration experience and his cultural expectations.

Video 10: It gets kind of confusing (2:41)

The interview illustrates some of the complexities of identity that may affect a patient's clinical presentation. Knowledge about her cultural identity is essential for treatment.

Video 11: You still show up on Sunday (3:26)

The patient's answers to core CFI questions reveal important values as well as conflicts about his sense of himself that stem from the role of spirituality and religion in his life.

Video 12: Ties that bind (3:35)

The clinician's prompts elicit the patient's description of feelings of anger and social isolation and her conflictive family situation in relation to the disclosure of her sexual orientation identity.

Video 13: I don't have a problem (3:00)

Through the interview, the patient's various coping strategies are revealed.

Video 14: Planning for something better (1:59)

Using the core CFI, the clinician explores the patient's expectations and perceived barriers to treatment, and the patient explains what could help her more effectively.

Video 15: In my own language (0:42)

How the core CFI question on the patient-clinician relationship can yield useful concrete information to guide treatment planning even during an intake visit is demonstrated.

Video 16: After the fall (4:00)

Questions from the supplementary module Older Adults highlight how developmental experiences around aging are a source of dynamic cultural meaning-making during an illness.

Video 17: Getting back on my feet (3:46)

The interviewer transitions to the domain of the supplementary module on the quality and nature of social supports and caregiving by asking how recovery has changed relationships with friends and family.

Video 18: I've been feeling really frustrated (4:20)

The interview shows how the core CFI functions well in a situation of acute symptomatology in the emergency department.

Video Credits

The senior video content and production editor was Ravi DeSilva M.D., M.A. The video examples of CFI interviews created for this book were developed and produced by a core interdisciplinary team of physicians and social workers committed to improving cultural competence training and education for all clinicians. The CFI video writing, production, and editing team consisted of Ravi DeSilva M.D., M.A.; Matthew Pieh M.D.; Courtney Flint, LMSW; Linda Gregory, LMSW; and Carlos Benítez, M.S.W.

Special thanks go to the cast of these films who generously gave their time and talents to bring these scenarios to life, highlighting the many ways in which culture impacts clinical care. The video cast members are Neil Krishan Aggarwal, Cándida C. Batista, Carlos Benítez, Enrico Castillo, Ravi DeSilva, Bruce Dohrenwend, Courtney Flint, Linda Gregory, Sheldene Gorovitzc, Myunghoon Kim, Roberto Lewis-Fernández, Lee Lovejoy, Hamna Mela, Matthew Pieh, Paul Reardon, and Lianna Valdez.

Note. The clinical cases portrayed are fictional. Any resemblance to real persons is purely coincidental. The videos feature the work of volunteer clinicians and actor patients who agreed to demonstrate commonly used interview techniques.

Introduction

Roberto Lewis-Fernández, M.D., M.T.S.

Neil Krishan Aggarwal, M.D., M.B.A., M.A.

Laurence J. Kirmayer, M.D.

Culture shapes every aspect of patient care in psychiatry, influencing when, where, how, and to whom patients narrate their experiences of illness and distress (Kirmayer 2006), the patterning of symptoms (Kleinman 1977), and the models clinicians use to interpret and understand symptoms in terms of psychiatric diagnoses (Kleinman 1987). Culture also shapes patients' perceptions of care, including what types of treatment are acceptable and for how long (Lewis-Fernández et al. 2013). Even when patients and clinicians share similar cultural, ethnic, or linguistic backgrounds, culture impacts care through other influences on identity, such as gender, age, class, race, occupation, sexual orientation, and religion (Lu et al. 1995). Cultural contexts and expectations frame the clinical encounter for every patient, not only for underserved minority groups, and cultural formulation therefore is an essential component of any comprehensive psychiatric assessment.

But how is cultural assessment to be carried out? What are its components? Can only experts perform it, or can it be learned by any practicing clinician and implemented in routine practice? How comprehensive must it be to be useful for mental health care? Is it possible to develop a standard assessment approach for everybody, or does every cultural group need its own method and content? Can the assessment itself yield enough information, or is it necessary for the clinician to start out with some background knowledge?

This handbook takes up many of these questions, marshaling the available evidence in support of a standardized approach to cultural assessment, the DSM-5 (American Psychiatric Association 2013) Cultural Formulation Interview (CFI). A product of the 2007–2013 DSM revision process, the CFI is composed of three types of semistructured interviews that offer clinicians concrete ways to carry out the cultural assessment of a patient and his or her entourage according to a revision of the Outline for Cultural Formulation (OCF), first published in DSM-IV (American Psychiatric Association 1994). The three components of the CFI are a core 16-item questionnaire; the CFI–Informant Version, which is used to obtain information from caregivers; and 12 supplementary modules that expand on these basic assessments. (The core CFI and CFI–Informant Version are published in DSM-5 and are available online along with the supplementary modules at www.psychiatry.org/practice/ dsm/dsm5/online-assessment-measures. In addition, the core CFI, CFI–Informant Version, and 12 modules are included in the appendixes of this handbook.) The developers of the CFI, the DSM-5 Cross-Cultural Issues Subgroup (DCCIS), envisioned the use of the CFI as a telescoping process, beginning with the core CFI, a basic assessment that can be conducted with any patient in any mental health setting and that can be learned and implemented with fidelity by any clinician. For some clinical situations, this level of assessment may be sufficient. If used routinely to frame the intake interview, the core CFI can help establish a foundation of person-centered information on the patient's context and perspective, as well as a working alliance, on which to build the rest of the diagnostic interview and treatment negotiation process.

If additional cultural information is needed, the other components of the CFI can be called into play. When collateral information is desired, the CFI–Informant Version can supplement what the patient reports, or it may become the primary source of information when the patient is unable to participate actively in his or her care, such as in the case of some young children or individuals with cognitive impairment or florid psychosis. If the clinician sees the need for additional information, the supplementary modules expand on the content obtained from the core assessments. Use of all of the modules and the CFI–Informant Version along with the core CFI constitutes a fairly comprehensive cultural assessment, particularly useful for situations involving the following:

- Difficulty in diagnostic assessment owing to significant differences in the cultural, religious, or socioeconomic backgrounds of clinician and the individual
- Uncertainty about the fit between culturally distinctive symptoms and diagnostic criteria
- Difficulty in judging illness severity or impairment
- Disagreement between the individual and clinician on the course of care
- Limited engagement in and adherence to treatment by the individual (American Psychiatric Association 2013, p. 751)

Three kinds of supplementary modules are included (see Chapter 3, "Supplementary Modules"): *Core CFI expansion* modules amplify key sections of the core CFI (e.g., the Explanatory Model); *specific populations* modules assess particular populations (e.g., older adults, refugees) who may have specific needs and experiences as a result of certain aspects of their background or identity; and *informant perspectives* modules clarify how individuals who assist the patient with his or her care and members of the patient's social network view the patient's situation. Although the CFI–Informant Version is not strictly one of the 12 supplementary modules, it can be considered an informant perspectives module because it helps the clinician obtain a fuller picture of the patient's situation when combined with the core CFI. The CFI telescoping approach means that the clinician can select how much information to obtain and therefore how much time to dedicate to each aspect of the interview for his or her particular purposes. Several components of the CFI can be obtained all at once, possibly during the initial interview, or at different points throughout the process of care.

Practical concerns were front and center in the work of the DCCIS. In current practice environments, the duration of the clinical visit is an important constraint for practitioners, administrators, and health plans. To be taken up widely, interventions must be feasible and cost-effective, or they risk remaining of academic interest only. In this respect, the DCCIS faced a dilemma: how to revise the OCF to increase its functionality for busy clinicians without weakening its role as a narrative, person-centered account of suffering that supplements the criteria-based diagnostic practice of contemporary psychiatry (Lewis-Fernández 2009). The cultural formulation approach operationalizes a more thorough evaluation of the sociocultural context in which illness experience is embedded. Without this systematic contextual assessment, the meaning of much of patients' illness behavior—including accurate calibration of symptom severity—may elude a busy provider, increasing the risk of clinical mismanagement, patient dissatisfaction, nonadherence, and poor treatment response. On the other hand, a long and complex cultural assessment approach that will not be implemented in actual practice is of little practical value. To escape both horns of the dilemma, the DCCIS developed the CFI to combine sufficient contextual depth with functionality and to facilitate dissemination by operationalizing the interview as a parsimonious, telescopic, but useful, set of questions (Lewis-Fernández 2009). The draft of the core CFI was revised based on clinician and patient feedback obtained in an international field trial prior to its inclusion in DSM-5. The field trial provided evidence of the CFI's feasibility, acceptability, and perceived clinical utility (R. Lewis-Fernández et al., Feasibility, acceptability and clinical utility of the core Cultural Formulation Interview: Results from the international DSM-5 field trial, manuscript in preparation, March 2015).

Although the CFI is designed to be integrated seamlessly into clinical practice, the CFI is also designed to advance what is, in effect, a radical agenda: to change the way clinicians conduct a diagnostic interview so that the perspective of the patient becomes at least as important as the signs and symptoms of disease identified by the clinician (Kleinman 1988; Mezzich and Appleyard 2010). The mission of the CFI is, in fact, to expand what counts as *data* in a clinical encounter (Marková and Berrios 2012; Nordgaard et al. 2013), encouraging the clinician—and the patient, who is empowered to recount his or her experience more fully—to attend to the experience of illness and the lifeworld (Aggarwal et al. 2015). This corresponds to the current person-centered turn in mental health care, in which the patient's voice—as well as that of the patient's family and other important people in his or her life—becomes a primary focus of the clinician's attention (Mezzich 2007; Stanghellini et al. 2013). The CFI helps to elaborate the patient's perspective within a specific *local world,* such as the views of the community—exemplified by the patient's social network—and the life context in which the problem presented emerges (Kleinman and Benson 2006). The CFI can help clarify what the patient is looking for in the clinical encounter, the various possibilities for treatment and other forms of self-coping and help seeking the patient can draw upon, and, very specifically, the ways in which treatment will be carried out. The greater understanding afforded to the clinician—paired with a fuller expression of the problem, preferences for care, and trust on the part of the patient—should facilitate a process of shared decision making (U.S. Department of Health and Human Services 2010), including negotiating and clarifying the subsequent concrete steps and decisions for both partners in the session. Our hope is that by making the CFI questions easier for clinicians to ask, the usefulness of the information and rapport elicited by these questions will encourage the routine use of the CFI in clinical care.

The CFI also carries forward another more challenging goal: to transmit a more sophisticated understanding of an individual's experience of culture as a dynamic, constantly changing distillation of multiple engagements with all the communities to which he or she belongs, whether based on gender, spirituality, age, language, race/ ethnicity, occupation, geographical region, leisure activities, national origin, or any other element of the person's background and collective life. In the CFI, *culture* is reflected in the cognitive, behavioral, and emotional predispositions as well as the commonsense, taken-for-granted knowledge that affect a person's values, thoughts, perceptions, intuitions, bodily experiences, and practices—in short, every aspect of the patient's life. This includes interpretations of what constitutes a clinical problem, what the patient's illness—if any—may be, how to cope, and what help to seek, including whether to access psychiatric care and what treatment to expect (Kleinman et al. 1978). This also includes the commonsense, taken-for-granted knowledge of clinicians in the health care system that should not be assumed for patients. In U.S. health care practice, notions of culture are frequently paired exclusively with racialized/ethnic categories, which may lead to the unintended consequence of stereotyping patients. As noted by Arthur Kleinman, M.D., in the foreword to this book, the CFI challenges this view, guiding clinicians to see the contextual frame of each patient's experience—seeking to use information about the collective to understand an individual's perspective and to clarify how local environments impinge on the person's situation, including how sociocultural contingencies help to pattern a set of events. The goal is to understand the patient's predicament—both the aspects of which the patient is aware and those that are outside his or her awareness. Recognizing that the patient may not be able to provide all of this background, the intent of the CFI is to raise these questions for clinicians to examine, possibly through additional sources of data, including collateral information from relatives; reading literature on the person's self-identified background group(s); reflection on the clinician's knowledge of the patient's culture(s); and consultations with culture brokers, interpreters, religious leaders, or other clinicians with relevant experience. The CFI enables clinicians to construct a cultural formulation genuinely based on the patient's self-identified group, freeing the clinician from the burden of incorrectly guessing group markers of identity—such as race and ethnicity—or offering treatment recommendations based on inaccurate stereotypes. As the above examples suggest, the CFI may be particularly revealing when it leads the clinician beyond the individual patient interview to a greater engagement with the patient's lifeworld, a gradual process that can enrich clinical care much beyond the focus on symptoms and disorders so prevalent in contemporary psychiatry. Although the clinician's past experience with particular groups can guide and enrich the interview process, the CFI can be implemented by clinicians with no explicit knowledge about the cultural backgrounds of their patients. In this sense, it is a self-contained instrument; however, its effectiveness is likely to increase with experience, both with the CFI itself and with specific groups and contexts.

Just how effective is the CFI? Research is actively examining various types of clinical usefulness. The potential research outcomes are legion: diagnostic accuracy;

level of patient participation and engagement; intrasession processual and communication dimensions; treatment effectiveness; patient satisfaction, retention, and adherence; cost-effectiveness; self-defined recovery; impact on level of care over time (e.g., rehospitalization rates); effect on quality of life and illness-related impairment; and so on. Chapter 2 ("The Core and Informant Cultural Formulation Interviews in DSM-5") presents the results of the DSM-5 international field trial in 14 sites across six countries that tested the core CFI's feasibility, acceptability, and clinical utility, as reported by patients and clinicians. This trial showed that both patients and clinicians found the core CFI to be feasible, acceptable, and useful. These findings may encourage clinicians to take up the CFI, patients to request its use, and educators to include the CFI at all levels of clinical training. As more research is conducted, it will be crucial to generate evidence that examines the impact of the CFI in order to determine the value of its widespread and sustained implementation.

Contents of the Handbook

This handbook is organized into six major chapters, two of which have multiple subchapters. Chapter 1 ("Cultural Formulation Before DSM-5") describes the foundations of the CFI: the OCF and the various semistructured instruments that were developed from it in North America and Europe prior to DSM-5. Chapter 2 ("The Core and Informant Cultural Formulation Interviews in DSM-5") introduces the core CFI and the CFI–Informant Version, explaining the intent of each question and providing guidelines for their use in clinical practice. As stated above, it also reviews key findings from the DSM-5 field trial on the feasibility, acceptability, and perceived clinical utility of an early draft of the core CFI that was revised into the final version in DSM-5 based on field trial results.

Chapter 3 ("Supplementary Modules") introduces the supplementary modules; each of 12 subchapters describes a module in detail, including guidelines for its use, exemplified with case vignettes. Figure 3–1 presents all of the modules and their relationship to the core CFI and the CFI–Informant Version. The subchapter on cultural identity focuses first on cultural identity in general and is then further subdivided, describing three major components of identity: national, ethnic, racial, language, and migration issues; spirituality, religion, and moral traditions; and gender identity and sexual orientation identity.

Chapter 4 ("Clinical Implementation of the Cultural Formulation Interview") is subdivided into three subchapters, addressing various aspects of the CFI implementation process in clinical care. Chapter 4 reviews how implementation strategies can facilitate uptake of novel interventions such as the CFI. It presents two possible CFI implementation strategies—one for clinicians and the other for organizational teams, the two groups of stakeholders ultimately responsible for delivering culturally competent care to patients. The chapter covers seven dimensions whose clarity would concretely operationalize implementation: the actors, the action, the action target, temporality, dose, implementation outcomes affected, and justification. The subchapter "Use of the Cultural Formulation Interview in Different Clinical Settings" documents issues that come up during the application of the CFI in diverse clinical settings: emergency departments, consultation-liaison services (i.e., inpatient medical and surgical units in general hospitals), outpatient clinics, and urban or rural community health centers. Each setting presents unique environmental and patient- and staff-related features that are reviewed and illustrated with clinical vignettes. The subchapter "Administrative Perspectives on the Implementation and Use of the Cultural Formulation Interview" discusses CFI implementation from the point of view of administrators in a busy multicultural clinic in San Francisco that participated in the DSM-5 field trial. Administrators present the "business case" for the CFI, addressing organizational purpose and need, use and benefits, implementation strategies, and implementation challenges and potential solutions related to CFI uptake. The subchapter "Application of the Cultural Formulation Interview in International Settings" describes the experience that various clinician investigators have had with the CFI questions in four international settings involved in the development of the CFI and/or the DSM-5 field trial. Work is presented from India, Kenya, the Netherlands, Sweden, and other Nordic countries and is illustrated by case vignettes. This subchapter also discusses how the CFI may need to be modified for international settings and what role psychiatric practice in other countries may play in continuing to refine the CFI.

Chapter 5 ("Cultural Competence in Psychiatric Education Using the Cultural Formulation Interview") reviews current regulations and published guidelines on the teaching of culturally appropriate assessment in medical student and resident training and continuing medical education and suggests how the CFI can be incorporated into these efforts. Finally, Chapter 6 ("Conclusion: The Future of Cultural Formulation") provides some directions for the future development of the CFI and of cultural formulation more generally, in terms of theory, research, and practice.

Conclusion

In summary, the CFI represents an important advance in cultural assessment for use in routine clinical care. The CFI seeks to enhance the person centeredness of diagnostic practice and treatment negotiation by focusing on the person's experiences, views, and expectations of illness and care as influenced by cultural background and context. The goal is to help clinicians and patients communicate as effectively as possible and overcome all barriers to the successful outcome of treatment. This handbook provides a starting point for the continued development and refinement of cultural assessment as a central pillar of mental health practice.

KEY CLINICAL POINTS

- The three components of the Cultural Formulation Interview (CFI)—core CFI, CFI–Informant Version, and supplementary modules—provide a flexible approach to cultural assessment that can be tailored by the clinician to the needs of the patient and the clinical situation.
- The handbook text and accompanying videos provide detailed guidance on how to use the CFI.

Questions

1. What is the rationale for including the CFI in DSM-5?

2. In what ways does the CFI represent an advance on previous approaches to cultural formulation?

3. How is culture defined in the CFI?

References

Aggarwal NK, DeSilva R, Nicasio AV, et al: Does the Cultural Formulation Interview for the fifth revision of the Diagnostic and Statistical Manual of Mental Disorders (DSM-5) affect medical communication? A qualitative exploratory study from the New York site. Ethn Health 20(1):1–28, 2015 25372242

American Psychiatric Association: Diagnostic and Statistical Manual of Mental Disorders, 4th Edition. Washington, DC, American Psychiatric Association, 1994

American Psychiatric Association: Diagnostic and Statistical Manual of Mental Disorders, 5th Edition. Arlington, VA, American Psychiatric Association, 2013

Kirmayer LJ: Beyond the "new cross-cultural psychiatry": cultural biology, discursive psychology and the ironies of globalization. Transcult Psychiatry 43(1):126–144, 2006 16671396

Kleinman AM: Depression, somatization and the "new cross-cultural psychiatry." Soc Sci Med 11(1):3–10, 1977 887955

Kleinman A: Anthropology and psychiatry. The role of culture in cross-cultural research on illness. Br J Psychiatry 151:447–454, 1987 3447661

Kleinman A: The Illness Narratives: Suffering, Healing, and the Human Condition. New York, Basic Books, 1988

Kleinman A, Benson P: Anthropology in the clinic: the problem of cultural competency and how to fix it. PLoS Med 3(10):e294, 2006 17076546

Kleinman A, Eisenberg L, Good B: Culture, illness, and care: clinical lessons from anthropologic and cross-cultural research. Ann Intern Med 88(2):251–258, 1978 626456

Lewis-Fernández R: The cultural formulation. Transcult Psychiatry 46(3):379–382, 2009 19837777

Lewis-Fernández R, Balán IC, Patel SR, et al: Impact of motivational pharmacotherapy on treatment retention among depressed Latinos. Psychiatry 76(3):210–222, 2013 23965261

Lu FG, Lim RF, Mezzich JE: Issues in the assessment and diagnosis of culturally diverse individuals, in American Psychiatric Press Review of Psychiatry, Vol 14: Assessment and Diagnosis. Edited by Oldham JM, Riba MB, Washington, DC, American Psychiatric Press, 1995, pp 477–510

Marková IS, Berrios GE: Epistemology of psychiatry. Psychopathology 45(4):220–227, 2012 22627668

Mezzich JE: Psychiatry for the person: articulating medicine's science and humanism. World Psychiatry 6(2):65–67, 2007 18235854

Mezzich JE, Appleyard J: Person-centered integrative diagnosis: conceptual basis and structural model. Can J Psychiatry 55:701–708, 2010

Nordgaard J, Sass LA, Parnas J: The psychiatric interview: validity, structure, and subjectivity. Eur Arch Psychiatry Clin Neurosci 263(4):353–364, 2013 23001456

Stanghellini G, Bolton D, Fulford WK: Person-centered psychopathology of schizophrenia: building on Karl Jaspers' understanding of patient's attitude toward his illness. Schizophr Bull 39(2):287–294, 2013 23314193

U.S. Department of Health and Human Services: Shared Decision-Making in Mental Health Care: Practice, Research, and Future Directions (HHS Publ No SMA-09-4371). Rockville, MD, Center for Mental Health Services, Substance Abuse and Mental Health Services Administration, 2010

Suggested Readings

Kirmayer LJ, Guzder J, Rousseau C (eds): Cultural Consultation: Encountering the Other in Mental Health Care. New York, Springer, 2014

Kleinman A, Benson P: Anthropology in the clinic: the problem of cultural competency and how to fix it. PLoS Med 3(10):e294, 2006

CHAPTER 1

Cultural Formulation Before DSM-5

Roberto Lewis-Fernández, M.D., M.T.S.

Neil Krishan Aggarwal, M.D., M.B.A., M.A.

Laurence J. Kirmayer, M.D.

The introduction of the Outline for Cultural Formulation (OCF) in DSM-IV (American Psychiatric Association 1994) marked a transition from an earlier period of general recommendations for conducting cultural assessments in psychiatry (Kleinman 1980) to the beginning of a series of efforts to systematize the application of cultural assessments in routine clinical practice. As an early attempt at systematization, the DSM-IV OCF was developed as a conceptual framework—a summary of the topics that should be included in a cultural assessment during a mental health evaluation to improve diagnostic accuracy and patient engagement in treatment planning. Over the last two decades, mental health clinicians, researchers, and social scientists in several countries have worked to refine the OCF and make it even more user-friendly for clinicians and mental health trainees by illustrating its application in questionnaires, protocols, and semistructured interviews. This work on operationalizing the cultural assessment process led to the Cultural Formulation Interview (CFI), a set of semistructured instruments included in DSM-5 (American Psychiatric Association 2013) that show how to collect information for the OCF (note usage of CFI to indicate multiple components and core CFI to indicate the 16-question interview). The CFI is composed of three parts: a core 16-item questionnaire (Appendix A in this handbook), an informant version of the core CFI to obtain information from caregivers (Appendix B), and 12 supplementary modules that expand on these basic assessments (Appendix C).

This handbook describes the development of the CFI, the content of each of its components, and recommendations for how to apply them in mental health care, including how to train clinicians in their use. This chapter takes a first step toward our

1

goal by describing the foundations of the CFI: the OCF and the various semistructured instruments that were developed from it in North America and Europe prior to
the publication of DSM-5. To summarize this foundational material, we combine two
sources of information: 1) findings from a series of literature reviews on the OCF domains conducted by members of the DSM-5 Cross-Cultural Issues Subgroup (DCCIS)
that were used to develop the CFI and 2) a summary of the main conceptual issues
raised by the DCCIS during the DSM revision process (Lewis-Fernández et al. 2014).

Outline for Cultural Formulation

The OCF is a conceptual framework that was developed to encourage clinicians to
identify the impact of culture on key aspects of an individual's clinical presentation
and care (Mezzich et al. 2009). According to the DSM-IV text, the OCF was "meant to
supplement the multiaxial diagnostic assessment and to address difficulties that may
be encountered in applying DSM-IV criteria in a multicultural environment" (American Psychiatric Association 1994, p. 843).

The DSM-IV OCF organized clinical information into four domains: 1) cultural
identity of the individual; 2) cultural explanations of the individual's illness; 3) cultural factors related to psychosocial environment and levels of functioning; and 4) cultural elements of the relationship between the individual and the clinician.
Information from these domains influencing diagnosis and treatment was summarized and synthesized in a fifth section to provide an overall formulation (American
Psychiatric Association 1994). Social theory and clinical-ethnographic research guided
the original delineation of the domains, including the role of identity in clinical presentation (domain 1), cultural meanings and explanatory models of illness (domain 2), social networks providing support or stressors affecting functional capacity (domain 3),
and the professional's reflections on the patient-clinician relationship (domain 4)
(Mezzich 2008). A key goal of the OCF has always been to yield an account of the patient's illness that captures his or her symptom experience along with personal and
cultural interpretations and the social contexts or circumstances of the illness. This information may help identify causal explanations and meanings of illness by the patient and by his or her family and community and extends a biopsychosocial
formulation into the realm of cultural assessment (Kleinman 1988; Lewis-Fernández
and Díaz 2002; Mezzich 1995).

The OCF was reprinted without revision in DSM-IV-TR (American Psychiatric Association 2000). In DSM-5, the OCF was revised by making the DSM-IV-TR text more
explicit in places. Examples of this clarification include the following: incorporating
elements of cultural identity not mentioned in DSM-IV-TR (e.g., religious affiliation,
sexual orientation); instructing clinicians to identify actual stressors and supports in
the patient's environment as well as how they are interpreted by the individual and
the clinician in relation to the social context; and mention of the potential impact of
racism and discrimination on the clinician-patient relationship. However, the content
of the OCF has remained roughly unchanged since 1994.

The OCF has been used worldwide. Educators have employed it in training programs in Canada, Denmark, India, the Netherlands, Norway, Spain, Sweden, the

United Kingdom, and the United States (e.g., Jadhav 2010a; Kirmayer et al. 2012; Lim 2006; Østerskov 2011). In the United States, the OCF is commonly part of psychiatric training. In a qualitative study with 20 preceptors of cultural psychiatry from U.S. adult psychiatry residency programs, 70% had at least one class on the OCF, usually during the first 2 years (Hansen et al. 2013). Similarly, centers providing outpatient mental health services to migrants and refugees in Sweden (Bäärnhielm and Scarpinati Rosso 2009) and the Netherlands (Rohlof et al. 2009) have used the OCF for standard clinical assessment.

The diagnostic utility of the OCF has been documented in numerous case reports and case series in various countries (e.g., Lewis-Fernández 1996; Rohlof et al. 2009). The most extensive literature beyond case studies comes from a cultural consultation service (CCS) at the Jewish General Hospital in Montreal, Quebec, Canada, that receives referrals from primary care clinicians and mental health practitioners seeking to address barriers to care that they attribute to cultural differences (e.g., failed rapport, poor adherence) (Kirmayer et al. 2003, 2014). The consultation procedure involves clinical assessment by a team including a psychiatrist or psychologist, an interpreter, and a culture broker and follows an interview guide based on an expanded version of the DSM-IV OCF developed by the CCS (Kirmayer et al. 2014). The assessment interviews typically involve one to three 1-hour sessions and usually include family members. The information collected through this interview process is integrated into a case formulation at a multidisciplinary case conference. *Culture brokers* are individuals with lived experience in the patient's cultural reference group(s)—frequently community members—who have been trained to bridge ("broker") potential communication gaps between local and professional perspectives (Miklavcic and LeBlanc 2014). At the CCS, findings from the OCF-based assessment are routinely discussed in a multidisciplinary case conference with all members of the cultural consultation team to develop a cultural formulation (Kirmayer et al. 2014).

Use of the OCF was well received by consultants and culture brokers working in the CCS. On a survey inquiring about their use of the DSM-IV OCF and the CCS version, 93% of them found the expanded OCF interview to be useful, although many were unfamiliar with the DSM-IV tool or had not used it before (Kirmayer et al. 2008b). In terms of diagnostic impact, use of the OCF resulted in substantial rates of rediagnosis: overall, cultural formulation led to a rediagnosis in about 60% of 400 cases seen by the service (Kirmayer et al. 2014). In one study, 49% of 70 patients with a referral diagnosis of psychotic disorder were rediagnosed as nonpsychotic after OCF-based assessment (Adeponle et al. 2012). Many of the patients misdiagnosed with a psychotic disorder were immigrants or refugees suffering from posttraumatic stress disorder, adjustment disorder, and other stress-related conditions. Rediagnosis from psychotic to nonpsychotic disorder was more likely among patients who had recently arrived in Canada and were referred from nonmedical sources (e.g., social workers or occupational therapists).

Although the OCF was found to be a useful clinical tool in much of this previous work, problems with its implementation have also been identified. Guidance has been lacking on when, with whom, and why to use the OCF (Cuéllar and Paniagua

2000). Clinicians have struggled to find ways to cover the many topics included in the four broad domains of the OCF within the time constraints of various practice settings (Lewis-Fernández 2009). Some subsections of the OCF may be imprecise and overlapping, and some important topics were absent in the DSM-IV version (Ton and Lim 2008). It is not clear which components of the OCF are particularly relevant for treatment planning and adaptation of clinical approaches and therefore should be emphasized in practice (Mezzich et al. 2009). Although the OCF is framed in terms of patients' knowledge and experience, the use of the OCF with children, immigrants and refugees, homeless populations, individuals with limited literacy, and the elderly may require collateral sources of information or local adaptations (Aggarwal 2010a, 2010b; Groen 2009b; Rohlof et al. 2009). The lack of a standard approach to the OCF has hindered generalizable research, and the lack of guidance on how to collect relevant information has limited clinical uptake (Mezzich et al. 2009).

Development of OCF-Related Interviews Prior to DSM-5

The concerns described in the section "Outline for Cultural Formulation" prompted efforts in various countries to make the OCF more user-friendly for clinicians by including lists of suggested questions, protocols for topics to be covered during OCF-based assessments, and semistructured interviews (Table 1–1). Interview approaches to the OCF were developed in Canada (Kirmayer et al. 2001), the Netherlands (Groen 2009a; Rohlof et al. 2002), Sweden (Bäärnhielm and Scarpinati Rosso 2009), the United States (Mezzich et al. 2009), the United Kingdom (Jadhav 2010a, 2010b), and Denmark (Østerskov 2011). All of these interviews were designed to enhance clinical assessment and treatment planning rather than to elicit research data. In related work, more detailed interviews were developed for research focusing on cultural variations in illness experience and explanatory models, including the Explanatory Model Interview Catalogue (Weiss 2001) and the McGill Illness Narrative Interview (Groleau et al. 2006). Developers of many of these interviews and instruments were members of the DCCIS, and their experience informed the preparation of the CFI.

In the sections that follow, we summarize work on each OCF domain and its operationalization prior to DSM-5. We also review challenges that emerged when implementing the OCF in clinical practice. Key themes and implications for the CFI in DSM-5 that emerged from the work of the DCCIS are summarized in Table 1–2. Each section below is based on the deliberations of the DCCIS and on English-language literature reviews since 1994, augmented by references from 1965 to 1994 and by additional material in Danish, Dutch, French, Norwegian, Spanish, and Swedish when appropriate (Lewis-Fernández et al. 2014).

TABLE 1–1. Inclusion of Outline for Cultural Formulation domains in question lists, assessment protocols, and semistructured clinical interviews prior to the Cultural Formulation Interview

	Canada[a]	Netherlands[b]	Sweden[c]	United States[d]	United Kingdom[e]	Denmark[f]
Cultural identity						
Cultural reference group(s)	√	√	√	√	√	√
Patient's and key relatives' cultural identifications (e.g., ethnic, religious, national)	√	√	√	√	√	√
Cultural identity of key members of social network (e.g., parents, relatives, friends)	√	√	√	√		√
Importance or meaning to patient/family of cultural identification		√	√	√	√	
Perceptions of patient's identity by others			√			√
Experience of multiple identities and/or changes of identity over time		√*	√		√	√
Relationship of cultural identity factor(s) to problem presented					√	
Characteristics of culture of origin and differences from host culture		√				
Language						
Language use by developmental period and setting (e.g., at home, in health care)	√	√	√	√	√	√
Language(s) in which patient is literate	√		√	√		√
Perceived fluency in language of host culture		√			√	
Cultural factors in development	√					

TABLE 1–1. Inclusion of Outline for Cultural Formulation domains in question lists, assessment protocols, and semistructured clinical interviews prior to the Cultural Formulation Interview *(continued)*

	Canada[a]	Netherlands[b]	Sweden[c]	United States[d]	United Kingdom[e]	Denmark[f]
Involvement with culture of origin (e.g., country of origin, migrants from same origin)	✓	✓	✓	✓		✓
Importance/frequency of involvement to patient		✓	✓	✓		✓
Perceptions of culture of origin	✓	✓*		✓		✓
Elements of culture of origin that are missed/relieved to have left		✓*	✓	✓		✓
Involvement with host culture (e.g., peers, food, news)	✓	✓	✓	✓	✓	✓
Perceptions of host culture (e.g., racism, values relative to culture of origin, opportunities)	✓	✓	✓	✓	✓	✓
Relationship of engagement with host culture to presenting problem					✓	
Migration history (e.g., reasons, route, journey experience, hopes, people left behind)	✓	✓	✓		✓[g]	✓
Cultural explanations of the individual's illness						
Predominant idioms of distress and illness categories, including illness/problem label	✓	✓	✓	✓	✓	✓
How patient describes problem to social network			✓			
How social network/culture of origin describes problem		✓	✓	✓	✓	✓
Most troubling aspect of problem to patient					✓	

TABLE 1–1. Inclusion of Outline for Cultural Formulation domains in question lists, assessment protocols, and semistructured clinical interviews prior to the Cultural Formulation Interview (*continued*)

	Canada[a]	Netherlands[b]	Sweden[c]	United States[d]	United Kingdom[e]	Denmark[f]
Meaning and severity of symptoms in relation to cultural norms	√	√	√	√	√	√
Patient's views (e.g., of severity)	√	√	√	√	√	√
Views of social network	√	√	√		√	√
In relation to norms of host culture (e.g., clinicians)	√	√	√			√
Impact on patient's life/biggest fear	√	√		√	√[h]	√
Perceived causes and explanatory models (e.g., illness mechanism[s], course, expected outcomes)	√	√	√	√	√	√
Views of social network (e.g., of causes)	√	√*	√	√	√	√
Prototypes (e.g., knowledge of anyone with same problem)	√	√*	√	√	√	√
Treatment expectations (e.g., preferred treatment, concerns)	√	√*	√	√	√	√
Help-seeking experiences and plans	√	√	√	√	√	√
Treatments sought or planned in formal health care system	√	√*	√	√	√	
Most useful treatment received		√*		√	√	
Help/treatment recommended in country of origin/by social network		√*	√			
Use of traditional healers and alternative services	√	√*	√	√	√	√

TABLE 1–1. Inclusion of Outline for Cultural Formulation domains in question lists, assessment protocols, and semistructured clinical interviews prior to the Cultural Formulation Interview *(continued)*

	Canada[a]	Netherlands[b]	Sweden[c]	United States[d]	United Kingdom[e]	Denmark[f]
Cultural factors related to psychosocial environment and levels of functioning						
Social stressors in relation to cultural norms	√	√*	√	√	√	√
Social network's perception of stressors	√			√		
Impact on patient		√	√	√	√	√
Relationship with partner		√				√
Social supports in relation to cultural norms	√	√	√	√	√	√
Role of religious/spiritual supports (e.g., prayer)		√	√	√		√
Barriers to receiving supports			√			
Levels of functioning and disability in relation to cultural norms	√		√	√	√	√
Views of social network and culture of origin on levels of functioning/disability				√		
Cultural elements of the relationship between the individual and the clinician						
Patient's views of the relationship		√	√		√	√
Experience of quality of communication/language use during interview		√*	√		√	√
Important topics not covered		√*	√		√	√
Perception of own role during interview (e.g., should I ask questions?)		√				
Importance to patient of match with clinician (e.g., gender, faith)		√			√	√

TABLE 1–1. Inclusion of Outline for Cultural Formulation domains in question lists, assessment protocols, and semistructured clinical interviews prior to the Cultural Formulation Interview *(continued)*

	Canada[a]	Netherlands[b]	Sweden[c]	United States[d]	United Kingdom[e]	Denmark[f]
Clinician's views of the relationship	√	√*	√	√	√	√
Experience of quality of communication/language use during interview	√	√*	√	√	√	√
Awareness of own culture/historical relationships of patient and clinician cultures of origin	√		√	√	√	
Impact of intercultural differences/similarities (e.g., on diagnosis, engagement, treatment plan)	√	√*	√	√	√	√

Note. The countries are presented following the order of publication of their respective instruments.

[a]Kirmayer et al. 2001 (English).

[b]Rohlof 2008, Rohlof et al. 2002 (items included in abbreviated version by Groen 2009a are noted with an asterisk; Dutch and English).

[c]Bäärnhielm et al. 2007, 2010a, 2010b (Swedish, English, Finnish, and Norwegian).

[d]Mezzich et al. 2009 (English).

[e]Jadhav 2010a, 2010b (English).

[f]Østerskov 2011 (Danish).

[g]Utilizes a map of the world to trace migration journey.

[h]Utilizes a schema of the human body to trace mechanisms of illness/treatment.

Source. From Lewis-Fernández et al. 2014. Reprinted with permission.

TABLE 1–2. Key themes and implications for DSM-5 related to the Cultural Formulation Interview (CFI) and its clinical implementation

CFI as an intervention

OCF domain	Key themes	Implications for DSM-5
Cultural identity of the individual	Patients' cultural identities should be assessed directly—rather than assigned by the clinician—including asking about how these change with context. Key aspects of identity from previous OCF instruments include patient's multiple cultural identifications, their meaning for the patient and the social network, language use, relationship of identity with presenting problem, and immigrants' separate involvement with culture of origin and host culture. Assessment of identity presents particular challenges for specific groups (e.g., youth, older adults, refugees).	The CFI includes open-ended questions that allow patients to narrate their own cultural identities. Cultural identity is conceptualized broadly to include culture, race, ethnicity, gender, religion, language, geographical origin, and sexual orientation. Inquiry about cultural identity is linked to its impact on the clinical problem, treatment choices, other aspects of care, and life problems in general. Supplementary modules for this topic and by patient population can be used for detail.
Cultural explanations of the individual's illness	Patients' narrations of illness present diversely, as logical explanations or as more metaphorical accounts, and may change with context. Eliciting the views of patients' friends and family may clarify which illness models are most relevant to care. Culture also affects patients' communication styles, engagement expectations, and preferences for care. Previous OCF operationalizations inquire about illness idioms, symptom meaning and perceived severity, causes, course, past care, and treatment expectations, usually from both the patient and close associates.	The CFI uses open-ended questions to elicit illness models from patients and their close associates, allowing for exploration of all types of illness models. Using patient illness terms as prompts may reveal cultural information and facilitate engagement. Attention to past experiences of care and current treatment preferences can improve patient engagement. Identifying potential barriers to care early in treatment may allow clinicians to address them. Supplementary models allow greater exploration of illness models as needed.

TABLE 1–2. Key themes and implications for DSM-5 related to the Cultural Formulation Interview (CFI) and its clinical implementation *(continued)*

CFI as an intervention

OCF domain	Key themes	Implications for DSM-5
Cultural factors related to psychosocial environment and levels of functioning	Assessment should combine patients' subjective experience of stressors, supports, and levels of functioning with clinicians' objective analysis of the social and cultural context.	The CFI follows the subjective-objective approach by emphasizing documentation of patient and clinician interpretations about social supports, stressors, and levels of functioning.
	Multiple social factors increase risk for psychopathology; diverse social groups face discrimination due to their devalued social status and should be assessed.	The CFI may be used with all patients, assessing experiences of diverse social groups.
	The impact of religion, spirituality, and moral traditions on coping is often neglected.	Open-ended questions assess supports, stressors, and the most troubling aspect of the presenting problem.
	Previous OCF instruments prioritize impact of stressors on the patient, role of spiritual support, and the views of close associates.	Supplementary modules for informants, levels of functioning, psychosocial stressors, special patient populations, and religion/spirituality/moral traditions can be used for detail.
Cultural elements of the relationship between the individual and the clinician	Facilitating clinician self-reflection via standardized questions on the clinician-patient relationship can help reduce unintended stereotyping and bias and increase rapport and engagement.	The CFI inquires about previous experiences with racism and discrimination in clinical care.
	Previous OCF instruments address this topic through questions aimed at the clinician, the patient, or both.	The CFI focuses on barriers to treatment, such as lack of resources or of culturally competent professionals or services that may impact the patient-clinician relationship.
	Raising these sensitive issues early in care (e.g., during intake) may show willingness to overcome past treatment barriers in the current therapeutic relationship.	The Patient-Clinician Relationship supplementary module contains additional questions for patients and clinicians to self-reflect on how their backgrounds and the health system affect care.

TABLE 1–2. Key themes and implications for DSM-5 related to the Cultural Formulation Interview (CFI) and its clinical implementation *(continued)*

Implementing the CFI in service settings

Implementation topic	Key themes	Implications for DSM-5
Contexts of use	Best-practice recommendations have varied as to when, where, and how to use the OCF (e.g., routine care with all patients vs. only for overcoming specific culture-related barriers).	The CFI is designed to initiate the standard clinical intake. The CFI can be used with all patients by all clinicians or adjunctive staff in all settings.
	There are advantages and disadvantages to having clinicians themselves or adjunctive staff obtain information using the OCF.	Special situations may be especially important for CFI use, as when clinicians are unfamiliar with the patient's culture or disagree with the patient's preferences and expectations of care.
Length and content	Length and content of previous OCF operationalizations have varied, reflecting the diverse clinical settings and cultural contexts of use.	To facilitate use, the core CFI consists of 16 questions for all patients. Supplementary modules can be used to balance the level of cultural information needed with clinical constraints on time and priorities of the clinical setting.
Training	Standardized training protocols are a necessary step in the large-scale implementation of the CFI.	The CFI has clear written guidelines for clinicians to follow during training.
	CFI training approaches may be guided by past efforts focused on the OCF, including case supervision, class presentations of formulated cases, didactic review, and more advanced experiential, self-reflective, and ethnographic methods.	A training video is currently in preparation. When it becomes available, it will be announced at www.nyspi.org/culturalcompetence. The CFI may respond to ACGME requirements for psychiatric residents and program directors to demonstrate cultural competence throughout different aspects of training.

Note. ACGME=Accreditation Council for Graduate Medical Education; OCF=Outline for Cultural Formulation.
Source. From Lewis-Fernández et al. 2014. Reprinted with permission.

Key Themes Related to the CFI as an Intervention

Cultural Identity of the Individual

Cultural psychiatrists regard understanding a patient's cultural identity as indispensable to evaluation. Much of what clinicians understand as *culture* relates to a person's identity: What is the patient's cultural background—for example, in terms of ethnicity, religion, socioeconomic status (SES), or nationality? What languages does the patient speak? What groups does the individual relate to regularly or, by contrast, avoid? What are the individual's values regarding, for example, health, health care, and spirituality? What aspects of the patient's experience, such as child-rearing practices or migration, have shaped his or her perception of self and possibly his or her illness?

Cultural identity can be ascribed to the person by others, on the basis of perceived characteristics, or can be self-defined (Kirmayer et al. 2008a). *Self-defined cultural identity* can be understood as the part of a person's self-construal that is related to the feeling of belonging to one or more cultural groups, including the history of one's past group affiliation(s) and future aspirations in relation to one's cultural group(s) (Weinreich 1986). *Ascriptions of identity by others* may be accepted or resisted by the person but will have an impact on his or her self-construal and social identity, as well as the response of others.

Cultural identity was included in several of the questionnaires, protocols, and interviews that operationalized the OCF prior to the CFI. Certain aspects were included in nearly all instruments: determining the cultural groups with which patients identify; establishing the importance and meaning ascribed by patients and their families to this identification; assessing language use, including by developmental period and setting; and determining the patients' involvement with the cultures of origin and resettlement for immigrants, including both positive and negative experiences (Table 1–1). These aspects of identity were prioritized in the CFI.

Several key points about identity emerge from work on the OCF. First, assessment of cultural identity should be comprehensive. Many aspects of experience shape the person's identity. Early guidelines on cultural assessment (Lu et al. 1995) suggested assessing cultural identity through an "interpersonal grid" (p. 483) documenting ethnicity, race, geographical origin, language, acculturation, gender, age, sexual orientation, religious or spiritual beliefs, socioeconomic class, and education. Cultural assessment must inquire about these aspects of identity directly, to avoid stereotyping patients or simplifying sociocultural phenomena based on a clinician's determination of the patient's identity (Lewis-Fernández 1996).

Second, cultural assessment must recognize that a person's identity may shift across time, context, and expectations. Identity is always framed in relation to the person's past history, current concerns, and future prospects. Moreover, the ways that people think about and describe their identity depend on the setting and the interlocutor. The OCF attempts to clarify how a person's cultural identity can change with context (e.g., with family members compared with strangers from a different ethnicity), including how the patient's own experience of identity is affected by his or her perception of the clinician's identity (Aggarwal 2012; Yilmaz and Weiss 2000). Sometimes a patient may emphasize, consciously or unconsciously, aspects of identity that are closer to his or her view of the clinician's background. An immigrant, for example, may stress his or her shared identity with the clinician (as an "American" or as a member of a particular ethnocultural, racial, or other group) rather than emphasizing their cultural differences (Laria and Lewis-Fernández 2015).

The third point is related to the second: a person's identity is never one-sided; people have many facets or strands to their identity. The various strands that contribute to one person's identity may come from very disparate sources—one or multiple religions, several ethnic or racial backgrounds in the family, different geographical displacements, the meaning ascribed in different places to belonging to a certain generation, or evolving gender and sexual orientation identities, to name just a few. Individuals who have undergone marked cultural shifts, such as immigrants and refugees, can experience their identity in complex ways, as different elements of their background come to the fore in response to particular developmental transitions, life choices, stresses, and social situations. Assessing this "hybrid" nature of identity is important, including how it changes over time and in relation to illness (Aggarwal 2010a). Conflicts over sense of identity can cause substantial internal and interpersonal distress and influence the person's clinical presentation.

Fourth, a comprehensive assessment of cultural identity should help the clinician recognize the influence of identity, distress, stigma, language, and other cultural factors on the patient's clinical presentation and concerns as well as modes of symptom expression, illness interpretation, and help-seeking expectations. Assessment of cultural identity in mental health must be attentive to the ways the person's identity interacts with other cultural and contextual influences to pattern multiple aspects of the person's problem in the context of care. All of these aspects of cultural identity are discussed further in the subchapter "Supplementary Module 6: Cultural Identity."

Assessment of cultural identity may involve challenges for particular populations. Refugees may be suspicious of questions about identity, and many migrants may not know how to describe or discuss their identities with clinicians unfamiliar with their geographical, political, and historical backgrounds (Rohlof et al. 2009). Children and adolescents may have different identities than their parents depending on mixed parentage, adoption (Rousseau et al. 2008), and acculturation as a result of migration (Aggarwal 2010a). The identity of older patients may be shaped by cultural meanings of old age based on social roles and status (Aggarwal 2010b). The CFI paid particular attention to the assessment of identity in these populations through the development of supplementary modules.

Cultural Explanations of the Individual's Illness

Comparing previously developed OCF instruments reveals that all include questions on illness-related idioms, symptom meaning (and usually severity) in relation to cultural norms, causes, expected course of illness, experiences with care, and treatment expectations (Table 1–1). These, as well as other commonly elicited domains, were included in the CFI (Lewis-Fernández et al. 2014).

The research on cultural explanations of illness most directly relevant to the CFI involves anthropological methods that are person centered (Kirmayer and Bhugra 2009). Medical and psychological anthropology have developed methods for eliciting and analyzing patients' explanatory models of illness, which may include experiences and ideas about onset, causes, mechanisms, course, and treatment expectations. Arthur Kleinman's seminal description of explanatory models emphasized information about causality, mechanisms, and anticipated outcomes (Kleinman 1980). Ethnographic fieldwork has shown that in everyday explanatory accounts of illness, people may use multiple types of knowledge and modes of narration. For example, patients may link symptoms to explanations based on *chain complexes* (Kirmayer et al. 1994; Young 1981, 1982) because they were closely connected in time and space (contiguity) or as a result of logical shortcuts to denote complex experiences (e.g., metonymy), such as using the term *nerves* to refer to the anatomical and functional aspects of the nervous system, including the feelings and sensations it mediates, much as journalists use the term *Washington* to refer to the entire U.S. government. People also commonly use *illness prototypes*—illness episodes, experienced previously by the individual or by others, that provide salient examples used to reason analogically about one's own experience (Young 1981, 1982). In effect, patients' illness narratives may combine models common to a cultural group, idiosyncratic assemblies of related or even disconnected events, and models based on past experiences (Kirmayer et al. 1994).

Illness models also change in response to context, including interviewer and location, as well as interactions with family, community, or health care system; during the adaptation or acculturation of immigrants to new cultural contexts; and even over the span of a long interview, as trust is established and memories are evoked. Furthermore, culture also influences elicitation of illness models. Cultural norms affect patient communication with providers, family, and friends. Eliciting the experiences, views, and expectations of illness (*illness representations*) of the patient's family members, friends, or close associates can clarify the range of views influencing the illness experience. The organization of health care services may also determine attitudes toward disease, diagnosis, and treatment; for example, patients may emphasize physical symptoms and expect somatic remedies when working with physicians as opposed to nonmedical therapists (Kirmayer and Bhugra 2009; Weiss and Somma 2007).

Eliciting past and current expectations of care are important goals of the OCF section "Cultural explanations of the individual's illness." Following broadly accepted cultural "scripts," illness representations may be associated with specific types of self-coping and help seeking, including the perceived relevance and efficacy of mental health treatments (L.J. Kirmayer, L. Ban, V. Fauras, et al., "Illness Explanations in the Cultural Formulation," paper prepared for DSM-5 Work Group, Culture and Mental Health Research Unit, Montreal, 2012.). For example, the cultural script for psychiatric distress understood as the result of sinful behavior and loss of religious faith is likely to include more frequent prayer, revitalization of church attendance, and increased involvement with one's faith community rather than use of psychiatric medication. Cultural adaptations of treatment interventions that incorporate cultural scripts or explanations may enhance patient engagement and outcomes, indicating the value of identifying cultural models and meanings before treatment (Griner and Smith 2006). Nonmedical forms of self-coping and help seeking are common and merit clinical attention because they may complement or conflict with psychiatric care. Barriers to service utilization also reflect cultural priorities for care, family values and interactions, and local health system factors affecting access.

Earlier OCF guidelines (Lu et al. 1995) included culture-bound syndromes in the section on cultural explanations of illness. In DSM-5, the term *culture-bound syndrome* has been replaced by three newer terms: *cultural syndromes, cultural idioms of distress,* and *cultural explanations* (American Psychiatric Association 2013). In reviewing the literature for DSM-5, members of the DCCIS recognized that few disorders around the world are truly "bound" to one culture; cases are found in other cultural contexts with similar illness models, and sporadic cases are found across very diverse societies. Moreover, all disorders—including those described in North America—are influenced by the cultural context of the patient. Also, many cultural concepts or illness terms do not refer to "syndromes"—that is, they do not reference a relatively invariant pattern of co-occurring symptoms. To avoid confusion, these newer terms distinguish among culturally shaped or influenced symptom clusters (*syndromes*); common modes of expressing distress (*idioms*), which may not involve specific symptoms; and explicit causal models, attributions, or explanations. Patient clinical presentations may be influenced by these cultural concepts and modes of expression. Although the same illness term may be used with all three meanings at times, it is clinically useful to understand how the term or construction is functioning for a given patient.

Cultural Factors Related to Psychosocial Environment and Levels of Functioning

The OCF directs clinicians to clarify cultural interpretations of the stressors and supports associated with a patient's illness and the fears and hopes affecting levels of functioning. The goal is a description of the context in which the illness emerged and the current situation through the perspectives of the patient and others close to him or her.

The pre–DSM-5 OCF instruments assess stressors, supports, and levels of functioning in different ways. Alternatives include focusing on the impact of stressors on the patient, the views of the social network, the role of the person's partner and/or of spiritual support, barriers to receiving help, and the views of the social network on resulting levels of functioning. Pre–DSM-5 instruments used open-ended questions to obtain a richer picture of these topics.

The illness experience of the patient and the responses of family members or others in the social network are important because stress and support are strongly influenced by cultural meanings and practices, which shape the perceived centrality, magnitude, and tractability of the problem (Bäärnhielm and Scarpinati Rosso 2009). As part of personal coping styles or culturally influenced modes of self-presentation, patients may minimize or amplify stress, social support, and level of functioning; hence, collateral information from family members or others in their entourage can clarify clinically relevant aspects of the psychosocial environment. During assessment, the person's *internal,* subjective experience is interpreted through the clinician's *external* analysis of the social and cultural context. Like evaluating stress and social support, the functional assessment of activities of daily living includes the interpretations of patients and their social networks in relation to cultural norms of functioning (see subchapter "Supplementary Module 4: Psychosocial Stressors").

Ethnocultural minorities and racially identified groups may face distinctive stressors associated with their social status. Migration status is a potent social determinant of health for refugees independent of premigratory trauma (Kirmayer et al. 2011). Factors most associated with risk for psychopathology include low SES, poor housing, unemployment or underemployment, lack of residency, linguistic barriers, limited social networks, discrimination, role strain, family conflict, status loss, acculturative stress, nostalgia, and bicultural tension (Bhugra 2004; Finch and Vega 2003; Hovey and Magaña 2002; Tartakovsky 2007). Discrimination affects various social groups, such as religious minorities, lesbian-gay-bisexual-transgender-queer persons, and low-SES and disability communities, whose subjective experience of stress and coping should be assessed. Questions may need adaptation to address the experience of discrimination, social position, and specific predicament of the patient.

To adequately assess social stressors and supports, an operationalized OCF needs to obtain collateral information from the patient's social network; this is important for all patients but is especially so for children and adolescents and older adults. Similarly, there is a need for guidance on obtaining information through medical interpreters and culture brokers (Mezzich et al. 2009; Rohlof et al. 2009; Rousseau et al. 2008).

Finally, any assessment of help seeking must consider the fact that patients often turn to religion, spirituality, and moral traditions to understand and respond to mental illness. There is a "religiosity gap" between clinicians trained in positivistic scientific methods who may disparage religion and patients who search for holistic treatments and are invested in religious beliefs and practices (Lukoff et al. 1992). Cultural assessment thus should attend to the meanings and practices associated with religion in illness experience, especially when a religious community provides support (Whitley 2012). Such information can help to mobilize support that contributes to recovery.

Cultural Elements of the Relationship Between Individual and Clinician

The relationship between patient and clinician is influenced by the expectations, role definitions, and resources each brings to the encounter. Evaluating this interaction is an important dimension of cultural assessment and requires self-reflection on the part of the clinician. Many OCF case studies illustrated challenges in providing cross-cultural care. These included tensions between biomedical treatment and other forms of healing (Barrett 1997), the failure of health systems to provide interpreters (Bucardo et al. 2008), and difficulties in communication (Yilmaz and Weiss 2000). Many of these are structural issues, but some reside primarily in the quality of the clinical relationship and communication. In several studies (e.g., Groen 2009b), clinicians discussed tensions between considering the patient individually and considering him or her as part of a social group. Despite clinicians' best efforts, the medical encounter may be influenced by stereotyping, discrimination, racism, and subtle forms of bias.

Existing instruments address this domain differently (Table 1–1). Some focus on the clinician, providing queries to consider rather than questions addressed to the patient. The Montreal CCS interview (Kirmayer et al. 2001) includes questions on the mutual perceptions of power and positioning of the patient and clinician, including historical relations between their respective cultural groups. The concepts of *cultural transference* and *cultural countertransference* are thus mobilized to analyze patient-physician relationships (Comas-Díaz and Jacobsen 1991; Mezzich et al. 2009). Other instruments suggest questions for the patient, including on the quality of communication, the need for interpreters, topics missed during the interview, the impact of cultural matching with the clinician, and the role of the patient. Open inquiry into the sensitive topics of negative treatment experiences and potential miscommunications early in care (e.g., during intake) may facilitate rapport and engagement because it conveys a commitment to overcome treatment barriers; it also acknowledges from the beginning that both patients and clinicians bring their cultural perspectives to bear on the clinical encounter and that these perspectives may evolve and interact over the course of care.

Key Themes Related to Implementation of the CFI

By the time of the DSM-5 revision, multiple implementation questions had arisen regarding the operationalization of the OCF. These included questions about the contexts of its use, the length and content of the interview, and the training required to learn to administer it. The CFI development group came up with suggested solutions for these questions, as described in the three subsections that follow. Although these solutions are useful, they are based on expert consensus rather than research data. More empirical research and clinical experience are needed to clarify many of the following implementation issues.

Contexts of Use

Obstacles to wider use of the OCF have included the lack of detail on when, where, and how culturally focused assessment should be used, including for which patients, for what purposes, by which staff members, and at which point in the course of clinical care (Cuéllar and Paniagua 2000). There are differing opinions, which may reflect different contexts of practice. For example, Jadhav (2010a, 2010b), working in an inpatient setting in the United Kingdom, recommended using the OCF to engage all patients. Caballero-Martínez (2009) has suggested reserving the OCF for patients whose presentation includes cultural content unfamiliar to the clinician. It is also necessary to clarify what roles the OCF can play in ongoing treatment beyond the initial evaluation (Lewis-Fernández 2009). Additionally, whereas most published case studies have featured patients from cultural backgrounds unfamiliar to the treating clinician, such as immigrants or ethnic minorities, some have also included reports of culturally similar patients and clinicians, illustrating how the OCF can be used to clarify intracultural issues (Aggarwal 2010a).

Guidance is also needed on the clinical training and skills needed to conduct cultural assessment and produce a cultural formulation. In most published case reports, the treating clinician was the interviewer. However, the OCF may also be used by nonmedical cultural experts attached to the clinical team, such as a culture broker or anthropologist (Kirmayer et al. 2008b; Rohlof et al. 2009) who may prepare a report based on OCF data that can be integrated with routine clinical findings. In Montreal's CCS, both clinicians and nonmedical culture brokers found the OCF to be useful, and psychologists tended to find it more useful than did physicians (Kirmayer et al. 2008b). Dinh et al. (2012) showed that the OCF changed the dynamics of a multidisciplinary group by increasing the participation of nonmedical professionals (e.g., social workers and others) who could contribute to understanding the patient's social world. Assigning the task of cultural assessment to specialized experts may enhance the cultural information gathered but poses challenges for integrating the formulation into clinical care.

Views differed about whether or not OCF-based questions should be integrated into routine clinical assessment. Some authors suggested that the assessing clinician could incorporate portions of the OCF into the clinical evaluation—for example, by including questions about the history of the present illness in the domain of cultural explanations of the individual's illness (Aggarwal 2010b; Caballero-Martínez 2009; Jadhav 2010a). This approach may encourage attention to this aspect of the OCF without a full interview for every patient. To ensure comprehensive assessment of complex cases, the Montreal CCS conducts a combined clinical-cultural assessment over one to three visits that include the patient as well as key people in his or her social network (Kirmayer et al. 2003). Other clinicians in refugee clinics in Sweden and the Netherlands conduct supplementary interviews after the intake assessment (Bäärnhielm and Scarpinati Rosso 2009; Rohlof et al. 2009).

Although cultural formulation is potentially relevant and useful for any patient, the DSM-5 OCF group identified five main situations in which assessment of cultural factors may be especially relevant for patient care: 1) when the clinician's unfamiliarity with the patient's culture leads to difficulties in diagnostic assessment, 2) when the clinician is uncertain about how diagnostic criteria fit with the patient's symptoms, 3) when the clinician is having difficulties judging illness severity or impairment, 4) when the patient and clinician disagree about the appropriate course of care, and 5) when the patient demonstrates limited treatment adherence and engagement (American Psychiatric Association 2013). Future work will likely identify other situations in which the CFI can be useful.

Length and Content

The lengths of the various OCF interviews, questionnaires, and protocols described in Table 1–1 vary from 30 to 90 minutes. The practical dilemma is how to balance brevity with sufficient depth. Kirmayer et al. (2008b) found that 27% of clinicians working with the CCS felt that the interview failed to assess important information and 30% found it too lengthy. The lengths of cultural assessment interviews vary widely based on the complexity of the cases; for example, complicated migration history and past illness experience take longer to review.

The literature is divided on which section(s) of existing interviews could be shortened or eliminated. A study of patients referred for cultural consultation found that the OCF domain cultural explanations of the individual's illness contributed less to final formulations than did other domains, including psychosocial environment, cultural identity, and clinician-patient relationship. This might be because systemic issues are most important but also because many patients have several concurrent models of illness and are reluctant to offer views that diverge from what they believe the clinician expects (Kirmayer et al. 2003), a finding replicated elsewhere (Bäärnhielm and Scarpinati Rosso 2009). Rohlof et al. (2009) suggested that the domain cultural elements of the relationship between the individual and the clinician could be subsumed elsewhere. Others, however, supported an elaboration of this section to establish rapport, promote engagement, and uncover information around cultural factors related to psychosocial environment and levels of functioning, such as discrimination and acculturation (Jadhav 2010a, 2010b). As mentioned earlier in this section, these differing suggestions may reflect the diverse clinical settings and cultural contexts in which the OCF has been used and suggest the need for flexible application in both the order of presentation and the depth of elaboration.

Training

Developing a standard training protocol is a necessary step in the large-scale implementation of any intervention, including assessment interviews such as the CFI. Typically, a training protocol consists of reviewing written guidelines with clinicians and answering any questions, observing the intervention through a video demonstration, and practicing the intervention through case-based simulations. Live supervision or review of videotaped interviews can be used to ensure that trainees are able to apply the interview protocol as intended. As measurement-based care becomes more widespread, CFI implementation may be assessed through instruments that rate fidelity of use after training, a topic covered within Chapter 4 (see discussion in "Planning and Assessment").

The DSM-5 CFI has several of the elements needed to develop a standard training protocol. The sample interview questions in the core CFI and CFI-Informant Version are accompanied by guidelines indicating the rationale and goal for each item, which can be reviewed by clinicians. Video simulations similar to those developed for the DSM-5 field trial of the CFI have been prepared for this handbook (see "Video Guide") and for a training video in collaboration with the New York State public mental health system (the availability of this video will be posted on the Web site of the New York State Center of Excellence for Cultural Competence at www.nyspi.org/ culturalcompetence). The Psychiatry Milestone Project, a joint endeavor of the Accreditation Council for Graduate Medical Education and the American Board of Psychiatry and Neurology, requires psychiatry residents to evaluate cultural factors in psychiatric formulation and differential diagnosis, patient development across the life span, knowledge of psychopathology, and clinical ethics. The CFI may address these needs, and future work could investigate the reception of CFI training by residency directors, course leaders, and trainees; the challenges of including the CFI within the curriculum; and the extent to which trainees use the CFI after graduation. The development of training videos and evaluation materials would help residency directors and service administrators assess clinician skill in using the CFI. Training models in cultural psychiatry aimed at medical students and residents illustrate how to teach the OCF, including didactic review and journal club discussion of OCF domains, case illustration by preceptors, and supervised case formulation and class presentations by trainees; these approaches are sometimes combined with experiential learning (e.g., community visits), cultural self-reflection exercises, and basic ethnographic techniques (e.g., simple field notes), especially by preceptors cross-trained in the social sciences (Hansen et al. 2013; Kirmayer et al. 2012). These OCF-focused methods may help guide CFI training and are described in Chapter 5 ("Cultural Competence in Psychiatric Education Using the Cultural Formulation Interview"). The same approaches can be extended to continuing education and in-service training for multidisciplinary teams to ensure adequate training of current practitioners.

Conclusion

The OCF in DSM-IV generated substantial international interest as a potential way of improving the cultural validity of diagnosis and treatment planning. With the development of the CFI in DSM-5, the considerations of culture and context introduced in DSM-IV have been greatly expanded. The literature reviews conducted for DSM-5 and the experience of the DCCIS supported the value of the OCF framework and guided the design of the CFI as a tool for facilitating cultural aspects of assessment and treatment planning in clinical practice.

The challenge faced in developing the CFI was how to increase the use of the OCF by shortening the assessment process so that it is practical in busy clinical settings while still eliciting crucial information about what is at stake for the patient and promoting the dialogue necessary for person-centered care (Kleinman and Benson 2006). The contextual understanding facilitated by the OCF is a complement to the decontextualized, criteria-based diagnostic assessment that is the focus of much of DSM. To follow the OCF, clinicians must more thoroughly assess the sociocultural context of patients' illness experience. Without this systematic contextual assessment, the meaning of patients' illness behavior and experience—including accurate calibration of their symptom severity, stressors, and level of functioning—may elude the practitioner, increasing the risk of clinical mismanagement and of patient dissatisfaction, nonadherence, and poor treatment response. The ways in which the CFI attempts to strike a balance between depth and concision in clinical assessment are described in Chapter 2 ("The Core and Informant Cultural Formulation Interviews in DSM-5").

KEY CLINICAL POINTS

- The DSM-IV Outline for Cultural Formulation (OCF) provides a conceptual framework for the topics that should be included in a cultural assessment during a mental health evaluation to improve diagnostic accuracy and patient engagement in treatment planning.

- Implementation gaps hindering widespread adoption of the OCF have included limited guidance on how to turn the OCF conceptual framework into an interview for use with patients; lack of guidelines on when, with whom, and why to implement the OCF; need for adaptation for use with certain populations (e.g., children); and missing topics useful in practice (e.g., barriers to treatment access).

- The DSM-5 Cultural Formulation Interview (CFI) was developed to help bridge these implementation gaps.

- The CFI is composed of three parts: a core 16-item questionnaire, an informant version of the core CFI to obtain collateral information from close associates of the patient, including caregivers, and 12 supplementary modules that expand on these basic assessments.

- The four domains of the OCF were included in the development of the CFI, which also addressed several implementation barriers identified in research and clinical practice with the OCF since 1994.

Questions

1. What are the four domains of the OCF?

2. To what extent has the OCF been taken up by clinicians and mental health educators?

3. What evidence exists on the clinical utility of the OCF?

4. What are some of the clinically relevant features assessed by each domain of the OCF?

5. Which implementation barriers were addressed in the development of the CFI?

References

Adeponle AB, Thombs BD, Groleau D, et al: Using the cultural formulation to resolve uncertainty in diagnoses of psychosis among ethnoculturally diverse patients. Psychiatr Serv 63(2):147–153, 2012 22302332

Aggarwal NK: Cultural formulations in child and adolescent psychiatry. J Am Acad Child Adolesc Psychiatry 49(4):306–309, 2010a 20410723

Aggarwal NK: Reassessing cultural evaluations in geriatrics: insights from cultural psychiatry. J Am Geriatr Soc 58(11):2191–2196, 2010b 20977437

Aggarwal NK: Hybridity and intersubjectivity in the clinical encounter: impact on the cultural formulation. Transcult Psychiatry 49(1):121–139, 2012 22218399

American Psychiatric Association: Diagnostic and Statistical Manual of Mental Disorders, 4th Edition. Washington, DC, American Psychiatric Association, 1994

American Psychiatric Association: Diagnostic and Statistical Manual of Mental Disorders, 4th Edition, Text Revision. Washington, DC, American Psychiatric Association, 2000

American Psychiatric Association: Diagnostic and Statistical Manual of Mental Disorders, 5th Edition. Arlington, VA, American Psychiatric Association, 2013

Bäärnhielm S, Scarpinati Rosso M: The Cultural Formulation: a model to combine nosology and patients' life context in psychiatric diagnostic practice. Transcult Psychiatry 46(3):406–428, 2009 19837779

Bäärnhielm S, Scarpinati Rosso M, Pattyi L: Kultur, kontext och psykiatrisk diagnostik. Manual för intervju enligt kulturformuleringen i DSM-IV [Culture, context and psychiatric diagnosis: Interview manual according to DSM-IV], Translated by Wicks S, Bäärnhielm S. Stockholm, Transkulturellt Centrum, 2007

Bäärnhielm S, Scarpinati Rosso M, Pattyi L: Kulttuuri ja psykiatrinen diagnostiikka. Käsikirja kulttuuriseen haastatteluun psykiatriassa, Translated by Halla T. Helsinki, Duodecim, 2010a

Bäärnhielm S, Scarpinati Rosso M, Pattyi L: Kultur, kontekst og psykopatologi. Manual for diagnostisk intervju baseret på kulturformuleringen fra DSM-IV [Culture, context and psychiatric diagnosis: Interview manual according to DSM-IV], Translated by Kale E, Jareg K. Oslo, NAKMI (Nasjonal kompetanseenhet for minoritetshelse), Norsk psykiatrisk forening, den Norske legerforening och Norsk psykologforening fra DSM-IV, 2010b

Barrett RJ: Cultural formulation of psychiatric diagnosis. Sakit Gila in an Iban longhouse: chronic schizophrenia. Cult Med Psychiatry 21(3):365–379, 1997 9352169

Bhugra D: Migration and mental health. Acta Psychiatr Scand 109(4):243–258, 2004 15008797

Bucardo JA, Patterson TL, Jeste DV: Cultural formulation with attention to language and cultural dynamics in a Mexican psychiatric patient treated in San Diego, California. Cult Med Psychiatry 32(1):102–121, 2008 18188683

Caballero-Martínez L: DSM-IV-TR cultural formulation of psychiatric cases: two proposals for clinicians. Transcult Psychiatry 46(3):506–523, 2009 19837784

Comas-Díaz L, Jacobsen FM: Ethnocultural transference and countertransference in the therapeutic dyad. Am J Orthopsychiatry 61(3):392–402, 1991 1951646

Cuéllar I, Paniagua FA: Handbook of Multicultural Mental Health: Assessment and Treatment of Diverse Populations. Orlando, FL, Academic Press, 2000

Dinh NM, Groleau D, Kirmayer LJ, et al: Influence of the DSM-IV Outline for Cultural Formulation on multidisciplinary case conferences in mental health. Anthropol Med 19(3):261–276, 2012 22309357

Finch BK, Vega WA: Acculturation stress, social support, and self-rated health among Latinos in California. J Immigr Health 5(3):109–117, 2003 14512765

Griner D, Smith TB: Culturally adapted mental health intervention: a meta-analytic review. Psychotherapy (Chic) 43(4):531–548, 2006 22122142

Groen S: Brief Cultural Interview 2009 (BCI-2009). Available at: http://www.mcgill.ca/iccc/files/iccc/Interview.pdf, 2009a. Accessed July 2, 2013.

Groen S: Recognizing cultural identity in mental health care: rethinking the cultural formulation of a Somali patient. Transcult Psychiatry 46(3):451–462, 2009b 19837781

Groleau D, Young A, Kirmayer LJ: The McGill Illness Narrative Interview (MINI): an interview schedule to elicit meanings and modes of reasoning related to illness experience. Transcult Psychiatry 43(4):671–691, 2006 17166953

Hansen H, Dugan TM, Becker AE, et al: Educating psychiatry residents about cultural aspects of care: a qualitative study of approaches used by U.S. expert faculty. Acad Psychiatry 37(6):412–416, 2013 24185288

Hovey JD, Magaña CG: Psychosocial predictors of anxiety among immigrant Mexican migrant farmworkers: implications for prevention and treatment. Cultur Divers Ethnic Minor Psychol 8(3):274–289, 2002 12143104

Jadhav S (producer): The Bloomsbury Cultural Formulation Interview [motion picture]. London, University College London, 2010a. Available at: http://www.ucl.ac.uk/ccs/specialist-services/#bcf-lightbox. Accessed July 1, 2013.

Jadhav S: Testing the clinical efficacy of Cultural Formulations in acute mental health: a randomized controlled trial (UKCRN ID 5251). London, National Forensic Mental Health R&D Programme, 2010b

Kirmayer LJ, Bhugra D: Culture and mental illness: social context and explanatory models, in Psychiatric Diagnosis: Patterns and Prospects. Edited by Salloum IM, Mezzich JE. New York, John Wiley and Sons, 2009, pp 29–37

Kirmayer LJ, Young A, Robbins JM: Symptom attribution in cultural perspective. Can J Psychiatry 39(10):584–595, 1994 7828110

Kirmayer LJ, Rousseau C, Rosenberg E, et al: Development and Evaluation of a Cultural Consultation Service in Mental Health. Montreal, Canada, Culture and Mental Health Research Unit, Institute of Community and Family Psychiatry, Sir Mortimer B. Davis-Jewish General Hospital, 2001. Available at: http://www.mcgill.ca/tcpsych/research/cmhru/working-papers/. Accessed June 15, 2013.

Kirmayer LJ, Groleau D, Guzder J, et al: Cultural consultation: a model of mental health service for multicultural societies. Can J Psychiatry 48(3):145–153, 2003 12728738

Kirmayer LJ, Rousseau C, Jarvis GE, et al: The cultural context of clinical assessment, in Psychiatry, 3rd Edition. Vol 1. Edited by Tasman A, Kay J, Lieberman JA, et al. Chichester, UK, Wiley-Blackwell, 2008a, pp 54–66

Kirmayer LJ, Thombs BD, Jurcik T, et al: Use of an expanded version of the DSM-IV outline for cultural formulation on a cultural consultation service. Psychiatr Serv 59(6):683–686, 2008b 18511590

Kirmayer LJ, Narasiah L, Muñoz M, et al: Common mental health problems in immigrants and refugees: general approach in primary care. CMAJ 183(12):E959–E967, 2011 20603342

Kirmayer LJ, Fung K, Rousseau C, et al: Guidelines for training in cultural psychiatry. Can J Psychiatry 57(3):1–17, 2012

Kirmayer LJ, Guzder J, Rousseau C (eds): Cultural Consultation: Encountering the Other in Mental Health Care. New York, Springer, 2014

Kleinman A: Patients and Healers in the Context of Culture: An Exploration of the Borderland Between Anthropology, Medicine, and Psychiatry. Berkeley, University of California Press, 1980

Kleinman A: The Illness Narratives: Suffering, Healing, and the Human Condition. New York, Basic Books, 1988

Kleinman A, Benson P: Anthropology in the clinic: the problem of cultural competency and how to fix it. PLoS Med 3(10):e294, 2006 17076546

Laria AJ, Lewis-Fernández R: Issues in the assessment and treatment of Latino patients, in Clinical Manual of Cultural Psychiatry, 2nd Edition, Edited by Lim RF, Washington, DC, American Psychiatric Publishing, 2015, pp 183–249

Lewis-Fernández R: Cultural formulation of psychiatric diagnosis. Cult Med Psychiatry 20(2):133–144, 1996 8853962

Lewis-Fernández R: The cultural formulation. Transcult Psychiatry 46(3):379–382, 2009 19837777

Lewis-Fernández R, Díaz N : The Cultural Formulation: A method for assessing cultural factors affecting the clinical encounter, Psychiatr Q 73(4):271–295, 2002 12418357

Lewis-Fernández R, Aggarwal NK, Bäärnhielm S, et al: Culture and psychiatric evaluation: operationalizing cultural formulation for DSM-5. Psychiatry 77(2):130–154, 2014 24865197

Lim RF (ed): Clinical Manual of Cultural Psychiatry. Washington, DC, American Psychiatric Publishing, 2006

Lu FG, Lim RF, Mezzich JE: Issues in the assessment and diagnosis of culturally diverse individuals, in American Psychiatric Press Review of Psychiatry, Vol 14: Assessment and Diagnosis. Edited by Oldham JM, Riba MB. Washington, DC, American Psychiatric Press, 1995, pp 477–510

Lukoff D, Turner R, Lu F: Transpersonal psychology research review: psychoreligious dimensions of healing. Journal of Transpersonal Psychology 24:41–60, 1992

Mezzich JE: Cultural formulation and comprehensive diagnosis. Clinical and research perspectives. Psychiatr Clin North Am 18(3):649–657, 1995 8545273

Mezzich JE: Cultural formulation: development and critical review, in Cultural Formulation: A Reader for Psychiatric Diagnosis. Edited by Mezzich JE, Caracci G. Lanham, MD, Jason Aronson, 2008, pp 87–92

Mezzich JE, Caracci G, Fabrega H Jr, et al: Cultural formulation guidelines. Transcult Psychiatry 46(3):383–405, 2009 19837778

Miklavcic A, LeBlanc MN: Culture brokers, clinically applied ethnography, and cultural mediation, in Cultural Consultation: Encountering the Other in Mental Health Care. Edited by Kirmayer LJ, Guzder J, Rousseau C. New York, Springer, 2014, pp 115–137

Østerskov M: Kulturel Spørgeguide [Cultural Interview Guide, in Danish]. Copenhagen, Denmark, Videnscenter for Transkulturel Psykiatri, 2011

Rohlof H: The cultural interview in the Netherlands: The Cultural Formulation in your pocket, in Cultural Formulation: A Reader for Psychiatric Diagnosis. Edited by Mezzich JE Caracci G. Lanham, MD, Jason Aronson, 2008, pp 203–213

Rohlof H, Loevy H, Sassen L, et al: Het culturele interview [The cultural interview], in Cultuur, Classificatie en Diagnose: Cultuursensitief Werken met de DSM-IV [Culture, Classification, and Diagnosis: Culture-Sensitive Work With DSM-IV]. Edited by Borra R, van Dijk R, Rohlof H. Houten, The Netherlands, Bohn Stafleu Van Loghum, 2002, pp 251–260

Rohlof H, Knipscheer JW, Kleber RJ: Use of the cultural formulation with refugees. Transcult Psychiatry 46(3):487–505, 2009 19837783

Rousseau C, Measham T, Bathiche-Suidan M: DSM IV, culture and child psychiatry. J Can Acad Child Adolesc Psychiatry 17(2):69–75, 2008 18516309

Tartakovsky E: A longitudinal study of acculturative stress and homesickness: high-school adolescents immigrating from Russia and Ukraine to Israel without parents. Soc Psychiatry Psychiatr Epidemiol 42(6):485–494, 2007 17502976

Ton H, Lim RF: The assessment of culturally diverse individuals, in Clinical Manual of Cultural Psychiatry. Edited by Lim RF. Arlington, VA, American Psychiatric Publishing, 2008, pp 3–31

Weinreich P: The operationalisation of identity theory in racial and ethnic relations, in Theories of Race and Ethnic Relations. Edited by Rex J, Mason D. Cambridge, UK, Cambridge University Press, 1986, pp 299–320

Weiss MG: Cultural epidemiology: an introduction and overview. Anthropol Med 8:5–29, 2001

Weiss MG, Somma D: Explanatory models in psychiatry, in Textbook of Cultural Psychiatry. Edited by Bhugra D, Bhui K. Cambridge, UK, Cambridge University Press, 2007, pp 127–140

Whitley R: Religious competence as cultural competence. Transcult Psychiatry 49(2):245–260, 2012 22421686

Yilmaz AT, Weiss MG: Cultural formulation: depression and back pain in a young male Turkish immigrant in Basel, Switzerland. Cult Med Psychiatry 24(2):259–272, 2000 10885789

Young A: When rational men fall sick: an inquiry into some assumptions made by medical anthropologists. Cult Med Psychiatry 5(4):317–335, 1981 7326949

Young A: Rational men and the explanatory model approach. Cult Med Psychiatry 6(1):57–71, 1982 7105790

Suggested Readings

Kirmayer LJ, Guzder J, Rousseau C (eds): Cultural Consultation: Encountering the Other in Mental Health Care. New York, Springer, 2014

Lewis-Fernández R, Aggarwal NK, Bäärnhielm S, et al: Culture and psychiatric evaluation: operationalizing cultural formulation for DSM-5. Psychiatry 77:130–154, 2014

McGill University: CCS Cultural Formulation. Available at: http://www.mcgill.ca/iccc/resources/cf. Accessed June 15, 2013. Web site on how the CFI's precursor, the OCF, has been implemented in different service settings around the world.

Mezzich JE, Caracci G, Fabrega H Jr, et al: Cultural formulation guidelines. Transcult Psychiatry 46(3):383–405, 2009

New York State Office of Mental Health, Center of Excellence for Cultural Competence: Cultural Formulation Interview Project. Available at: http://nyculturalcompetence.org/research-initiatives/initiative-diagnosis-engagement/cultural-formulation-interview-project/. Accessed September 4, 2014. Web site hosts publications, videos, and training modules on the Cultural Formulation Interview.

CHAPTER 2

The Core and Informant Cultural Formulation Interviews in DSM-5

Neil Krishan Aggarwal, M.D., M.B.A., M.A.

Oscar Jiménez-Solomon, M.P.H.

Peter C. Lam, M.P.H.

Ladson Hinton, M.D.

Roberto Lewis-Fernández, M.D., M.T.S.

In this chapter, we introduce the DSM-5 (American Psychiatric Association 2013) core Cultural Formulation Interview (CFI) and the CFI–Informant Version. We begin with a theoretical description of the core CFI. The CFI comprises three tools for clinicians to complete a cultural assessment: 1) the core CFI of 16 questions with associated prompts for direct patient interviewing; 2) the CFI–Informant Version that can be administered to close associates of the patient, such as family, friends, caregivers, and other social supports; and 3) the 12 CFI supplementary modules that expand the number of questions by cultural domain or include topics of additional interest for certain populations. All of these tools share a common theoretical foundation, and our aim in this chapter is to describe this foundation through detailed descriptions of the core CFI and the CFI–Informant Version; Chapter 3 ("Supplementary Modules") covers the supplementary modules in greater depth.

In addition, in this chapter we review key findings from the DSM-5 field trial that tested an earlier version of the core CFI consisting of 14 items. The field trial results were taken into account in the final revised core CFI that is included in DSM-5. More details on field trial recruitment, inclusion and exclusion criteria, assessment instruments, and analytical strategies can be found elsewhere (Aggarwal et al. 2013; Lewis-Fernández and Aggarwal 2013). Here, we focus on three themes that may convince clinicians and administrators to implement the CFI: 1) its feasibility, acceptability, and perceived clinical utility as reported by patients and clinicians (Lewis-Fernández et al., Feasibility, acceptability and clinical utility of the core Cultural Formulation Interview: Results from the international DSM-5 field trial, manuscript in preparation, March 2015); 2) its beneficial effects on patient-clinician communication (Aggarwal et al. 2015); and 3) suggestions for overcoming barriers to implementing the CFI in clinical practice (Aggarwal et al. 2013). Clinicians are more likely to implement interventions with a robust evidence base than interventions without such empirical support (Aarons 2004; Damschroder et al. 2009), and we hope to make the case here that the CFI possesses a strong and expanding evidence base.

Development of the CFI

The three components of the CFI were developed by the DSM-5 Cross-Cultural Issues Subgroup (DCCIS) based on a review of the scientific literature since the publication of the Outline for Cultural Formulation (OCF) in DSM-IV (American Psychiatric Association 1994) and previous attempts to operationalize the OCF by researchers around the world, many of whom also served on the DCCIS (Bäärnhielm and Scarpinati Rosso 2009; Groen 2009; Kirmayer et al. 2014; Lewis-Fernández et al. 2014; Mezzich et al. 2009; Østerskov 2011; Rohlof 2008; Rohlof et al. 2002; van Dijk et al. 2012). Mental health professionals have long recognized the need to conduct accurate cultural assessments of patients to prevent misdiagnosis and promote treatment engagement. However, as explained in Chapter 1 ("Cultural Formulation Before DSM-5"), there have been many ways to conduct such assessments, and few have attempted to analyze their similarities and differences or harmonize their content. The CFI was developed as a consensus approach to guide clinicians in how to obtain the information requested by the OCF directly from patients and members of their entourage. Conceptual and practical problems in the use of the OCF that could benefit from further attention were identified through the DCCIS literature review and discussed in committee meetings. In the case of the core CFI, this resulted in an initial draft to be tested in the DSM-5 field trial (Lewis-Fernández et al. 2014). The process of conducting a comprehensive literature review to identify areas for revision, with revisions tested systematically in a field trial with human subjects, has been the revision process for DSM-5 (Kraemer et al. 2010; Kupfer et al. 2002). Owing to time and financial constraints, the CFI–Informant Version and the supplementary modules were not included in the field trial.

The core CFI consists of 16 questions with associated instructions for clinicians to use in conducting a patient-centered cultural assessment. The DCCIS also recommended that all clinicians begin every standard clinical assessment with the core CFI. This tool has been designed for use with patients of all diagnoses and in all inpatient, outpatient, emergency, and transitional settings. This broad approach acknowledges that all patients and clinicians come from cultural backgrounds that can affect clinical care, rather than assuming that culture is only a pertinent factor in the care of racial and ethnic minorities (Aggarwal 2010; Kleinman and Benson 2006). Instructions for the core CFI have therefore addressed the gap in implementation guidelines for cultural assessments in general and for the OCF in particular.

The DCCIS also deliberated over the order of questions in the core CFI. Several cultural domains of the DSM-IV OCF had been criticized for being too indistinct and overlapping (Ton and Lim 2008), often leading to redundant information (Caballero-Martínez 2009). It was unclear whether clinicians were to obtain information under these domains in the specific order listed in the OCF. DCCIS members decided to reorganize the OCF domains to facilitate use of the core CFI at the beginning of every clinical assessment. For example, whereas the OCF starts with consideration of the patient's cultural identity, the core CFI initiates the assessment with the cultural elements of the patient's and social network's definition of the clinical problem. This parallels a routine mental health evaluation, in which establishing the patient's presented complaint helps the clinician organize the rest of the interview. Patients may otherwise find it odd to lead off with questions about their cultural identity prior to an assessment of the current problems that cause them to seek care. Appendix A presents the core CFI that appears in DSM-5 and is based on revisions from the version used in the field trial.

The core CFI is intended to obtain cultural views and practices in a patient-centered way. For example, the introduction to the core CFI reiterates that "there are no right or wrong answers." This acknowledgment emphasizes that the patient has a right to narrate his or her illness experience. This introduction also affirms that the patient's understanding of illness may differ from the clinician's biomedical understanding of the disease process (Eisenberg 1977).

Content of the Core CFI

The core CFI is divided into four main domains. The first domain, "Cultural Definition of the Problem," consists of the first three questions. Question 1 is meant to be a broad and open-ended inquiry about the patient's presenting concerns. The prompt invites the patient to describe his or her problems and emphasizes an understanding of the patient's illness narrative (Kleinman 1988), even if these descriptions are "similar to or different from how doctors describe the problem." Question 2 seeks to clarify further the patient's description of the problem as he or she would discuss it with close associates such as family or friends, a recognition that culture can influence how information is shared differentially depending on audience and social context (Kirmayer 2006). At this early point in the interview, patients may be reticent to describe the problem in ways that the clinician might find unusual and therefore may consciously or inadvertently censor nonmedical descriptions. By framing the question in relation to the person's social network, the goal is to facilitate the patient's report of as wide a range of descriptions of the situation as is salient in his or her immediate social environment. Question 3, which asks what troubles the patient most about the problem, is designed to explore what is most at stake for the individual during the illness experience (Kleinman and Benson 2006).

Questions 4–10 are grouped in the second core CFI domain, "Cultural Perceptions of Cause, Context, and Support." Questions 4, 6, and 7 focus the interview on the patient's explanatory models regarding the causes of the problem (Kleinman 1980; Kleinman et al. 1978), social supports that make the problem better, and social stressors that contribute to the problem (Mezzich et al. 2009). Question 4 includes the placeholder "[PROBLEM]," which is designed to solicit the patient's own terms and phrases for how a problem is framed in the clinical setting—these are known as *idioms of distress* (Nichter 1981). The interviewer can then substitute the patient's vocabulary for the placeholder throughout the interview, which helps to build rapport and bridge linguistic differences in patient and clinician understandings of illness. In some cases, the patient might use biomedical vocabulary, such as when a patient says, "I might have depression." In other cases, the patient might use a more psychosocial description, such as "I worry about my rent, my electricity, my phone bill." Terms that communicate the problem presented may vary greatly, and the CFI can reveal how patients frame issues so that clinicians can tailor treatment strategies most effectively.

Additionally, question 5 asks the patient to consider what friends, family, and close associates might understand as the cause of illness; this question is included to explore one understanding of culture—that is, as the meanings and viewpoints transmitted within social groups (American Psychiatric Association 2013). In this instance, the meanings being transmitted are the understandings of illness, and the social group is the patient's network of close associates. As with question 2 on the definition of the problem, framing the inquiry in terms of the social network encourages patients to report a fuller range of explanations in their social environment that may be influencing their explanatory models. For example, in video 1, *Full CFI*, that accompanies this book, when asked about her "inability to relate to others," the patient answers, "They just don't understand what's going on.... They just think that I'm crazy." This information suggests that the patient's presented problem is not culturally normative within her social network.

 Video Illustration 1: Full CFI (6:57)

One understanding of culture in DSM-5 is "the influence of family, friends, and other community members (the individual's *social network*) on the individual's illness experience" (p. 750). The relationship between the individual and her social network is on display in the video illustrating use of the core CFI, which includes segments of a full CFI evaluation. The video begins with the interviewer asking the open-ended, first question, "What brings you here today?" The woman also responds in an open-ended manner, discussing concerns about starting college as context before conveying that she hears the voice of her deceased grandmother. "She keeps telling me to go to Panama and just start my life over," the woman says. The interviewer continues by asking how the patient would describe the problem to others in her social network, and the patient answers that she cannot discuss this problem with them. In response to what troubles her most about the problem, she says, "Nobody is taking me seriously." Just from these initial questions, we learn that the patient experiences significant distance from her social network with respect to her problem.

Next, the interviewer transitions into questions about the patient's explanations for her current experiences. In responding to a question on associated stressors, she says, "Now I have the answer that I need. My grandmother is telling me what I need to do.... I guess what's stressing me out now is I need to figure out how to get to Panama." Here the CFI assists the clinician in interpreting degrees of social impairment.

Afterward, the CFI questions on identity invite the patient to share experiences about her background. In response to a question about how her background or identity relates to the problem, the patient answers that she used to be close to her family and specifically names her brothers and grandmother. When considered in relation to earlier answers, we learn that hearing her grandmother's voice may contribute to her present sense of estrangement from her family. Notably, the family unit is central to her sense of self and its relationship to the problem she presents. Despite being a woman of Panamanian background, she does not identify gender, ethnicity, or geographical origin as the social groups that most influence her illness experience. These markers of background and identity may be important in other situations but do not seem pertinent in this health care setting. Therefore, the CFI is able to clarify that the family unit is the group she regards as most clinically relevant.

Finally, the interviewer asks about the patient's past and present forms of coping and help seeking. We learn that the patient has tried to write as a form of self-coping upon encouragement from others, but this has not been particularly successful. She has also sought help from her family, who, in turn, have said, "Go talk to a therapist." The examiner asks about barriers to care, and the patient answers, "Everyone...Nobody understands what is happening.... I can't trust anybody." She remains focused on moving to Panama and obeying the wishes of her grandmother in response to what would best help her now. "The people that I tried to confide in don't understand me.... I need someone who will take me seriously." Interpersonal problems appear to distress her, and the CFI has now uncovered two clinical problems that could be addressed in the future: 1) her relationship to her social network and 2) hearing the voice of her deceased grandmother. A standard interview could also provide information on hearing voices, but it is unlikely that details about the social network would be obtained unless an extensive social history was obtained. With this foundation, the clinician can use the CFI supplementary module on the social network with the patient or the CFI–Informant Version with key members from the patient's social network—with patient consent—to better understand their perspectives.

Questions 8, 9, and 10 also belong to this second domain, but they orient the interview toward the patient's cultural identity. Question 8 is preceded by a brief introduction that clinicians can use to clarify the meaning of *cultural background or identity* as relevant to the health care context. The introduction also provides examples of identities that may be important for the patient, such as language, ethnicity, religion, and sexual orientation. Question 8 then asks the patient directly about the most important aspects of background or identity. This method of allowing the patient to name his or her cultural identity departs from previous models of cultural competence that have often made assumptions about patient identities based on a group affiliation such as race or ethnicity without accounting for their importance to the individual (Aggarwal 2012). For example, one patient in the field trial initially named his identity as Cuban but then explained that identifying as a Christian was more helpful in understanding his suffering existentially. In his case, a model of cultural competence that assumed ethnicity was the patient's most important group affiliation—without accounting for his self-ascribed identity—might have overlooked the role of religion in providing meaning to the illness experience. Question 9 then asks the patient how this identity may impact the current illness experience, predicament, or other patient-centered definition of the clinical problem. Question 10 asks the patient to consider how identity may cause other problems throughout life that may not initially come to mind as related to the illness but may, nonetheless, be important for clinicians to understand, such as problems with migration, gender roles, or intergenerational conflict.

Questions 11, 12, and 13 form the third domain, "Cultural Factors Affecting Self-Coping and Past Help Seeking." The goal of this domain is to encourage patients to share past forms of self-coping and help seeking, a recognition that most forms of help are sought outside of the biomedical health care system (Rogler and Cortés 1993). Question 11 addresses the patient's coping practices, and question 12 considers help seeking broadly, to include help within and outside of the biomedical system (e.g., religion-based support, support groups). One patient, for example, mentioned that going to church meetings that were specifically tailored to his age group provided the most comfort during exacerbations of auditory hallucinations. An additional prompt for question 12 clarifies the types of help that have been most and least helpful. This information may aid the clinician in developing a treatment plan for the current illness episode. Question 13 asks about past barriers to treatment. This information may also prove useful in devising the current treatment plan around available resources.

The final three questions of the CFI constitute the last domain, "Cultural Factors Affecting Current Help Seeking." Question 14 asks the patient about current treatment preferences, and question 15 explores treatment preferences that may be expressed by close associates. As with the questions on patient terms for illness or other self-definitions of the clinical situation, and their causes, this question on treatment preferences is examined at the individual and social levels. Finally, question 16 is preceded by an open-ended statement for the patient to anticipate how any perceived differences with the clinician can adversely affect care. By asking the patient directly about this potential barrier, the clinician can validate patient concerns and work to resolve such differences. Even if the question is not answered directly during the initial visit, the clinician's openness to the topic may empower the patient to raise concerns about the patient-clinician relationship later in the treatment.

In summary, the core CFI adopts an ecological approach to culture by first asking the patient about the illness, moving outward to the role of social supports and stressors, and then finishing broadly with the illness in relation to the health care system.

Development of the CFI–Informant Version

The purpose of the CFI–Informant Version is to assist clinicians in conducting a cultural assessment of the presenting clinical problem from the perspective of a key informant, such as a spouse, other family member, or friend who may be present during the clinical encounter. Patients are often accompanied by family or other potential informants during clinic visits, providing clinicians with the opportunity to include these close associates in the process of psychiatric diagnosis and treatment planning. The mental health literature has documented the many ways that social relationships can have profound effects—both positive and negative—on pathways to and through mental health treatment, including decisions about when or whether to seek care, participation in clinic visits, and implementation of treatment plans in the home, including adherence to medication (Jenkins and Karno 1992; Lefley 1996). As mentioned in the section "Development of the CFI," the expected roles of close associates and these individuals' perspectives on illness and treatment are rooted in culture. In this section, we describe the rationale for the CFI–Informant Version, clinical situations when this version may be useful, and issues for the clinician to anticipate when using the CFI–Informant Version in clinical practice. We do not explain each question of the CFI–Informant Version because it shares the same theoretical basis as the core CFI. The CFI–Informant Version is reproduced in Appendix B.

To be most effective, psychiatric diagnosis and treatment planning often require consultation with relatives or friends of individuals with mental illness. Certain aspects of culture may be shared among patients and others within the social network, but there may be important and unexpected differences even within families. For example, an older Vietnamese man who is depressed and most comfortable speaking Vietnamese may be accompanied by an adult child who speaks English and has adopted Anglo-European cultural values. In such cases, the patient and the informant may have quite different explanatory models for the patient's depression or view of treatment. In such situations, the CFI–Informant Version can assist in eliciting the cultural perspectives of key informants, enabling a deeper understanding of the patient's illness and the interpersonal dimensions of care. These varieties of perspective can open up opportunities for negotiation and the development of shared understandings of illness and goals for treatment.

After the decision has been made to conduct a cultural assessment, administration of the CFI–Informant Version can play an important role in clinical care in several types of clinical situations when an informant is available. In some instances, the informant may be the primary or sole source of information that is needed to assess the role of cultural factors in psychiatric diagnosis and treatment. This may occur, for example, when the clinician is assessing someone who is not able to give a meaningful or coherent history because of conditions such as severe cognitive impairment (e.g., due to a neurodegenerative brain process such as Alzheimer's disease or a head injury), catatonia, severe paranoia, or agitation. Similarly, if the patient is a young child, it may be necessary to conduct a cultural assessment of the parent's or another caregiver's perspective. In other cases, the clinician may seek clarification from the informant when the patient's responses to the CFI are ambiguous or partial (e.g., when asking the patient about how others in his or her cultural group would view the symptoms). The clinician may also choose to administer the CFI–Informant Version if there is an identified family member or friend who is perceived to be influential and active in the patient's clinical care and decision making. In certain situations, decisions about care may reside fully with a family member or other significant person in the patient's life. In these situations, conducting a cultural assessment of the informant's perspective may help to negotiate and implement a treatment plan. Finally, the CFI–Informant Version may be useful when treatment hits an impasse and a fuller assessment of the social context may identify underlying causes. The following is a summary of the types of clinical situations in which use of the CFI–Informant Version may be helpful: 1) the patient is unable to give a coherent account of illness (e.g., because of significant cognitive impairment); 2) the patient's history is vague, contradictory, or ambiguous, and collateral information would be beneficial for clarification; 3) the informant plays a significant role in health care decision making and/or caregiving; 4) the patient has a strong preference for including the family member in the cultural assessment (e.g., for cultural or other reasons); and 5) diagnostic or treatment challenges emerge later in the course of treatment, and additional collateral information may be useful.

In choosing whether to use the CFI–Informant Version, the clinician should ponder several issues. Initially, it is critical for the clinician to discuss the involvement of an informant with the patient and to respect the patient's desire for autonomy and privacy. Patients may have many different reasons for not wanting a family member involved, including concerns about burdening family members, shame about certain aspects of the problem, or discomfort with discussing conflicts with the informant that are contributing to the patient's problem. In these situations, the clinician may need to negotiate family involvement over time, after the patient and clinician have established rapport. In other situations, such as when the patient insists on having family members present during the clinical encounter and defers to them, the clinician may need to negotiate time during the visit to meet individually with the patient to provide an opportunity for sensitive issues to be discussed that might involve family members (e.g., conflict, abuse). After the informant interview, the clinician may need to decide whether to reinterview the family member (or other informant) in the presence of the patient and vice versa. Ultimately, this decision should be based on the preferences of the patient.

A related issue is that the clinician may find important differences between the views of patients and informants (e.g., in their illness explanatory models or in the extent to which behavior is viewed as normative for their cultural group). One possible approach to such situations is to present the different perspectives in a nonjudgmental way, together with the biomedical view of illness, and then to try to negotiate a partially shared understanding of illness and treatment (Hinton and Kleinman 1993). When multiple perspectives cannot be resolved in this way, at least documenting the differences may assist the clinician in seeking additional information to clarify diagnostic issues or help in anticipating obstacles to implementing the treatment plan.

It is also essential to note that the clinician has flexibility in the timing and administration of the CFI–Informant Version. For example, the clinician can decide whether to use the Informant Version at the initial visit or later in the course of treatment. In addition, the clinician may choose to use all of the Informant Version or only the part that seems most relevant to clinical care. Third, in situations with multiple family members or caregivers, the clinician needs to make pragmatic decisions about whom to interview based on patient preference as well as the informant's knowledge of the patient and the extent to which he or she is involved in day-to-day caregiving. Finally, the supplementary modules may be useful in conjunction with the CFI–Informant Version, particularly the Caregivers supplementary module, which explores in greater depth the role of cultural factors in the experience and enactment of caregiving.

Key Findings From the DSM-5 Field Trial

Having introduced the core CFI and the CFI–Informant Version, we now turn to findings from the international DSM-5 field trial. The field trial tested an earlier version of the core CFI, and data analyses conducted midway led to the revision of the core CFI that is now included in DSM-5. We briefly present an overview of the study design to help clinicians contextualize key results.

Overview

The international composition of the DCCIS allowed us to expand the scope of the DSM-5 field trials beyond the United States. Between 2011 and 2012, field trials were conducted in 14 sites across six countries (5 in the United States, 1 in Peru, 2 in Canada, 3 in the Netherlands, 1 in Kenya, and 2 in India). Table 2–1 lists all participating sites by country, along with local primary investigators.

Apart from the three clinics in the Netherlands that agreed to act as a single consortium site, all other individual sites sought to enroll at least 30 patients and five clinicians to test the core CFI's feasibility (Is it doable?), acceptability (Do people like it?), and perceived clinical utility (Is it helpful?). Patients were recruited by treating clinicians who made study referrals to research staff at each site. Appreciating that many clinicians work in busy service settings, the DCCIS created the core CFI so that it could be completed in 15–20 minutes, reasoning that a full cultural and clinical assessment could be completed within 1 hour. Our assumption was that core CFI questions would reduce the need to obtain redundant information with respect to the history of present illness, past psychiatric history, and social history. Clinicians and patients completed questionnaires before and after the CFI session on experiences with the core CFI.

Study Participants

Patients ages 18–80 years were enrolled because patients in this age group can directly provide informed consent. We enrolled patients of any race or ethnicity in recognition that all people—not only individuals from racial and ethnic minority groups—have a culture. To reduce any bias arising from cultural information obtained by interpreters, all patients and clinicians were matched by language. Patients with all psychiatric diagnoses were enrolled, and these psychiatric diagnoses were determined by referring clinicians.

TABLE 2–1.	All participating sites by country in the DSM-5 core Cultural Formulation Interview field trial
Country	**Local institutions (site investigators)**
Canada	McGill University (Laurence Kirmayer)
	University of Toronto (Monica Scalco)
India	Dr. Ram Manohar Lohia Hospital (Smita Deshpande and Sushrut Jadhav)
	KEM Hospital Research Centre (Vasudeo Paralikar and Mitchell Weiss)
Kenya	University of Nairobi (David Ndetei)
Netherlands	Centrum '45 (Hans Rohlof)
	De Evenaar Centre for Transcultural Psychiatry North Netherlands (Simon Groen)
	Parnassia Bavo Groep (Rob van Dijk)
Peru	Universidad Peruana Cayetano Heredia (Renato Alarcón and Johann Vega-Dienstmaier)
United States	Columbia University and the New York State Psychiatric Institute (Roberto Lewis-Fernández and Neil Krishan Aggarwal)
	Richmond Area Multi-Services (Kavoos Bassiri)
	University of California–Davis (Sergio Aguilar-Gaxiola and Oanh Meyer)
	University of Minnesota (Joseph Westermeyer)
	Yale University (Esperanza Díaz)

We excluded patients who were acutely suicidal or homicidal at the time of the interview for safety reasons, as well as patients with conditions that could interfere with the interview process (e.g., acute substance intoxication or withdrawal, dementia, florid psychosis, mental retardation). As with other DSM-5 field trials that tested new diagnoses or revisions to diagnoses from DSM-IV, all patients and clinicians who volunteered were enrolled (Clarke et al. 2013). A total of 314 patients were included.

All clinicians in the field trial were already on staff at each site and possessed a terminal degree (MD, MSW, PhD, or a local equivalent) that allowed them to practice independently. Clinicians accepted into the field trial had to agree to attend a 2-hour training session on the core CFI. During the session, the core CFI and its guidelines were reviewed, a video was shown of the core CFI in a simulated scenario, and role-playing exercises were conducted in which clinicians practiced questions with each other. All clinicians were asked to complete the core CFI in its entirety before transitioning into their usual diagnostic assessment. Interviews were recorded only with patient and clinician consent. A total of 75 clinicians were included.

Main Results

Feasibility, Acceptability, and Perceived Clinical Utility of the Core CFI

Patients and clinicians completed surveys on their perceptions of the feasibility, acceptability, and clinical utility of the core CFI after every encounter. Items were scored

TABLE 2–2.   Feasibility, acceptability, and clinical utility subscores by patients and clinicians participating in field trial

	Patients		Clinicians	
	Mean	Standard deviation	Mean	Standard deviation
Feasibility	1.33	0.57	0.77	0.89
Acceptability	1.27	0.71	1.01	0.72
Clinical utility	1.30	0.52	0.93	0.72

Note.   Numerical range from which patients and clinicians chose scores for feasibility, acceptability, and clinical utility: –2=strongly disagree; –1=disagree; 1=agree; 2=strongly agree.

on a four-point scale: –2 (strongly disagree), –1 (disagree), 1 (agree), and 2 (strongly agree). Scores on the negative half of the scale indicated greater disagreement with the core CFI as feasible, acceptable, or clinically useful, whereas positive scores indicated greater agreement on those factors. We assessed feasibility, acceptability, and perceived clinical utility as separate subscales.

Although survey length and wording differed between the patient and clinician versions, the fundamental concepts ascertained by the survey subscales were considered comparable. Psychometric analyses were performed on the survey subscales to generate Cronbach α, as a measure of internal consistency (Cronbach 1951). For the clinician version of the subscales, these analyses showed adequate internal consistency: feasibility $\alpha=0.77$, acceptability $\alpha=0.78$, and clinical utility $\alpha=0.89$. For the patient version of the survey, removal of one negatively worded item from the feasibility and acceptability subscales that demonstrated poor correlation with the rest of the subscale items led to acceptable internal consistency: feasibility $\alpha=0.45$ and acceptability $\alpha=0.46$. The patient clinical utility subscale scores demonstrated good internal consistency ($\alpha=0.82$), and no item was removed from this subscale for analytical purposes. These data suggest that the scales created for the DSM-5 field trial had adequate to good internal consistency.

Table 2–2 lists the mean scores and standard deviations of these final subscales for patients and clinicians. Patients generally rated each construct with higher scores than did clinicians, but both groups appear to appreciate the core CFI as feasible, acceptable, and clinically useful (no negative mean values).

CFI's Effects on Medical Communication

To understand why patients and clinicians reported that the core CFI was feasible, acceptable, and clinically useful, we analyzed debriefing questionnaires given to all participants after the CFI session. Case reports on the OCF have suggested that cultural questions help clinicians overcome communication barriers and improve patient satisfaction (Groen 2009; Caballero-Martínez 2009). Therefore, we sought to assess clinician and patient perspectives of the core CFI's effects on medical communication.

A team of three people from the New York State Psychiatric Institute coded all of the New York interviews to explore how participants believed the core CFI affected medical communication based on a framework widely used in medical education (Lazare et al. 1995). This framework suggests that the medical interview has three main functions: 1) to determine and monitor the problem presented; 2) to develop, maintain, and conclude the therapeutic relationship; and 3) to carry out patient education and implementation of treatment plans. Each task is further divided into specific tasks. Table 2–3 presents code rankings from patient and clinicians interviews.

Patients and clinicians thought that the main functions of the core CFI were 1) to determine and monitor the nature of the problem and 2) to develop, maintain, and conclude the therapeutic relationship. They also responded most positively to four main tasks within these functions: eliciting data, eliciting the patient's perspective, perceiving data at multiple levels, and enhancing rapport through satisfaction with the interview. We expected high scores for the first two tasks because the core CFI was created to obtain patient experiences of illness. Our analysis observed fewer themes for the third function, patient education and implementation of treatment plans. This may be due to the nature of our study, in which patients and study clinicians met once in order to test the interview. Patients were not educated about diagnoses, and treatment plans were not implemented.

Our most significant finding was our code for a new theme that did not appear in the original medical communication framework (Lazare et al. 1995). We defined this theme as "enhancing patient-clinician rapport through satisfaction with the CFI." Patients believed that the core CFI itself possessed communication properties that were therapeutic, independent of the clinician's ability to establish rapport. The coding team included this theme under the function of developing, maintaining, and concluding the therapeutic relationship. These data suggest that the actual structure of the core CFI may elicit positive communication. The CFI invites patients to participate actively throughout the clinical encounter via the use of a nonjudgmental introduction, open-ended questions on illness experience, patient-clinician word matching, and a patient-centered approach to how culture is relevant for the individual's illness. We hypothesize that these communication strategies may be responsible for increased satisfaction, although more studies on patient-clinician communication exchange through the core CFI are necessary to isolate exact linguistic properties. More studies are also needed on whether increased patient satisfaction through use of the core CFI improves overall treatment response, such as symptom reduction or improvements in quality of life. Nonetheless, these results build the evidence base that the core CFI may operate successfully at the level of content through the elicitation of patient cultural views and at the level of process through improved patient-clinician communication.

Barriers to Implementing the Core CFI in Clinical Practice

Finally, we wanted to understand how patients and clinicians reported limitations in the core CFI's feasibility, acceptability, and clinical utility. We analyzed the same debriefing interviews for problems with the core CFI. We used another framework on the barriers encountered when new interventions are introduced in clinical settings (Gearing et al. 2011), which differentiates problems related to the intervention from problems associated with its implementation. For example, problems related to the

TABLE 2–3. Core Cultural Formulation Interview's (CFI's) effects on medical communication as coded in debriefing interviews

	Patient rank[a]	Clinician rank[a]
Determining and monitoring the nature of the problem		
Diseases and disorders: The CFI helps clinicians make a biomedical diagnosis.	7	7
Psychosocial issues: The CFI illustrates how patients respond to their condition before entering medical care.	9	6
Eliciting data: The CFI encourages communications skills by letting patients tell their own stories, facilitating narration, easing flow of the interview, using appropriate questions, or summarizing information.	2	2
Perceived data at multiple levels: The CFI helps clinicians use their five senses and their own personal responses.	4	2
Generating and testing hypothesis: The CFI helps clinicians create or test hypotheses based on patient data.	Last	5
Developing, maintaining, and concluding the therapeutic relationship		
Defining the relationship: The CFI helps clinicians clarify their exact role in the patient's care.	8	8
Communicating expertise: The CFI helps clinicians demonstrate scientific competence and wisdom in their judgment and decisions.	Last	9
Communicating care: The CFI helps clinicians communicate positive emotions such as rapport, interest, respect, support, and empathy.	3	4
Recognizing communication barriers: The CFI helps clinicians recognize and resolve communication problems with patients by openly discussing differences, overcoming patient psychological barriers, providing emotional support, or negotiating communication differences.	5	4
Eliciting the patient's perspective: The CFI elicits the patient's perspective on definition, causes, mechanisms, fears, and goals related to the problem.	4	1
Enhancing rapport through satisfaction with the interview: The CFI increases rapport among patients and clinicians.	1	3
Patient education and implementation of treatment plans		
Determining areas of difference: The CFI helps clarify where patients and clinicians may disagree about ideas regarding patient's sickness.	6	5
Communicating diagnostic significance: The CFI helps clinicians communicate the significance of the problem from a biomedical perspective, taking into account the patient's concerns, beliefs, and fears.	Last	Last
Negotiating diagnostic procedures and treatment: The CFI helps clinicians discuss diagnosis and treatment options.	Last	10
Negotiating preventive measures: The CFI helps clinicians negotiate and recommend preventive measures.	Last	Last
Enhancing coping: The CFI helps clinicians work with patients to discuss coping strategies related to worsening social and psychological functioning from the illness or treatment.	8	9

Note. [a]Tied rank is based on number of references in all interviews.
Source. Adapted from Aggarwal et al. 2015.

intervention could include its complexity, lack of clarity, and problems with standardization, whereas problems related to organizational or clinician factors could include frequent clinician turnover, training costs, and difficulties with scheduling that make implementation difficult. Table 2–4 presents barriers to implementing the core CFI as reported by patients and clinicians.

Notably, more clinicians than patients reported barriers for each theme, perhaps because clinicians are responsible for implementation of the CFI. The highest-ranked barrier reported by clinicians was that they could not see how the core CFI responds to the need for a cultural assessment. To overcome this barrier, the DCCIS made the following revisions in the final core CFI version included in DSM-5: defined culture in the core CFI guidelines, provided specific indications for when a cultural assessment is necessary, and explained the purpose of each question. The second barrier is lack of motivation based on patient and clinicians responses combined. For example, the field trial version of the core CFI included a question on the patient-clinician relationship that troubled some clinicians: "Is there anything about my own background that might make it difficult for me to understand or help you with your [PROBLEM]?" Many clinicians reported that this question was too direct and could lead to negative emotions such as discomfort or awkwardness. Consequently, this question was revised to question 16 in the final version of the core CFI: "Sometimes doctors and patients misunderstand each other because they come from different backgrounds or have different expectations. Have you been concerned about this and is there anything that we can do to provide you with the care you need?" With awareness of this reported barrier, the DCCIS was able to improve the core CFI in order to increase its feasibility, acceptability, and clinical utility.

Three responses tied for the third most-reported barriers to the core CFI. Some clinicians found the field trial version of the core CFI to be too repetitive. This concern also became apparent for the OCF during the DCCIS systematic literature review (Lewis-Fernández et al. 2014). Subsequently, the DCCIS revised the core CFI during the field trial to ensure that cultural topics would be unique and not repetitive. Finally, some clinicians raised doubts about whether the core CFI could be used in its entirety during the initial diagnostic assessment and whether certain illnesses such as psychotic disorders would render the core CFI difficult to use.

Conclusion

In this chapter, we introduced the core CFI, the CFI–Informant Version, and the CFI evidence base through key findings from the DSM-5 field trial. We hope that clinicians and administrators will find the scholarship on the CFI convincing and will attempt its implementation in their service settings (as discussed in Chapter 4, "Clinical Implementation of the Cultural Formulation Interview"). Research is ongoing on the best ways to use all three components and the extent to which their use affects illness outcomes. The CFI represents the state of the art in cultural assessment throughout the mental health professions. Widespread use of the CFI—especially the core CFI—by clinicians and administrators is expected to help close the research-practice gap in cultural assessment and inform the next round of revisions for future DSMs.

TABLE 2–4. Barriers to implementing the core Cultural Formulation Interview (CFI) in clinical practice

Theme	Patient reported (n=32)	Clinician reported (n=32)	Barrier rank (of 64 interviews)
Internal barriers to using the core CFI			
Repetition: Parts of the CFI may be too repetitive	—	20	3[a]
Drift in procedures: Doubts about using the CFI in its entirety at the beginning of the evaluation	—	20	3[a]
Lack of motivation/buy-in: Negative attitudes or emotions regarding the CFI (such as questions on past illnesses or on religion)	8	14	2
Severity of the individual's illness: Concerns that the patient's illness presentation would affect CFI implementation	1	19	3[a]
External barriers to using the core CFI			
Lack of conceptual relevance between the CFI and culture: Comments that the purpose of the CFI or specific questions lacked clarity	—	31	1

Note.   Dash indicates none reported.
[a]The rankings are based on total references in patient and clinician interviews combined.
Source.   Adapted from Aggarwal et al. 2013.

KEY CLINICAL POINTS

- The core and informant versions of the Cultural Formulation Interview (CFI) constitute a state-of-the-art cultural assessment in mental health that builds off the existing evidence base in the social and clinical sciences.
- The core CFI is a semistructured questionnaire of 16 questions that can be used with all patients to assess relevant cultural variables in every clinical encounter. The CFI–Informant Version obtains similar information from a collateral historian.
- Patients and clinicians found the core CFI generally to be feasible, acceptable, and useful for practice. Field trial data were used to revise the core CFI questions for inclusion in DSM-5.
- The CFI improves medical communication.

Questions

1. How does the DSM-5 CFI differ from the DSM-IV OCF?

2. With what patient populations can the core CFI and CFI–Informant Version be used?

3. What are some of the core CFI effects on medical communication?

4. What kinds of barriers can be anticipated so that the core CFI is more feasible, acceptable, and useful in clinical practice?

5. In what clinical settings can the core CFI be used?

References

Aarons GA: Mental health provider attitudes toward adoption of evidence-based practice: the Evidence-Based Practice Attitude Scale (EBPAS). Ment Health Serv Res 6(2):61–74, 2004 15224451

Aggarwal NK: Reassessing cultural evaluations in geriatrics: insights from cultural psychiatry. J Am Geriatr Soc 58(11):2191–2196, 2010 20977437

Aggarwal NK: Hybridity and intersubjectivity in the clinical encounter: impact on the cultural formulation. Transcult Psychiatry 49(1):121–139, 2012 22218399

Aggarwal NK, Nicasio AV, DeSilva R, et al: Barriers to implementing the DSM-5 Cultural Formulation Interview: a qualitative study. Cult Med Psychiatry 37(3):505–533, 2013 23836098

Aggarwal NK, DeSilva R, Nicasio AV, et al: Does the Cultural Formulation Interview for the fifth revision of the Diagnostic and Statistical Manual of Mental Disorders (DSM-5) affect medical communication? A qualitative exploratory study from the New York site. Ethn Health 20(1):1–28, 2015 25372242

American Psychiatric Association: Diagnostic and Statistical Manual of Mental Disorders, 4th Edition. Washington, DC, American Psychiatric Association, 1994

American Psychiatric Association: Diagnostic and Statistical Manual of Mental Disorders, 5th Edition. Arlington, VA, American Psychiatric Association, 2013

Bäärnhielm S, Scarpinati Rosso M: The Cultural Formulation: a model to combine nosology and patients' life context in psychiatric diagnostic practice. Transcult Psychiatry 46(3):406–428, 2009 19837779

Caballero-Martínez L: DSM-IV-TR cultural formulation of psychiatric cases: two proposals for clinicians. Transcult Psychiatry 46(3):506–523, 2009 19837784

Clarke DE, Narrow WE, Regier DA, et al: DSM-5 field trials in the United States and Canada, part I: study design, sampling strategy, implementation, and analytic approaches. Am J Psychiatry 170(1):43–58, 2013 23111546

Cronbach LJ: Coefficient alpha and the internal structure of tests. Psychometrika 16:297–334, 1951

Damschroder LJ, Aron DC, Keith RE, et al: Fostering implementation of health services research findings into practice: a consolidated framework for advancing implementation science. Implement Sci 4:50, 2009 19664226

Eisenberg L: Disease and illness. Distinctions between professional and popular ideas of sickness. Cult Med Psychiatry 1(1):9–23, 1977 756356

Gearing RE, El-Bassel N, Ghesquiere A, et al: Major ingredients of fidelity: a review and scientific guide to improving quality of intervention research implementation. Clin Psychol Rev 31:79–88, 2011

Groen S: Brief Cultural Interview, 2009 (BCI-2009). Available at: http://www.mcgill.ca/iccc/files/iccc/Interview.pdf. Accessed February 4, 2014.

Hinton L, Kleinman A: Cultural issues and international psychiatric diagnosis, in International Review of Psychiatry, Vol 1. Edited by Costa e Silva JA, Nadelson C. Washington, DC, American Psychiatric Press, 1993, pp 111–129

Jenkins JH, Karno M: The meaning of expressed emotion: theoretical issues raised by cross-cultural research. Am J Psychiatry 149(1):9–21, 1992 1728192

Kirmayer LJ: Beyond the 'new cross-cultural psychiatry': cultural biology, discursive psychology and the ironies of globalization. Transcult Psychiatry 43(1):126–144, 2006 16671396

Kirmayer LJ, Groleau D, Rousseau C: Development and evaluation of the Cultural Consultation Service, in Cultural Consultation: Encountering the Other in Mental Health Care. Edited by Kirmayer LJ, Guzder J, Rousseau C. New York, Springer SBM, 2014, pp 12–45

Kleinman A: Patients and Healers in the Context of Culture: An Exploration of the Borderland Between Anthropology, Medicine, and Psychiatry. Berkeley, University of California Press, 1980

Kleinman A: The Illness Narratives: Suffering, Healing, and the Human Condition. New York, Basic Books, 1988

Kleinman A, Benson P: Anthropology in the clinic: the problem of cultural competency and how to fix it. PLoS Med 3(10):e294, 2006 17076546

Kleinman A, Eisenberg L, Good B: Culture, illness, and care: clinical lessons from anthropologic and cross-cultural research. Ann Intern Med 88(2):251–258, 1978 626456

Kraemer HC, Kupfer DJ, Narrow WE, et al: Moving toward DSM-5: the field trials. Am J Psychiatry 167(10):1158–1160, 2010 20889660

Kupfer DJ, First MB, Regier DE: Introduction, in A Research Agenda for DSM-5. Edited by Kupfer DJ, First MB, Regier DA. Washington, DC, American Psychiatric Publishing, 2002, pp xv–xxiii

Lazare A, Putnam S, Lipkin M: Three functions of the medical interview, in The Medical Interview: Clinical Care, Education, and Research, Edited by Lipkin M, Putnam S, and Lazare A. New York, Springer-Verlag, 1995 pp 3–19

Lefley HP: Family Caregiving in Mental Illness (Family Caregiver Applications Series, Vol 7). Thousand Oaks, CA, Sage Publications, 1996

Lewis-Fernández R, Aggarwal NK, Culture and psychiatric diagnosis. Adv Psychosom Med 33:15–30 2013 23816860

Lewis-Fernández R, Aggarwal NK, Bäärnhielm S, et al: Culture and psychiatric evaluation: operationalizing cultural formulation for DSM-5. Psychiatry 77(2):130–154, 2014 24865197

Mezzich JE, Caracci G, Fábrega H Jr, et al: Cultural formulation guidelines. Transcult Psychiatry 46(3):383–405, 2009 19837778

Nichter M: Idioms of distress: alternatives in the expression of psychosocial distress: a case study from South India. Cult Med Psychiatry 5(4):379–408, 1981 7326955

Østerskov M: Kulturel Spørgeguide [Cultural Interview Guide]. Copenhagen, Denmark, Videnscenter for Transkulturel Psykiatri, 2011

Rogler LH, Cortés DE: Help-seeking pathways: a unifying concept in mental health care. Am J Psychiatry 150(4):554–561, 1993 8465869

Rohlof H: The cultural interview in the Netherlands: the cultural formulation in your pocket, in Cultural Formulation: A Reader for Psychiatric Diagnosis. Edited by Mezzich JE, Caracci G. Lanham, MD, Jason Aronson, 2008, pp 203–213

Rohlof H, Loevy H, Sassen L, et al: Het culturele interview [The cultural interview], in Cultuur, Classificatie en Diagnose: Cultuursensitief Werken met de DSM-IV [Culture, Classification and Diagnosis: Culture-Sensitive Work With DSM-IV]. Edited by Borra R, van Dijk R, Rohlof H. Houten, The Netherlands, Bohn Stafleu, Van Loghum, 2002, pp 251–260

Ton H, Lim RF: The assessment of culturally diverse individuals, in Clinical Manual of Cultural Psychiatry. Edited by Lim RF. Washington, DC, American Psychiatric Publishing, 2008, pp 3–31

van Dijk R, Beijers H, Groen S: Het Culturele Interview [The Cultural Interview]. Utrecht, The Netherlands, Pharos, 2012

Suggested Readings

Mezzich JE, Caracci G (eds): Cultural Formulation: A Reader for Psychiatric Diagnosis. Lanham, MD, Jason Aronson, 2008. Explains the development of the OCF.

New York State Office of Mental Health, Center of Excellence for Cultural Competence: Cultural Formulation Interview Project, 2013. Available at: http://nyculturalcompetence.org/research-initiatives/initiative-diagnosis-engagement/cultural-formulation-interview-project/. Accessed September 15, 2014. A Web site with ongoing research on the Cultural Formulation Interview.

CHAPTER 3

Supplementary Modules

Overview

Devon E. Hinton, M.D., Ph.D.

Ladson Hinton, M.D.

The main goal of all of the components of the Cultural Formulation Interview (CFI; American Psychiatric Association 2013) (i.e., the core CFI, the CFI–Informant Version, and the supplementary modules) is to contextualize the problem that the patient presents in a complex multidimensional way—within the context of the person's sociocultural world, sense of identity, and ways of experiencing and understanding psychological distress. This ecological examination of the patient helps the clinician to select the appropriate treatment approach in collaboration with the patient, to enhance the patient's engagement in care (from session attendance to medication use), to improve the therapeutic bond, to promote positive expectancy, and to accomplish other key treatment goals (Hinton and Lewis-Fernández 2010).

To illustrate the value of this approach, we consider the case of a patient with a main complaint of "being depressed." The CFI focuses particularly on the patient's "illness," in the sense of a certain lived reality of the experience of suffering. The person is an active agent in dealing with her illness, has a set of understandings about her experience (including about the contribution of any underlying biomedical "disease" involving, e.g., abnormally functioning brain circuits), and is embedded in a particular sociocultural "local world" (Eisenberg 1977; Kleinman et al. 1978). These various dimensions of experience influence her behavioral strategies and adaptations to illness and treatment in a way that is directly relevant to clinical care—for example, by shaping her interpretation of the diagnosis and her expectations regarding medication taking. To neglect these various dimensions is to commit an "error of decontextualization" (Hinton and Good, in press; Weiner et al. 2010), whether these dimensions include the patient's understanding of the "problem," her life situation (e.g., income, employment), her sense of belonging to a set of social groups (e.g., elder adults, migrants), or the views about the problem held by others in her social world. Put another way, neglecting these factors is to commit a *dynamism error*—that is, the failure to examine how the patient reacts to and deals with the problem in various ways as influenced by a certain identity and sociocultural context.

The supplementary modules of the CFI—along with the CFI–Informant Version— help the clinician conduct a more comprehensive cultural assessment of the patient, which attempts to locate the person in his or her sociocultural context. As indicated in Figure 3–1, there are three kinds of supplementary modules: 1) core CFI expansion modules, to amplify key sections of the core CFI (e.g., the explanatory model); 2) special populations modules, to assess particular populations (e.g., refugees) who may have specific needs and experiences as a result of certain aspects of their background or identity; and 3) informant perspectives modules, to clarify how individuals who assist the patient with his or her care and members of the patient's social network view the patient's situation. Although the CFI–Informant Version is not strictly one of the 12 supplementary modules, it is included in this listing because it helps the clinician obtain a fuller picture of the patient's situation when combined with the core CFI. In this chapter, we discuss the clinical utility, types, and structure of these three types of modules to help clinicians choose among them when conducting a cultural assessment.

Uses of the Supplementary Modules: Research, Clinical Work, and Training

The core CFI is a basic tool for cultural assessment, but at times the clinician needs to use all or some of the supplementary modules to obtain more information. This may be because the core CFI either does not address certain assessment domains or assesses them too succinctly for the current situation or treatment need or because the clinician may not wish to administer the full core CFI but to focus, rather, on some of its domains, either because the core CFI has already been administered or because only a more limited assessment is currently necessary. For example, the clinician may wish to use one or more of the core CFI expansion modules to elicit information on the patient's understanding of his or her problem and related explanatory model or to learn more about the person's experience of, for example, spirituality, religion, and moral traditions and how they relate to the problem. Alternatively, the clinician may want to use one or more of the special populations modules because aspects of the person's identity (e.g., as an adolescent and immigrant) cause certain questions that are not part of the core CFI to become relevant. Finally, the clinician may turn to the informant perspectives modules to clarify the interviewee's views on the patient's problems because the interviewee helps to provide care to the patient or is a key member of the person's support system.

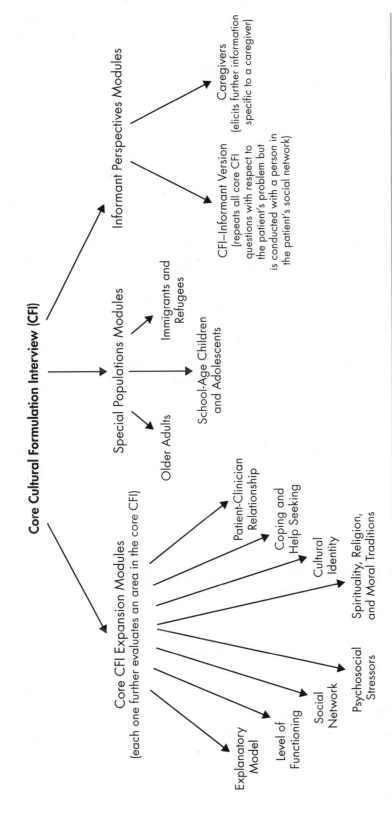

FIGURE 3–1. Decision tree showing possible further evaluations using the CFI–Informant Version and the supplementary modules after giving the core Cultural Formulation Interview.

We describe, as an example, how using the modules may improve the care of refugees or immigrants. The Immigrants and Refugees module would be a logical module to administer, but other modules can also become relevant. For example, a person may belong to an immigrant or refugee group that frequently describes certain mood, somatic, or other symptoms that may be unfamiliar to the clinician; these can be assessed through the Explanatory Model module and/or the Coping and Help Seeking module. Specifically, traumatized refugees often present with somatic complaints (e.g., shortness of breath or trembling among Caribbean Latinos or dizziness among Chinese and Southeast Asian populations) and can report culturally specific idioms of distress (e.g., complaints of "*nervios*" among Latinos or "neurasthenia" among Chinese populations) (Guarnaccia et al. 2003; Hinton and Lewis-Fernández 2011; Kleinman 1986). Moreover, the Caregivers module might be of great use if an immigrant or refugee is being cared for by a relative or an informally arranged care provider (e.g., a community member who receives compensation from the family). The Psychosocial Stressors module might also be helpful because of the key role of current life problems in generating distress (e.g., among traumatized refugees) (Hinton et al. 2011; Miller and Rasmussen 2010). Other modules can also be useful.

These examples suggest how the 12 supplementary modules can be used in conjunction with the core CFI and the CFI–Informant Version or as part of a stand-alone interview. In addition, the supplementary modules are invaluable tools for education and research. In psychiatry residency programs, for example, when residents are taught about cultural identity, the role of the social network in care, or explanatory models, they could be assigned interviews with a certain number of patients using the pertinent module(s) as further training in the relevant assessment area (for more information, see Chapter 5, "Cultural Competence in Psychiatric Education Using the Cultural Formulation Interview"). In terms of research, the modules are particularly suited for qualitative studies profiling key themes on either particular topics (e.g., caregiving practices) or specific patient groups. For example, the Coping and Help Seeking module could be used to study patients with a particular diagnosis or complaint. These reported diagnoses or complaints might include a range of categories, biomedical as well as local: "first-episode psychosis," "demoralization," "*nervios*," or "hyperactivity." The special populations modules could help ascertain key topics in the care of the group(s) in question—immigrants, older adults, and so on. As these examples suggest, the supplementary modules are a valuable tool for clinicians, trainees, educators, and researchers.

Types of Supplementary Modules

The three types of supplementary modules are described in the subsections and in Figure 3–1 and Tables 3–1 and 3–2. All of the supplementary modules are included in Appendix C. (These modules are also available online at www.psychiatry.org/practice/dsm/dsm5/online-assessment-measures).

TABLE 3–1. Core Cultural Formulation Interview (CFI) expansion modules

Module	Module subdomains	Items in module	Related core CFI questions
Explanatory Model	General understanding of the problem	14	1–5
	Illness prototypes		
	Causal explanations		
	Course of illness		
	Help seeking and treatment expectations		
Level of Functioning	Each question assesses an area of functioning (e.g., work)	8	3
Social Network	Composition of social network	15	5, 6, 12, 15
	Social network understanding of problem		
	Social network response to problem		
	Social network as a stress/buffer		
	Social network in treatment		
Psychosocial Stressors	Most questions assess a particular aspect of stressors (e.g., how the patient copes, how the stressor can be changed)	5	7, 9, 10, 12
Spirituality, Religion, and Moral Traditions	Spiritual, religious, and moral identity	16	6–12, 14, 15
	Role of spirituality, religion, and moral traditions		
	Relationship of this subdomain to the problem		
	Potential stresses or conflicts related to spirituality, religion, and moral traditions		

TABLE 3–1. Core Cultural Formulation Interview (CFI) expansion modules (*continued*)

Module	Module subdomains	Items in module	Related core CFI questions
Cultural Identity	National, ethnic, and racial background	34	6–10
	Language		
	Migration		
	Spirituality, religion, and moral traditions		
	Gender identity		
	Sexual orientation identity		
Coping and Help Seeking	Self-coping	13	6, 11, 12, 14, 15
	Social network		
	Help and treatment seeking beyond social network		
	Current treatment episode		
Patient-Clinician Relationship	Questions for the patient	12	16
	Question for the clinician after the interview		

TABLE 3–2.   Special populations modules

Module	Module subdomains	Items in module	Related core CFI questions
School-Age Children and Adolescents	Feeling of age appropriateness in different settings	20	8–10
	Age-related stressors and supports		
	Age-related expectations		
	Transition to adulthood/maturity		
	Addendum for parents' interview		
Older Adults	Conceptions of aging and cultural identity	17	5, 6–10, 12, 13, 15, 16
	Conceptions of aging in relationship to illness attributions and coping		
	Influence of comorbid medical problems and treatments on illness		
	Quality and nature of social supports and caregiving		
	Additional age-related transitions		
	Positive and negative attitudes toward aging and clinician-patient relationship		
Immigrants and Refugees	Background information	18	7–10, 13
	Premigration difficulties		
	Migration-related losses and challenges		
	Ongoing relationship with country of origin		
	Resettlement and new life		
	Relationship with problem		
	Future expectations		

Note.   CFI=Cultural Formulation Interview.

Core CFI Expansion Modules

The core CFI expansion modules help the clinician examine eight key domains of the core CFI in more depth. Table 3–1 lists the eight expansion modules, as well as the subdomains assessed, the total number of items in each supplementary module, and the core CFI questions that are related to each module. The core CFI expansion modules assess aspects of the person and the clinical encounter, such as the patient's social support system, the patient's cultural identity, and the clinician-patient relationship, with a particular focus on the problem that brought him or her to care. Often the modules overlap, assessing closely related domains. For example, the person's experience of spirituality (module 5, Spirituality, Religion, and Moral Traditions) may affect his or her understanding of the problem (module 1, Explanatory Model) and what help to seek for it (module 7, Coping and Help Seeking). Most modules expand beyond the focus on the problem presented, aiming for a broader contextualization of the clinical situation. As the 12 subchapters illustrate, the domains of the core CFI (e.g., explanatory model, self-coping, identity) further explored in the core CFI expansion modules are profoundly influenced by cultural factors.

Special Populations Modules

Three modules help elicit information from specific types of patient populations. Two are age-specific modules (module 9, School-Age Children and Adolescents, and module 10, Older Adults) and one focuses on immigrants and refugees (module 11). Table 3–2 describes the special populations modules and the subdomains assessed in each. These modules provide key information about these groups that affects care. For example, with respect to the age-specific modules, there is considerable cultural variation in how age-related transitions and challenges are experienced and negotiated at either end of the age spectrum. Also, with respect to the Immigrants and Refugees module, the person's background as an immigrant or refugee affects many domains, such as identity (e.g., language-based identity) and specific stressors (e.g., those related to traumatic events and acculturation).

Informant Perspectives Modules

The CFI–Informant Version asks all of the questions in the core CFI but of someone other than the patient. In this sense, the CFI–Informant Version can be considered an additional supplementary module of the core CFI. For a discussion of the CFI–Informant Version, see Chapter 2, "The Core and Informant Cultural Formulation Interviews in DSM-5." In addition, supplementary module 12, Caregivers, obtains information from an informant specifically regarding his or her role as a caregiver. The core CFI questions that are related to module 12 are 6, 12, and 14. Patients often have caregivers, who may be family members, friends, or paid workers. A caregiver's assistance may involve taking a patient to appointments, arranging medication, or even more intense care, such as assisting with all daily functions, including feeding and bathing. The purpose of this module is to examine cultural aspects of the caregiving experience, including the nature of the caregiving relationship, nature and impact of caregiving activities, and expectations of clinical care. For example, how caregivers interpret and respond to mental health problems and the treatment system, approach their day-to-day caregiving activities, and experience burden and gratification within the context of the caregiving role will be shaped by their own cultural orientations as well as other aspects of their identity (Flores et al. 2009; Hinton et al. 2008).

Structure of the Supplementary Modules

All of the supplementary modules share a similar format. They begin by indicating any questions from the core CFI that are repeated in the module. Instructions for administering the module are then provided, followed by an introduction that the clinician orally presents to the patient to frame the module questions. Most modules are organized in terms of specific subdomains, and each subdomain is assessed by several questions. For example, in the Cultural Identity module, the subdomains include language ability and migration history, assessed by six and nine questions, respectively.

Like the core CFI, the supplementary modules are problem focused in most cases, in the sense that they try to elicit how the module topic relates to the clinical problem presented by the patient. Some, like the Cultural Identity module, focus more on aspects of the patient's identity than on a problem per se, although the module still includes questions about how cultural identity affects the problem. Other modules, such as the Explanatory Model and the Coping and Help Seeking modules, are focused exclusively on the presented problem.

In some cases, questions central to one module are also assessed in another because those questions relate to both modules. For example, the Explanatory Model module includes an assessment of coping and help seeking because this line of questioning allows the interviewer to learn more about the person's explanatory model through the types of care and assistance sought for the problem.

Conclusion

A subchapter is devoted to each supplementary module. Figure 3–1 and Tables 3–1 and 3–2 help in navigating the succeeding chapters by clarifying how a given supplementary module relates to the other modules and the core CFI. We describe the modules in more detail in these chapters and provide case examples to illustrate how these tools can help contextualize a patient's presentation in terms of his or her explanatory model of illness, level of functioning, social support, or history of coping with and help seeking for that complaint. Figure 3–1 in particular shows the analytic lenses the clinician can bring to bear to evaluate a patient. This might be considered a form of multiaxial analysis, in which the clinician remains acutely aware of potential analytic dimensions that should always be kept in mind as possible "tools," just as a clinician may have in mind certain areas of questioning during the initial evaluation of a patient. These various means of contextualization can be employed not only during initial assessment but throughout treatment.

KEY CLINICAL POINTS

- The supplementary modules and the Cultural Formulation Interview–Informant Version help the clinician avoid errors of decontextualization that result from neglecting the patient's life situation, sense of belonging to one or more social groups, and understanding of the "problem" and how to obtain help for it, as well as the views on these issues held by the patient's close associates.

- Various types of supplementary modules can expand on the basic assessment obtained with the core Cultural Formulation Interview (CFI). Core CFI expansion modules further evaluate an area already in the core CFI, special populations modules provide key information about particular groups (e.g., refugees), and the informant perspectives modules assess the patient's problem as perceived by another person in the patient's social network (e.g., a caregiver).

Questions

1. What are some of the domains that are ignored as part of a decontextualization error?

2. What are the types of supplementary modules?

3. What are examples of CFI expansion modules?

4. What are examples of informant perspectives modules?

5. What are examples special populations modules?

References

American Psychiatric Association: Diagnostic and Statistical Manual of Mental Disorders, 5th Edition. Arlington, VA, American Psychiatric Association, 2013

Eisenberg L: Disease and illness: distinctions between professional and popular ideas of sickness. Cult Med Psychiatry 1(1):9–23, 1977 756356

Flores YG, Hinton L, Barker JC, et al: Beyond familism: a case study of the ethics of care of a Latina caregiver of an elderly parent with dementia. Health Care Women Int 30(12):1055–1072, 2009 19894151

Guarnaccia PJ, Lewis-Fernández R, Marano MR: Toward a Puerto Rican popular nosology: nervios and ataque de nervios. Cult Med Psychiatry 27(3):339–366, 2003 14510098

Hinton DE, Good BJ: Culture and PTSD: Trauma in Historical and Global Perspective. Philadelphia, University of Pennsylvania Press, in press

Hinton DE, Lewis-Fernández R: Idioms of distress among trauma survivors: subtypes and clinical utility. Cult Med Psychiatry 34(2):209–218, 2010 20407812

Hinton DE, Lewis-Fernández R: The cross-cultural validity of posttraumatic stress disorder: implications for DSM-5. Depress Anxiety 28(9):783–801, 2011 21910185

Hinton DE, Nickerson A, Bryant RA: Worry, worry attacks, and PTSD among Cambodian refugees: a path analysis investigation. Soc Sci Med 72(11):1817–1825, 2011 21663803

Hinton L, Tran JN, Tran C, et al: Religious and spiritual dimensions of the Vietnamese dementia caregiving experience. Hallym Int J Aging HIJA 10(2):139–160, 2008 20930949

Kleinman A: Social Origins of Distress and Disease: Depression, Neurasthenia, and Pain in Modern China. New Haven, CT, Yale University Press, 1986

Kleinman A, Eisenberg L, Good B: Culture, illness, and care: clinical lessons from anthropologic and cross-cultural research. Ann Intern Med 88(2):251–258, 1978 626456

Miller KE, Rasmussen A: War exposure, daily stressors, and mental health in conflict and post-conflict settings: bridging the divide between trauma-focused and psychosocial frameworks. Soc Sci Med 70(1):7–16, 2010 19854552

Weiner SJ, Schwartz A, Weaver F, et al: Contextual errors and failures in individualizing patient care: a multicenter study. Ann Intern Med 153(2):69–75, 2010 20643988

Suggested Readings

Eisenberg L: Disease and illness: distinctions between professional and popular ideas of sickness. Cult Med Psychiatry 1(1):9–23, 1977 756356

Hinton DE, Lewis-Fernández R: Idioms of distress among trauma survivors: subtypes and clinical utility. Cult Med Psychiatry 34(2):209–218, 2010 20407812

Hinton L, Tran JN, Tran C, et al: Religious and spiritual dimensions of the Vietnamese dementia caregiving experience. Hallym Int J Aging HIJA 10(2):139–160, 2008 20930949

Supplementary Module 1: Explanatory Model

Devon E. Hinton, M.D., Ph.D.

Roberto Lewis-Fernández, M.D., M.T.S.

Laurence J. Kirmayer, M.D.

Mitchell G. Weiss, M.D., Ph.D.

The concept of the illness explanatory models was introduced in psychiatry by Arthur Kleinman (1980). The concept is based on ethnographic research that indicated the clinical value of eliciting patients' models or explanations of their symptoms and afflictions. Research in medical sociology and psychology on illness behavior and commonsense illness representations supported the importance of such models as determinants of symptom experiencing and symptom-related coping and help seeking (Leventhal et al. 1980; Mechanic 1972).

Kleinman (1980) proposed eight simple questions that clinicians could ask to get a sense of patients' understanding of their problems, expectations, and concerns (see also Kleinman et al. 1978). This approach to explanatory models of illness has been highly influential in medical training, as well as in both clinical practice and research in cultural psychiatry (Weiss and Somma 2007). An illness explanatory model typically includes a patient's ideas about the causes of the problem; about its psychological, somatic, social, and/or spiritual effects over time; and about what would be the most appropriate and effective treatment. Patients' explanatory models of their symptoms and complaints may differ markedly from those of the treating clinician (Helman 1985), and this difference can profoundly influence help seeking, treatment adherence, clinical course, and outcome.

The models that patients use to make sense of their experience are not only personal but are also influenced by and shared with those around them. Each patient lives in one or more particular "cultural contexts," which shape the problem he or she presents and the experience of illness and its meaning—that is, how the patient interprets the problem's significance and what the patient perceives to be the cause of the clinical problem. These conceptualizations shape the particular concerns and ideas about what to do (Kirmayer and Bhugra 2009; Kleinman 1988). For the purposes of this book, we consider *culture* broadly to include ethnic or national group, religious group, gender-based identity, and work group (e.g., the "culture" of the U.S. veterans who were deployed to Iraq).

Explanatory models may vary with the type of complaint presented, and patients may have multiple concerns that they link to a single explanatory model or multiple explanatory models for the same complaint. The problem that a patient presents may include a relationship issue, a mood disturbance (e.g., anxiety or hopelessness), and somatic complaints. The complaints presented may also be a cultural concept of distress, such as an idiom of distress; for example, English speakers in the United States may refer to "being stressed," which invokes a popular model of symptom production (Young 1980). DSM-5 (American Psychiatric Association 2013) describes various cultural concepts of distress. For example, people from many cultural groups may present with symptoms that they describe in terms of the idiom of "thinking too much": Latino patients may refer to this as *pensar mucho,* Zimbabwean individuals may speak of *kufungisisa,* Mandarin-speaking Chinese patients may mention *xiang tai duo,* and Cambodian refugees may refer to *kut caraeun* (Hinton et al., in press; Patel et al. 1995; Yang et al. 2010; Yarris 2011). Or in South Asia, patients may explain a wide range of symptoms as due to their loss of *dhat,* a bodily humor identified with semen and associated with vital energy for which patients may expect tonics or other restorative treatment (Sumathipala et al. 2004).

In this subchapter, we review several approaches to assessing explanatory models. We then detail the approach adopted in the Cultural Formulation Interview (CFI) and provide examples of how the information so gained can be used clinically. We also summarize how administering the CFI helps to accomplish five key clinical tasks.

Measures to Assess Explanatory Models

The DSM-IV (American Psychiatric Association 1994) Outline for Cultural Formulation suggested examining certain aspects of explanatory models of illness (e.g., perceived causes) but did not specifically show how to elicit all of its dimensions. For research studies, various instruments have been developed to more systematically assess the construct. The Explanatory Model Interview Catalogue (EMIC) is an approach based on use of a semistructured interview that can be adapted to different contexts (Weiss 1997). EMIC interviews have a structure that enables comparison of the distribution of categories of illness-related experience, meaning, and behavior— that is, a cultural epidemiology (Weiss 2001)—elaborated and integrated with complementary narratives. Some other approaches, such as the Short Explanatory Model Interview (Lloyd et al. 1998), rely primarily on patients' narrative accounts of their problems. The McGill Illness Narrative Interview (MINI) is a semistructured protocol to identify explanatory models as one component of a broader exploration of illness experience (Groleau et al. 2006). The MINI is based on evidence that people use multiple types of models in thinking about illness. The interview aims to elicit three types of illness models or representations: chain complexes (implicit models structured by contiguity or metonymy), prototypes (models structured by analogies to salient images or exemplars), and causal explanations. Although usually woven together in a narrative, these different types of model or representation can be reliably identified in research data coding (Stern and Kirmayer 2004). Self-report checklists have also been used to study explanatory models (Bhui et al. 2006). Finally, there have been initial efforts to examine implicit models through indirect assessments because of concerns about distortions influenced by social desirability and other limitations in patients' responses to direct questions (Ghane et al. 2012).

Overview of the Supplementary Module

The Explanatory Model supplementary module can be found in Appendix C of this volume. All questions of the Explanatory Model module refer to the problem presented by the patient. The 14 questions of the module are divided into five sections, as described in the following subsections. In the description of the five sections, we also discuss the clinical importance of the questions, but we address clinical utility in more detail in the section "Why Assessing the Patient's Explanatory Models Is Important."

General Understanding of the Problem

Questions 1 and 2 are general probes to elicit the patient's understanding of the problem, setting the stage for the questions that follow to elaborate aspects of the explanatory model. For example, the first question asks, "Can you tell me more about how you understand your [PROBLEM]?"

Illness Prototypes

Questions 3–5 identify illness prototypes—that is, the patient's ideas about the condition based on knowledge of others with the condition, media attention to the problem, or the patient's own past experience with a similar situation (Kirmayer and Bhugra 2009). Patients are asked about the source(s) of information that shaped their understanding of the disorder. For example, one question asks, "Do you know anyone else, or heard of anyone else, with this [PROBLEM]? If so, please describe that person's [PROBLEM] and how it affected that person. Do you think this will happen to you?" This multipart question aims to evoke a patient's expectations about the problem presented and what might happen subsequently. For example, a patient may have a relative who was hospitalized for psychiatric illness, and the patient may assume that his or her own condition "runs in the family" and requires the same treatment. Similarly, in many parts of the world, serious mental disorders are associated with long-term institutionalization, and patients labeled with any psychiatric diagnosis may fear this outcome. A frequent example in the United States involves the impact that media coverage of attention-deficit/hyperactivity disorder (ADHD) has on many adolescents and their parents. Increased cultural awareness of this illness prototype is leading youth to present for treatment from mental health professionals for many kinds of school and behavior difficulties that they, their parents, or school officials mistakenly attribute to ADHD (Batstra et al. 2014).

Video 2 demonstrates the identification of a patient's illness prototype.

 Video Illustration 2: What does that have to do with my lungs? (4:26)

In this video, a consultation-liaison psychiatrist illustrates how to use some questions from the Explanatory Model to supplement a core CFI assessment with an African American woman who is hospitalized in a general hospital ward. The consultation aims to elucidate possible psychiatric aspects of her lung complaints and, in particular, her reasons for refusing indicated tests. The clinician appropriately frames the interview, stating that his questions aim to advance care and that there are no right or wrong answers. When asked about her understanding of her lung problems and the connection to smoking, the patient states that her husband had lung complaints, entered the hospital, and died; she asserts that the doctors killed him by subjecting him to a lot of unnecessary tests. She says she just wants to get something to help her breathing so she can go home and expresses being upset at having to see a psychiatrist. She also does not want any testing. Since her husband had the same tests, she is afraid the doctors will kill her, like her husband, through the tests.

The patient thus demonstrates having an illness prototype—namely, a certain understanding of her complaint ("I can't breathe") and an expected treatment course in the hospital based on the experience of someone she knew (her husband) with the same complaint. The interviewer tries to explore whether there are other sources of the illness prototype by questioning her further about her breathing problems, specifically inquiring about the Internet or television programs. The patient's answers confirm that the main source of her illness prototype is her husband's experience: "He came into the hospital, he had a problem breathing, he came into the hospital. They killed him. And they took his lungs, and they took his heart, and they took everything else."

The clinician's use of the Explanatory Module provides useful information. The interview reveals that the patient has catastrophic cognitions about her illness course that originate from her understanding of her husband's hospital experience. She believes the tests given at the hospital, possibly with the goal of harvesting her organs, will kill her rather than advance her care.

As the interviewer completes the Explanatory Model module, he can explore the patient's core complaint further. What does she think caused her difficulty breathing? What does she think her illness course will be? What treatment would be best? This information can also help answer another clinical question raised by the patient's fears of medical experimentation: Is she psychotic, or is her fear the result of nonpsychotic-level mistrust of hospital care possibly combined with low health literacy and insufficient explanation by her treatment team? More information about her presented complaint can help answer these questions and guide the clinician's explanation for the planned assessments and their treatment implications. This is called *explanatory model bridging*: the negotiation of the two explanatory models present in the clinical encounter—that of the patient and that of the clinician. Through this bridging process, the patient's illness prototype is further elucidated, helping to resolve a clinical impasse. For example, more information on the patient's explanatory model could help explain how the patient thinks the tests killed her husband. This may help to address her catastrophic cognitions about planned assessments and treatments, possibly optimizing her treatment engagement and positive expectancy.

Causal Explanations

Questions 6–9 elaborate on perceived causes of a problem to determine how a patient understands its source, reasons, and consequences. For example, "Can you tell me what you think caused your [PROBLEM]?" and "How do you think your [PROBLEM] affects your body? Your mind? Your spiritual well-being?" These questions get at the patient's ideas of how the problem "works"—that is, its causal mechanisms, including pathophysiology, psychology, and social, spiritual, or other processes. Frequently, these questions also elicit concerns related to self-stigmatization and anticipated social stigmatization associated with the problem (i.e., ideas about how the disorder is a shameful condition and will provoke negative social responses). For example, patients may consider their anxiety to be the result of committing moral or religious sins or transgressions. Very commonly, a patient may describe the cause as "stress" but have specific culturally influenced ideas about the causes and negative consequences of the condition. Such information provides the clinician an opportunity to address stigma (e.g., by describing the condition as a common condition amenable to appropriate treatment), to modify catastrophic cognitions (e.g., by explaining that the symptoms are caused by anxiety rather than some intrinsic fault or inexorable mechanism), to optimize adherence and positive expectations (e.g., by framing the treatment as addressing the conditions of concern and potential social responses), and to build rapport (e.g., by enhancing empathy and helping to make a patient feel understood). Other questions in the section on causal explanations clarify whether someone's explanatory model has changed over time, whether multiple and even conflicting explanatory models coexist, and whether others in the patient's social network have alternative explanatory models. The clinician may find that certain explanatory models of others in the family or social network have strongly influenced a patient's experience and illness behavior. The clinician may need to acknowledge or respond to these explanations if they cause concern, are harmful or stigmatizing, or jeopardize effective treatment.

Videos 3 and 4 illustrate the use of the Explanatory Model supplementary module.

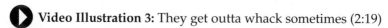 **Video Illustration 3:** They get outta whack sometimes (2:19)

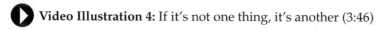 **Video Illustration 4:** If it's not one thing, it's another (3:46)

In videos 3 and 4, which are two parts of the same session, a mental health clinician illustrates the use of the Explanatory Model supplementary module through an interview with a 30-year-old Jewish woman referred for recurrent depression and past suicidal ideation. Video 3, titled *They get outta whack sometimes*, shows the patient's answers to the first three questions of the supplementary module. Video 4, *If it's not one thing, it's another,* contains the patient's answers to questions 6–8 of the module.

The interviews in videos 3 and 4 occur after the core CFI has taken place. The therapist appropriately couches the questions in the patient's own words for describing her depressive illness, which she labels "feeling down" and being "moody." The patient's general understanding of the illness is that it results from "chemicals in the brain…[that] get outta whack," so that "some people are just wired to not be happy all the time." Initially, she says that her symptoms have little relationship with actual events, but as the interview progresses—particularly as she describes her family's ideas about what causes her illness—she discusses stressors associated with her condition, such as feeling frustrated with her job and with her lack of a romantic relationship. The second question in the module —What did you know about feeling down before it affected you?—elicits some information about her illness prototype: an aunt who was known to have "down time" and who suffered the "weeps." Question 3 continues to explore past influences on her illness explanations. Here she adds that her mother used to label her as being "too moody" and took her for psychiatric intervention in adolescence. The patient saw a "shrink" for 10 years and thought it very helpful. However, the therapist became ill, leading to cessation of treatment. Questions 6 and 7 on causes go on to elicit information about how the patient tries to cope with her symptoms and her frustration at the limited effectiveness of the coping mechanisms. She also talks about her past exacerbations, including her suicidal ideation in college, her difficulties engaging the support of several members of her family, and the stresses of her work situation.

The interviewer moves in order through the domains of the Explanatory Model supplementary module, indicating the value of a systematic approach to the topic. By continuing to pursue the module, he can now explore several aspects of her Explanatory Model in more depth. The initial information on her aunt could be followed up with questions about that relative's illness course and what treatments she received. This could lead naturally to the questions in the module on the course of the patient's own illness. What does she expect from this course? How serious is her condition? What is its prognosis? Does the fact that the problem involves "brain chemicals" mean that it is permanent, or is it amenable to change? How does her condition compare to her aunt's? Did her aunt actually receive treatment? What was the outcome? Subsequent sections of the module can also explore her help seeking and treatment expectations, building on the information already provided about the patient's previous successful experience with her high school therapist. This information can help the clinician clarify what the patient expects from her current treatment and what potential areas of shared understanding and intervention can be expected going forward in care.

Course of Illness

Questions 10–12 ask about how patients understand what happens to people with conditions like their own and what to expect. These expectations may be based on causal explanations, self-image, past experience, or salient prototypes. For example, one question asks, "What usually happens to people who have this [PROBLEM]? In your own case, what do you think is likely to happen?" Some patients have more positive views of potential outcome than do their clinicians, especially those patients with milder conditions or those who do not seek help from mental health practitioners. In primary care, for example, patients may believe that the symptoms that the clinician has diagnosed as part of major depression are simply "problems of living," which will improve over time if only the precipitating difficulties improve. Other patients, however, may anticipate dire consequences, such as the idea that their "sadness" will never end and will ultimately progress to a vegetative-like state. Both situations indicate potential for a mismatch between the expectations of patients and clinicians, which if unaddressed can undermine a collaborative approach to care. Eliciting the views of others in the patient's social network helps to determine if such ideas need to be addressed. For example, if an influential person in the patient's social network, such as a parent, has an unduly negative or positive view of the expected course, this should be addressed to ensure realistic expectations and appropriate support.

Help Seeking and Treatment Expectations

Questions 13 and 14 explore what patients and others close to them regard as the most appropriate treatment for the problem. For example, one question asks, "What do you think is the best way to deal with this kind of problem?" The patient's explanation may provide a rationale for specific types of coping or intervention. This information may help a clinician to choose what treatment approaches to suggest and to begin a process of negotiation and shared decision making. For example, the clinician may encourage the patient to combine psychotherapy with other ways of dealing with the problem, such as prayer, other forms of supportive spiritual practice, exercise, or other activities. Accepting, or at least becoming aware of, the patient's preferred modes of coping and healing may result in better rapport and effectiveness. The clinician may also discover that the patient misunderstands the treatment available at the clinic, and this provides a chance to clarify. The questions in the help-seeking and treatment expectations section also give the clinician an opportunity to link the suggested treatment with the patient's presented complaint.

Why Assessing Patients' Explanatory Models Is Important

Exploring the patient's explanatory model can help accomplish five key clinical tasks, which were suggested by some of the examples provided in the preceding discussion of the content of the CFI (Hinton and Lewis-Fernández 2010). These tasks are described in the following sections.

Maximizing Treatment Engagement and Adherence

The clinician promotes engagement and adherence by describing the recommended treatment in a way that makes clear to a patient how treatment will address the problem presented. This requires linking the treatment to the patient's explanatory model in some way; this might be called *explanatory model bridging*. Simply taking the time to learn what the patient thinks causes the presented problem conveys a sense that the clinician understands and cares about the patient's concerns, which gives greater credence to subsequent treatment proposals. Eliciting explanatory models of problems that arise during care, such as medication side effects, may also contribute to clinical effectiveness. For example, a mild medication-induced tremor may be interpreted by a Caribbean Latina patient as a worrisome sign of impending "alteration of the nerves," possibly resulting in nervous system collapse and loss of motor function (Lewis-Fernández 2014).

Increasing Positive Expectancy

A large literature indicates that treatment effectiveness is increased when the patient has positive expectancy. This effect is found for both psychological interventions and medication treatment (Rutherford and Roose 2013; Tsai et al. 2014). Positive expectancy effects account for a substantial amount of variance in studies of psychological and psychopharmacological treatments. To increase positive expectancy, the treatment should be framed in ways that address a patient's key concerns to make the value of treatment more credible. Understanding the patient's explanatory model makes this possible. For example, patients from several Asian groups may attribute many psychological disorders and problems—and their associated somatic symptoms—to physical, mental, and/or spiritual weakness. In China, for instance, local models of neurasthenia may relate complaints of weakness to concepts of energy loss or imbalance (Kleinman 1986). Thus, in treating a person of Chinese origin with somatic symptoms of weakness, nervousness, or irritability, a clinician may use the CFI to clarify how symptoms are related to the person's explanatory model. Having ascertained the patient's explanation of "weakness" through the CFI, the clinician can then use similar terms to explain how the treatment works, for instance, by noting that antidepressants may increase a sense of energy by improving sleep and appetite or through direct effects on the nervous system. Alternatively, if the CFI shows that a patient regards bodily and psychological distress as a result of inner heat—as is seen, for example, among certain African populations (Thompson 2011)—the medication could be described as "cooling." In general, the aim is to frame the medicine and explain its action in ways that are both consistent with its known effects and intelligible to patients in terms of their personal and cultural explanatory models.

Building Empathy and Therapeutic Alliance

Explicit attention to the patients' own understanding of their problems is an indication of a clinician's empathy, which strengthens the clinical alliance. Explanatory models may link patients' concerns to past or current ideas about causes and future consequences, which have their own personal, social, and moral implications. A full and practical appreciation of patients' concerns therefore benefits from tracing the paths of causal influence, identifying salient prototypes, and exploring their personal and cultural meanings. This enhanced understanding can improve the empathic bond and thus increase the treatment alliance, adherence, and the effectiveness of interventions (Kirmayer 2013).

Addressing Catastrophic Cognitions

Explanatory models of a problem influence a person's cognitive-emotional response. In particular, attributions of symptoms to potentially serious or life-threatening causes may lead to excessive worry and give rise to catastrophic cognitions. For example, some Latino patients may be concerned that worry will permanently impair memory. Understanding such concerns can help a clinician address misunderstandings or misinterpretations of their problems that contribute to patients' distress. Social contexts give rise to explanations for health problems that circulate in society and influence ways of thinking and explaining problems. For example, a veteran of the war in Iraq may consider poor concentration resulting from anxiety to be an indicator of traumatic brain injury (Boehnlein and Hinton, in press). If the patient is troubled by this core concern, then explaining the link between poor concentration and anxiety may be reassuring and motivate adherence to treatment. Similarly, explanations of somatic complaints may refer to local cultural physiology (ethnophysiology), including links between social stressors and physiology (sociosomatics) (Groleau and Kirmayer 2004; Hinton et al. 2011; Kirmayer et al. 2004). For instance, among Cambodian refugees, dizziness is often attributed to an abnormal flow of *khyâl* in the body, called a *khyâl* attack, which may be caused by worry, among other causes (a sociosomatic explanation), and this interpretation often leads to catastrophic cognitions about somatic sensations, resulting in frequent panic attacks (Hinton et al. 2010). Modifying those catastrophic cognitions will have great therapeutic effect.

Addressing Stigmatization

Certain groups may consider particular symptoms or types of illness as shameful and stigmatizing. Veterans, for example, often consider having posttraumatic stress disorder to be a "weakness," and they are therefore reluctant to seek services. They may refuse treatment for fear of being labeled "crazy" and weak (Finley 2011). Similarly, police officers in the United States may be loath to report psychological difficulties in coping with a job-related traumatic event, so they might thereby avoid the anticipated stigmatization by their peer group for a mental health referral. Such stigma may have consequences. Affected persons may be regarded as emotionally unstable, have their weapons removed, and be assigned to desk duty. For certain Asian groups, mental illness in a family member may be viewed as a defect shared by or transmitted to others in the family and their offspring. In many South Asian communities, this belief may complicate the family duty of arranging a daughter's marriage. Understanding the social implications of an explanatory model and its associated stigma provides awareness and an opportunity to address stigma in treatment (Yang et al. 2014), which may, in turn, facilitate negotiation of treatment options, adherence, and better outcomes.

Conclusion

In this subchapter, we have tried to illustrate the clinical value of eliciting explanatory models of the presented problem as done in the Explanatory Model supplementary module. We have discussed how the information gleaned from the module—illness prototypes, causal explanations, expected course of illness, help seeking, and treatment expectations—can help the clinician accomplish key clinical and therapeutic tasks.

The Explanatory Model module can help the clinician to explore patients' understanding of their problems and to illuminate those problems within the context of the patients' social world. The module helps in understanding the way the person makes sense of his or her situation by using meaning systems shared with his or her family, friends, and immediate social network, as well as knowledge circulating in mass media. Many patients have multiple models that address different aspects of their problem, and many patients experience conflicts between their own explanations for their distress and the explanations favored by others around them. Attending to explanatory models, including the personal, social, and cultural sources of explanatory models and conflicts among competing explanatory models, is one way to avoid the error of *decontextualization*—the mistake of taking the presented problem out of its culturally shaped social and meaning context (Hinton and Good, in press; Weiner et al. 2010).

As we have tried to illustrate in this subchapter, patients understand their problems to have certain causes, consequences, and effects and mechanisms of action in the body, mind, and spiritual realm, and these conceptualizations may contribute to expectations for specific forms of healing and treatment. Clinicians must assess each patient's understanding of his or her presented complaint and related problems in his or her social and cultural context in order to accomplish key therapeutic tasks. The Explanatory Model module provides a way to begin this process.

KEY CLINICAL POINTS

- An illness explanatory model typically includes a patient's ideas about the causes of the problem; about the problem's psychological, somatic, social, and/or spiritual effects over time; and about what would be the most appropriate and efficacious treatment.
- Eliciting the patient's explanatory model(s) using the core Cultural Formulation Interview and the Explanatory Model supplementary module provides various types of potential clinical utility, such as improving adherence to treatment, building empathic rapport, addressing catastrophic cognitions, and allowing the bridging of the patient's and clinician's explanatory models.

Questions

1. What are explanatory models?

2. What clinical utility is provided by assessing the patient's explanatory model(s)?

3. How does eliciting the patient's explanatory model increase treatment engagement and adherence?

4. How does eliciting the patient's explanatory model increase positive expectancy?

5. What is explanatory model bridging?

References

American Psychiatric Association: Diagnostic and Statistical Manual of Mental Disorders, 4th Edition. Washington, DC, American Psychiatric Association, 1994

American Psychiatric Association: Diagnostic and Statistical Manual of Mental Disorders, 5th Edition. Arlington, VA, American Psychiatric Association, 2013

Batstra L, Nieweg EH, Pijl S, et al: Childhood ADHD: a stepped diagnosis approach. J Psychiatr Pract 20(3):169–177, 2014 24847990

Bhui K, Rüdell K, Priebe S: Assessing explanatory models for common mental disorders. J Clin Psychiatry 67(6):964–971, 2006 16848657

Boehnlein J, Hinton DE: From shell shock to posttraumatic stress disorder and traumatic brain injury: a historical perspective on responses to combat trauma, in Culture and PTSD. Edited by Hinton DE, Good B. Philadelphia, University of Pennsylvania Press, in press

Finley EP: Fields of Combat: Understanding PTSD Among Veterans of Iraq and Afghanistan. Ithaca, NY, ILR Press, 2011

Ghane S, Kolk AM, Emmelkamp PM: Direct and indirect assessment of explanatory models of illness. Transcult Psychiatry 49(1):3–25, 2012 22334241

Groleau D, Kirmayer LJ: Sociosomatic theory in Vietnamese immigrants' narratives of distress. Anthropol Med 11(2):117–133, 2004

Groleau D, Young A, Kirmayer LJ: The McGill Illness Narrative Interview (MINI): an interview schedule to elicit meanings and modes of reasoning related to illness experience. Transcult Psychiatry 43(4):671–691, 2006 17166953

Helman CG: Communication in primary care: the role of patient and practitioner explanatory models. Soc Sci Med 20(9):923–931, 1985 4012368

Hinton DE, Good BJ: Culture and PTSD: Trauma in Historical and Global Perspective. Philadelphia, University of Pennsylvania Press, in press

Hinton DE, Lewis-Fernández R: Idioms of distress among trauma survivors: subtypes and clinical utility. Cult Med Psychiatry 34(2):209–218, 2010 20407812

Hinton DE, Pich V, Marques L, et al: Khyâl attacks: a key idiom of distress among traumatized Cambodia refugees. Cult Med Psychiatry 34(2):244–278, 2010 20407813

Hinton DE, Nickerson A, Bryant RA: Worry, worry attacks, and PTSD among Cambodian refugees: a path analysis investigation. Soc Sci Med 72(11):1817–1825, 2011 21663803

Hinton DE, Reis R, de Jong JT: The "thinking a lot" idiom of distress and PTSD: an examination of their relationship among traumatized Cambodian refugees using the "Thinking a Lot" Questionnaire. Med Anthropol Q, in press

Kirmayer LJ: Embracing uncertainty as a path to competence: cultural safety, empathy, and alterity in clinical training. Cult Med Psychiatry 37(2):365–372, 2013 23539307

Kirmayer LJ, Bhugra D: Culture and mental illness: social context and explanatory models, in Psychiatric Diagnosis: Patterns and Prospects. Edited by Salloum IM, Mezzich JE. New York, Wiley and Sons, 2009, pp 29–40

Kirmayer LJ, Groleau D, Looper KJ, et al: Explaining medically unexplained symptoms. Can J Psychiatry 49(10):663–672, 2004 15560312

Kleinman A: Patients and Healers in the Context of Culture: An Exploration of the Borderland Between Anthropology, Medicine and Psychiatry. Berkeley, University of California Press, 1980

Kleinman A: Social Origins of Distress and Disease: Depression, Neurasthenia, and Pain in Modern China. New Haven, CT, Yale University Press, 1986

Kleinman A: Rethinking Psychiatry: From Cultural Category to Personal Experience. New York, Free Press, 1988

Kleinman A, Eisenberg L, Good B: Culture, illness, and care: clinical lessons from anthropologic and cross-cultural research. Ann Intern Med 88(2):251–258, 1978 626456

Leventhal H, Meyer D, Nerenz D: The common sense representation of illness dangers, in Medical Psychology, Vol 2. Edited by Rachman S. New York, Pergamon Press, 1980, pp 7–30

Lewis-Fernández R: Improving antidepressant engagement among depressed Latinos. Presented at Symposium 65, American Psychiatric Association Annual Meeting, New York, May 5, 2014

Lloyd KR, Jacob KS, Patel V, et al: The development of the Short Explanatory Model Interview (SEMI) and its use among primary-care attenders with common mental disorders. Psychol Med 28(5):1231–1237, 1998 9794030

Mechanic D: Social psychologic factors affecting the presentation of bodily complaints. N Engl J Med 286(21):1132–1139, 1972 4553340

Patel V, Simunyu E, Gwanzura F: Kufungisisa (thinking too much): a Shona idiom for non-psychotic mental illness. Cent Afr J Med 41(7):209–215, 1995 7553793

Rutherford BR, Roose SP: A model of placebo response in antidepressant clinical trials. Am J Psychiatry 170(7):723–733, 2013 23318413

Stern L, Kirmayer LJ: Knowledge structures in illness narratives: development and reliability of a coding scheme. Transcult Psychiatry 41(1):130–142, 2004 15171211

Sumathipala A, Siribaddana SH, Bhugra D: Culture-bound syndromes: the story of dhat syndrome. Br J Psychiatry 184:200–209, 2004 14990517

Thompson RF: Aesthetic of the Cool: Afro-Atlantic Art and Music. New York, Periscope Publishing, 2011

Tsai M, Ogrodniczuk JS, Sochting I, et al: Forecasting success: patients' expectations for improvement and their relations to baseline, process and outcome variables in group cognitive-behavioural therapy for depression. Clin Psychol Psychother 21(2):97–107, 2014 23280955

Weiner SJ, Schwartz A, Weaver F, et al: Contextual errors and failures in individualizing patient care: a multicenter study. Ann Intern Med 153(2):69–75, 2010 20643988

Weiss MG: Explanatory Model Interview Catalogue (EMIC): framework for comparative study of illness experience. Transcult Psychiatry 34:235–263, 1997

Weiss MG: Cultural epidemiology: an introduction and overview. Anthropol Med 8:5–29, 2001

Weiss MG, Somma D: Explanatory models in psychiatry, in Textbook of Cultural Psychiatry. Edited by Bhugra D, Bhui K. Cambridge, UK, Cambridge University Press, 2007, pp 127–140

Yang LH, Phillips MR, Lo G, et al: "Excessive thinking" as explanatory model for schizophrenia: impacts on stigma and "moral" status in Mainland China. Schizophr Bull 36(4):836–845, 2010 19193742

Yang LH, Lai GY, Tu M, et al: A brief anti-stigma intervention for Chinese immigrant caregivers of individuals with psychosis: adaptation and initial findings. Transcult Psychiatry 51(2):139–157, 2014 24318864

Yarris EY: The pain of "thinking too much": dolor de cerebro and the embodiment of social hardship among Nicaraguan women. Ethos 39:226–248, 2011

Young A: The discourse on stress and the reproduction of conventional knowledge. Soc Sci Med Med Anthropol 14B(3):133–146, 1980 7244678

Suggested Readings

Kirmayer LJ, Bhugra D: Culture and mental illness: social context and explanatory models, in Psychiatric Diagnosis: Patterns and Prospects. Edited by Salloum IM, Mezzich JE. New York, Wiley and Sons, 2009, pp 29–40

Kleinman A: Patients and Healers in the Context of Culture: An Exploration of the Borderland Between Anthropology, Medicine and Psychiatry. Berkeley, University of California Press, 1980

Weiss MG, Somma D: Explanatory models in psychiatry, in Textbook of Cultural Psychiatry. Edited by Bhugra D, Bhui K. Cambridge, UK, Cambridge University Press, 2007, pp 127–140

Supplementary Module 2: Level of Functioning

Smita Neelkanth Deshpande, M.D., D.P.M.

Triptish Bhatia, Ph.D.

Vishwajit Laxmikant Nimgaonkar, M.D., Ph.D.

Sofie Bäärnhielm, M.D., Ph.D.

Improving functional outcomes is an important goal of any intervention and thus a core component of psychiatric assessment. How can a clinician accurately estimate what constitutes a "normal" level and type of activity for a patient, while keeping in mind the person's social and cultural circumstances? The Level of Functioning supplementary module of the DSM-5 (American Psychiatric Association 2013) Cultural Formulation Interview (CFI) was developed to assist clinicians in taking culture into account when assessing the patient's level of functioning. Our goals in this subchapter are to describe the rationale for, contents of, and use of the Level of Functioning module in the clinical assessment and care of patients from diverse cultural backgrounds.

Rationale for the Supplementary Module

Culture and society define the value of every aspect of functioning—including personal care, housework activities, occupation, and income—as well as the meanings of terms that are commonly used to assess level of functioning. Culture and context influence patients' narratives as well as mental health workers' evaluation of symptoms and disability. In some cultures, successful functioning may be considered to be largely limited to paid employment activities that result in economic productivity and financial stability, whereas in other cultures, self-satisfaction rather than type of work may be perceived to be more important. Technologically developed cultures may value cognitive abilities above paid manual work.

Cultural background affects the expression of psychological distress, an important concept in DSM-5. With increasing migration of people all over the world, health care workers must be aware of cultural issues in the expression of symptoms and idioms of distress. For patients unfamiliar with a wide range of emotional or psychological terms, clinician awareness of how changes in level of function are related to cultural norms can be helpful for diagnostic evaluation. How a person functions in society in relation to work, interpersonal matters, coping, and self-esteem is one of the most important issues in assessing recovery.

Internationally used health assessment scales with appropriate cross-cultural adaptations and satisfactory psychometric properties that can accurately measure levels of cognition, mood, activities of daily living (ADLs), health-related quality of life, and loneliness may yet be insufficient for this purpose, and psychometric properties of many translated health assessment scales have not been fully tested (Uysal-Bozkir et al. 2013). Cross-cultural adaptation of scales of functioning must account for culture and belief systems—for instance, a level of functioning scale that is not gender sensitive may misclassify males who perform only household chores or women who are not permitted outdoor activities in their culture as inactive or impaired. In many Western societies, older citizens are expected to care for themselves independently, whereas in India, laws mandate that children take care of their aged parents (Maintenance and Welfare of Parents and Senior Citizens Act 2007). Thus, older adults would perforce appear to be more functional in Western cultures than in India, where they are "being cared for" and possibly mislabeled as impaired. Patients seeking health care in India are usually accompanied by the family caregiver, who assesses and reports their functioning. The expectations of the family may then determine reports on the person's level of functioning at any stage of life.

Disability may be a more quantifiable measure of functioning from a mental health perspective. The World Health Organization (2002) views *disability* as a contextual variable that is dynamic over time in relation to circumstances and defines it as the "gap between capacity and performance" and outcome (p. 13). The degree of disability is based on the interaction between the individual and his or her personal, institutional, and social environments. The assessment of disability should also be supplemented by information on the person's ability to engage in out rehabilitation plans.

Overview of the Supplementary Module

The Level of Functioning supplementary module (provided in Appendix C in this handbook) aims to address all areas of daily living likely to be affected by psychological distress. The module investigates several aspects of functioning through open-ended questions about each aspect, enabling the interviewer to focus on specific areas of concern as well as enabling further research in this area. Question 1 deals with ADLs; it touches on activities as well as responsibilities in a person's daily life. The focus on daily duties can be very specific to culture and gender, and therefore this question affords a good evaluation of the degree of deterioration. Changes in culture- and gender-patterned responsibilities, such as cooking, shopping, working outside the home, or independent living, provide good indicators not only of the person's participation in the usual cultural norms of his or her community but also of the patient's level of dysfunction. Although deficits in ADLs have been investigated extensively in dementia, ADLs are adversely affected in almost all mental disorders.

Question 3, on how the problem affects the patient's ability to work, starts to address the possibility of unemployment associated with serious mental illness. Although problems with employment may be the outcome of cognitive impairment and psychopathology, they are also strongly influenced by societal and economic pressures, availability of jobs, stigma, discrimination, and psychological and social barriers to working. The question about work also enables the clinician to broach the topic of other types of occupational activities, such as full-time or part-time study. Expectations regarding engagement in school are strongly influenced by cultural and contextual factors around the world; these factors include age, gender, socioeconomic status, and religion. Low social and family expectations about engaging in study and employment are strong barriers to active engagement in these activities, especially in the context of psychiatric illness. Question 4, which asks about the person's financial situation, is important because mental illness and poverty are intertwined, resulting in lower educational and socioeconomic outcomes for patients' families as well (Wolfe et al. 2014). Although loss of income may lead to mental distress or disorder, mental illness itself may be linked to subsequent poverty through many intervening factors (Chatterjee 2009; Draine 2013).

Social and community functioning is a multidimensional construct implying overall performance across everyday domains (Green 1996). The Level of Functioning module asks about the person's interactions with family and other members of his or her social network (question 2) and about how troubling disturbances in the patient's functioning are to them (question 8). Social functioning, social cognition, and social interaction, although most affected during episodes of active illness, often remain impaired during remissions, especially of serious mental illnesses. These concerns are addressed by question 5. Reinduction into social roles is an important aspect of recovery from severe mental illnesses (De Silva et al. 2013). Inability to experience pleasure in everyday activities is an important symptom of illness (question 6). Additionally, the module inquires about the aspect of lack of functioning that troubles the person to the greatest extent (question 7) and about the patient's ability to cope with the difficulties that arise day to day. Questions about community participation (question 5) and the family's concerns (question 8) help focus rehabilitation efforts on person-centered yet culturally grounded targets.

Video 5 demonstrates an assessment of the patient's level of functioning.

 Video Illustration 5: DWI (3:46)

This video illustrates how to use the CFI supplementary module on level of functioning to assess how a patient's drinking problem affects his work, earnings, life goals, and relationships. Substance use problems are universal and are often characterized by denial. Yet, in this video, by first focusing on the result of his drinking ("driving tickets"), the interviewer is able to elicit a good description of his drinking habits as well. The questions on level of functioning serve to define the presented problem and clarify the diagnosis.

The video begins after the module has been introduced by the clinician and the first question has already been asked. The interview illustrates how useful it is for the patient to describe how his drinking problem has affected not only his ability to earn a living but also his closest relationships. We learn that he drinks alone, he has no money, he has lost friends, and his parents have been hurt by his drinking. He no longer thinks of marrying because he has neither the time nor the money. Voicing these concerns can help the patient realize the extent of his problem and set goals for his recovery. Over time, following up on the answers to these questions could also help the clinician evaluate the effects of treatment.

On a deeper level, the module may help the interviewer and the patient develop an empathic rapport by demonstrating the clinician's willingness to explore the patient's daily concerns and to impart hope to the patient of achieving his life goals by taking control of his problem—helping his parents, getting married, and feeling less lonely and isolated. The standard psychiatric history and mental status examination can leave important areas of patient concern unexplored if done with a stereotyped, one-size-fits-all approach. By focusing on the patient's own assessment of the problem's impact, the Level of Functioning module can yield a personalized description of what is troubling the person the most about his or her situation, facilitating greater insight and engagement. This is evidenced in the video despite the patient's somewhat limited English-language proficiency. The interviewer's nonjudgmental approach when asking about the patient's functioning and relationships in daily life may also help the patient discuss the effects of his drinking as well as the possible benefits of change.

Guidelines for Clinical Use of the Module

The first two questions of the core CFI—about how the patient would describe the problem that triggered seeking care to the clinician and to his or her family—may not yield sufficient information on how the symptoms impair the patient's normal functioning as culturally perceived by the person and his or her community. Use of the Level of Functioning module may be considered when more information is required on the impact of symptoms and the effects of the illness on various day-to-day activities, while taking into account the individual's own cultural point of reference.

The module may be particularly useful when the clinician is unfamiliar with the social and cultural milieu of the patient and when patients are not accustomed to formulating suffering in the vocabulary of the clinician—for example, when the individual initially presents the impact of his or her suffering in terms of bodily idioms of distress, changed behavior, or impaired relations, but not in emotional or psychological terms. In many cultures, disturbances of mood and affect, as well as anxiety, may be viewed not as mental problems but instead as social and moral problems (Kirmayer 2001) and therefore may be described in terms of decreased activities and impaired relations. The Level of Functioning module can help clinicians clarify the level of impairment so as to formulate culturally sensitive management and treatment interventions.

Because the Level of Functioning module is short, with only eight open-ended questions, it can easily be combined with other instruments that provide a more itemized evaluation of disability, such as the World Health Organization Disability Assessment Schedule (WHODAS), version 2.0 (World Health Organization 2010). The open-ended approach of the Level of Functioning module complements the closed-ended, more decontextualized approach of instruments such as the WHODAS, potentially leading to a more culturally and contextually sensitive evaluation of level of functioning. Use of the closed-ended measures alone may not detect important differences in functioning across diagnostic groupings (Chakraborty et al. 2011). The following cases illustrate the clinical use of the Level of Functioning module.

Case Vignette 1

Psychiatric evaluation by a female psychiatrist of Greek origin did not reveal active psychotic symptoms in Johan, a 21-year-old unmarried man living with his family on a small farm in northern Sweden, who was referred for outpatient care after hospitalization for first-episode psychosis. Having left school earlier than expected in his social circle, Johan took various temporary jobs during the summers and did carpentry by himself at home during the winters. Six months after his initial evaluation, he participated in an interview with the Level of Functioning module. Johan appreciated the additional interview; he interpreted it as a sign of the psychiatrist's involvement in his care. During the interview, he revealed that he spent most of his time building a complicated wooden structure in a barn at the farm, guided by an invisible voice telling him what to do, speaking in Finnish, and calling him by the nickname his grandmother had given him. He stayed away from the family during these periods, as he felt they would question and tease him about this voice. Use of the module resulted in an improved therapeutic alliance with his psychiatrist, and the information obtained led the clinical team to realize that Johan was still living in a parallel psychotic world and was involved in daily activities very different from those of his local cultural setting.

Case Vignette 2

Songül, a 48-year-old Turkish immigrant to Sweden, was a mother of five children and a full-time housekeeping employee who complained of pain of uncertain origin since the birth of her youngest son. She had been treated with an antidepressant in primary care but showed poor adherence to medication and no improvement. The CFI, followed by the Level of Functioning module, was conducted by a male Swedish psychiatric resident with the help of a Turkish interpreter. Songül spoke of her unexplained physical pain and described how her capacity for doing things at home and at work had declined over the past year, especially in the mornings. On probing, she described other symptoms, including loss of appetite, loss of pleasure in her children's attentions and good academic performance, and growing social withdrawal. She was afraid that her acquaintances were gossiping about her, and she did not want her family in Turkey to know about her condition because they would become worried. Combined use of the CFI and the Level of Functioning module, particularly the questions on daily activities, helped to clarify that Songül had suffered from depression (which was associated with the symptoms she called "pain") for about a year, with substantial functional impairment. The focus on impairment at home and in her job enabled the patient to accept treatment that was focused on how to improve her daily functioning.

Conclusion

Assessing a patient's functional capacity and efficiency in conducting self-care, routine, and work-related activities is a cornerstone of psychiatric assessment. In usual practice, however, level of functioning receives much less attention than other aspects of psychopathology, such as symptoms. For patients and caregivers, however, impairment in functioning may be the most obvious manifestation of a psychiatric disorder. Clarification of the level of functioning may by itself help identify the diagnosis, as illustrated in the case vignettes.

Different aspects of functioning are important in diverse situations and indeed at different points in the life cycle. Although it may not be possible in a busy clinical setting to examine all of them, we expect that the Level of Functioning module will help focus attention on the most important aspects and help clinicians and patients arrive at a satisfactory outcome of care.

KEY CLINICAL POINTS

- Culture and society implicitly define the value of every aspect of functioning.
- Level of functioning is a core component of psychiatric assessment, and awareness of how changes in functioning are related to cultural norms can be helpful for diagnosis.
- The Level of Functioning module can help clarify the patient's level of impairment in order to formulate culturally sensitive management and treatment interventions.

Questions

1. How useful is it to evaluate a patient's level of functioning during routine psychiatric assessments?

2. In cross-cultural situations, what can interfere with the clinician's assessment of the patient's limitations in daily activities and responsibilities?

3. At which point during the process of psychiatric assessment will the Level of Functioning module be most useful in daily practice?

4. How important is it in a routine clinical assessment to ask what the patient enjoys doing?

5. From a cultural perspective, what are the advantages and disadvantages of exploring the patient's level of functioning with closed versus open questions?

References

American Psychiatric Association: Diagnostic and Statistical Manual of Mental Disorders, 5th Edition. Arlington, VA, American Psychiatric Publishing, 2013

Chakraborty S, Mehar H, Bhatia T, et al: Differences among major mental disorders in disability, quality of life and family burden: a short-term study. Indian J Soc Psychiatry 27:38–44, 2011

Chatterjee P: Economic crisis highlights mental health issues in India. Lancet 373(9670):1160–1161, 2009 19350704

De Silva MJ, Cooper S, Li HL, et al: Effect of psychosocial interventions on social functioning in depression and schizophrenia: meta-analysis. Br J Psychiatry 202(4):253–260, 2013 23549941

Draine J: Mental health, mental illnesses, poverty, justice, and social justice. Am J Psychiatr Rehabil 16:87–90, 2013

Green MF: What are the functional consequences of neurocognitive deficits in schizophrenia? Am J Psychiatry 153(3):321–330, 1996 8610818

Kirmayer LJ: Cultural variations in the clinical presentation of depression and anxiety: implications for diagnosis and treatment. J Clin Psychiatry 62 (suppl 13):22–28, discussion 29–30, 2001 11434415

Maintenance and Welfare of Parents and Senior Citizens Act. The Gazette of India, Vol DL-(N)04/0007/2003–07. New Delhi, Ministry of Social Justice and Empowerment, Government of India, 2007

Uysal-Bozkir Ö, Parlevliet JL, de Rooij SE: Insufficient cross-cultural adaptations and psychometric properties for many translated health assessment scales: a systematic review. J Clin Epidemiol 66(6):608–618, 2013 23419610

Wolfe B, Song J, Greenberg JS, et al: Ripple effects of developmental disabilities and mental illness on nondisabled adult siblings. Soc Sci Med 108:1–9, 2014 24607704

World Health Organization: Towards a Common Language for Disability, Functioning and Health—ICF. Geneva, Switzerland, World Health Organization, 2002

World Health Organization: Measuring Health and Disability: Manual for WHO Disability Assessment Schedule (WHODAS 2.0). Geneva, Switzerland, World Health Organization, 2010

Suggested Readings

Bäärnhielm S, Scarpinati Rosso M: The Cultural Formulation: a model to combine nosology and patients' life context in psychiatric diagnostic practice. Transcult Psychiatry 46:406–428, 2009

World Health Organization: The International Classification of Functioning, Disability, and Health. Geneva, Switzerland, World Health Organization, 2002

World Health Organization: WHODAS 2.0: World Health Organization Disability Assessment Schedule 2.0. Available at: http://www.who.int/classifications/icf/whodasii/en/

Supplementary Module 3: Social Network

Esperanza Díaz, M.D.

Tichianaa Armah, M.D.

Ladson Hinton, M.D.

Social networks often play a pivotal role in the onset, course, and outcomes of mental health conditions. *Social networks* are defined as all interpersonal relationships having an impact on a person's life (Speck and Attneave 1973). For the purposes of the DSM-5 (American Psychiatric Association 2013) Cultural Formulation Interview (CFI), the term encompasses "family, friends and other social contacts through work, places of prayer/worship or other activities and affiliations," as explained in the introduction to the Social Network supplementary module (see Appendix C in this handbook). Clinicians who understand the roles of the person's social network will be in a much better position to assess and treat persons with mental illness. The structure and qualities of social networks are, in turn, profoundly influenced by culture. For example, persons with mental illness may suffer as a result of being shunned or criticized by family or friends who hold culturally shaped and stigmatized views of mental illness. Alternatively, family or friends may seek to deflect stigma and social suffering by drawing on cultural explanations that normalize the patient's aberrant behaviors. The core CFI (see Appendix A in this handbook) includes several questions to elicit the cultural aspects of social networks as they impact mental health, but in some clinical situations, mental health providers may want to examine these issues in greater depth. In this subchapter, we examine the importance of assessing cultural dimensions of social networks as part of a cultural formulation, describe the Social Network supplementary module, and provide guidance to clinicians on when and how to use this module to conduct a more comprehensive cultural assessment of the impact of social networks on clinical care.

Social Networks, Mental Health, and Culture

There is a large body of work linking social connections to mental health that dates back to seminal sociological studies from the late 1800s (Durkheim 1951). Inclusion in a group may promote overall psychological well-being by creating a perception of order and belonging, fostering identity, and increasing self-worth (Smith and Christakis

75

2008; Speck and Attneave 1973). Individuals within social networks often share cultural orientations to health and illness, including perceptions of risk, illness explanatory models, constructs of health and well-being, strategies for managing symptoms, and patterns of care seeking (Kleinman 1987). A person's decisions about when and whether to seek care, for example, are often based on consultations with the people in his or her family and social group regarding the risk, level of perceived pathology, and seriousness of health-related changes, as well as observations of the actions and experiences of others in similar circumstances (Christakis and Fowler 2007; Malchodi et al. 2003; Shalizi and Thomas 2011). Social networks may also promote and/or impede mental health treatment (Hinton et al. 2014). For example, social ties through religious organizations can offer emotional support and assistance in coping with the symptoms of mental illness; depending on the orientation of the religious organization, faith-based social networks can also discourage help seeking in order to "leave all in God's hands" (Williams 2012).

Two models have been offered to explain the connection between social support and mental health outcomes: the *stress-buffering model* (Cohen and Wills 1985) and the *main effects model* (Lakey and Orehek 2011). The main effects model holds that inclusion and degree of integration in large social networks positively influence mental health independently of stressors. However, this embeddedness does not influence coping when the individual is confronted with stressful life events (Cohen and Wills 1985; Cohen et al. 2000; Thoits 2011). The stress-buffering model holds that social support impacts the pathway from stressful events to mental illness by influencing the interpretation of the stressful event and the behavioral and neuroendocrine responses. The perceived availability of interpersonal resources can influence the extent to which stressful events are perceived as threatening or stressful. Cultural assessment of social networks can help in formulating appropriate treatment recommendations, because individuals from different groups view relationships and the self in the context of social norms within their communities (Kim et al. 2008).

In summary, social networks may facilitate or impede access to help, mobilize resources to manage emotional problems, and provide concrete support such as basic needs (e.g., food), financial aid, counseling, and guidance (Greenblatt et al. 1982; Kogstad et al. 2013; Windell and Norman 2013). For example, the economic success of certain U.S. groups (e.g., Chinese, Cubans, Indians, Iranians, Jews, Lebanese, Mormons, Nigerians) is influenced by the level of affiliation within their social networks (Chua and Rubenfeld 2014). In other cases, social networks may trigger or amplify distress and impede treatment, such as by magnifying the perceived stigma of seeking psychiatric care (Hinton et al. 2014). The Social Network supplementary module aims to identify how the informal social network influences the problem.

Overview of the Supplementary Module

The overall goal of the Social Network module is to assist the clinician in assessing the influences of the social network on the patient's mental health problem, with a particular focus on the role of cultural factors. Prior work has documented both the stress-amplifying and stress-buffering effects of family, friends, and others on the experience of mental illness (Cohen and Wills 1985). The questions in this module may help clinicians map the specific roles of the patient's social network and may help clinicians navigate these sometimes complex interactions to promote more culturally competent care.

The Social Network module covers five domains. The questions in the first and second domains are designed to elicit a description of the key individuals in the patient's social network and their awareness and understanding of the mental health problem. The third domain examines the social and behavioral responses of those in the social network to the patient's mental health problems. These questions can, for example, help the clinician assess the role of cultural stigma (question 7: "Do your family, friends, and other people in your life treat you differently because of your [PROBLEM]?") and the role of the social network as a source of advice (question 6: "What advice have family members and friends given you about your [PROBLEM]?"). The fourth set of questions assesses the patient's perception of the extent to which those in the social network have made the mental health problem better or worse. The fifth domain examines the involvement of persons in the social network in the patient's mental health care, which may be of value to clinicians seeking to mobilize family members or friends to assist in an individual's mental health treatment.

Video 6 explores the role of the patient's family in her life.

 Video Illustration 6: The family (2:35)

In this video, the clinician is conducting the core CFI with a woman with postpartum depression who is quite engaged with the interviewer despite her obvious low mood. The video starts when the clinician is exploring the patient's supports (core CFI question 6). The patient describes the important role that her family members play in her social network. Her sense of belonging to her family is strong: "They're awesome, I love them. They come, they visit, they bring me food, they take care of the baby." She does not feel alone. Yet, the next question, on stressors, reveals the pressure she feels to fulfill her role as a family member. She fears her lack of a job outside the house will "drive us apart" given the more limited money to "meet the new demands" of the newborn. Despite their closeness ("They are my life"), she doubts her family's support will continue if they discover her postpartum depression: "I worry about my family and how they will react.... I don't know if I can tell them about what I am going through. That is probably the hardest part. What are they going to think of me? Are they going to judge me?" The questions on cultural identity highlight the terrible toll of her depressive illness, as it threatens the most important aspect of her identity, which is wrapped up in her intimate social network. It is clear from these initial questions that there are other aspects of her family relationships to explore.

The Social Network supplementary module could be very useful in this case. In particular, it is important to identify who among her relatives are the ones she trusts the most, whom she has told about her situation, whom she has not, and why. Asking directly what each key individual knows about depressive illness, their understanding of the problem, and what they think should be done about the situation would provide the clinician with essential data to help mobilize the patient's social network supports. In addition, exploring the types of advice the patient has received from her family is important to help decrease her anxiety and fear of stigmatization, for example, by first enlisting the help of some relatives rather than others. Inquiring about how the family makes the situation better or worse would help clarify how the social network would be most helpful in relieving her distress. Finally, learning about the family's expectations of treatment—and other forms of help seeking—is crucial for treatment planning.

Guidelines for Clinical Use of the Module

There are several entry points to the Social Network supplementary module. First, the clinician may become aware of social network–related information during administration of the core CFI (see Appendix A), particularly questions 5, 6, 12, and 15 (e.g., question 6: "Are there any kinds of support that make your [PROBLEM] better, such as support from family, friends, or others?"). The Social Network module can then be used in the same session or during a follow-up session to explore these issues further. Second, the clinician may choose to use the social support module when issues arise at any point over the course of treatment. The clinician can administer the module in its entirety or use only selected questions. Finally, other supplementary modules may also be relevant to the assessment of specific social network issues, such as the Psychosocial Stressors module (see subchapter on supplementary module 4) and the Spirituality, Religion, and Moral Traditions module (see subchapter on supplementary module 5).

It is important to ask the first set of questions in the Social Network module to identify whether a patient acknowledges having a social network. If no significant social networks are identified, the clinician and patient may decide to work together to identify potential social networks that the patient can engage. Alternatively, a patient's responses regarding social networks may be particularly helpful for planning care when the patient identifies strong ties to a network, such as an immigrant community, a religious group, or a group of family members.

Immigrant networks are linked together by the similarities of their migration experience, as modulated by the characteristics of the particular immigrant group, including those related to culture, ethnicity, gender, religion, language, and extent of discrimination. Immigrants from different ethnic or racial backgrounds can still develop strong ties due to their common experiences (Curran and Saguy 2001). Identifying these ties is important for developing a culturally informed treatment plan. For example, social network members can be included as supports during crises, potentially helping a patient to avoid a costly hospitalization. Immigrants often develop important connections to new friends, in addition to or instead of family members, as a result of the breakup of traditional family systems due to migration (Höllinger and Haller 1990). Use of the Social Network module can uncover these nontraditional social ties.

Religious group membership illustrates how the structural aspects of social support can impact physical and mental health. Religious communities typically vary in the extent to which they endorse use of mental health services; some offer alternative assistance and healing services. The CFI can help clinicians identify the importance of religion-related ties within a person's social network and the extent to which they affect his or her response to the problem. For example, patients who belong to religious organizations endorsing the view that life problems should be left in "God's hands" may be discouraged by their social networks from taking psychiatric medications and engaging in other forms of treatment (Bazler and Bazler 2002).

Conclusion

The exploration of social networks through the CFI has the potential to improve a patient's care by obtaining information about his or her social supports and ties to cultural communities and using this information to build appropriate recommendations. The CFI approach strives for congruence between treatment recommendations and the patient's understandings and values, in the context of his or her social network. Use of the Social Network supplementary module may contribute to research that analyzes the influence of social networks (Shalizi and Thomas 2011). The module also provides the opportunity to explore social determinants of mental health disparities, which if addressed can lead to improvement for individual patients. We encourage clinicians to use the module and provide feedback at www.dsm5.org/Pages/Feedback-Form.aspx.

KEY CLINICAL POINTS

- The level of a person's social support influences the pathway from stressful events to mental illness by affecting the interpretation of the event and the behavioral and endocrine responses.
- Exploring social networks may yield information about social supports and the person's ties to his or her cultural communities that can help the clinician develop culturally appropriate clinical recommendations.

Questions

1. Why is it useful to explore the person's social network?

2. What are the mental health advantages of belonging to a group?

3. What are some examples of types of social networks?

4. What can clinicians uncover by exploring an immigrant's social network?

5. Why is it useful to explore the person's social network?

References

American Psychiatric Association: Diagnostic and Statistical Manual of Mental Disorders, 5th Edition. Arlington, VA, American Psychiatric Association, 2013

Bazler L, Bazler R: Psychology Debunked: Revealing the Overcoming Life. Lake Mary, FL, Creation House, 2002

Christakis NA, Fowler JH: The spread of obesity in a large social network over 32 years. N Engl J Med 357(4):370–379, 2007 17652652

Chua A, Rubenfeld J: The Triple Package: How Three Unlikely Traits Explain the Rise and Fall of Cultural Groups in America. New York, Penguin Press, 2014

Cohen S, Wills TA: Stress, social support, and the buffering hypothesis. Psychol Bull 98(2):310–357, 1985 3901065

Cohen S, Underwood L, Gottlieb BHE: Social support measurement and intervention: a guide for health and social scientists. London, Oxford University Press, 2000

Curran SR, Saguy AC: Migration and cultural change: a role for gender and social networks. Journal of International Women's Studies 2:53–77, 2001

Durkheim E: Suicide. New York, Free Press, 1951

Greenblatt M, Becerra RM, Serafetinides EA: Social networks and mental health: on overview. Am J Psychiatry 139(8):977–984, 1982 7046481

Hinton L, Apesoa-Varano EC, Unützer J, et al: A descriptive qualitative study of the roles of family members in older men's depression treatment from the perspectives of older men and primary care providers. Int J Geriatr Psychiatry Aug 11, 2014 doi:10.1002/gps.4175. 25131709 [Epub ahead of print]

Höllinger F, Haller M: Kinship and social networks in modern societies: a cross-cultural comparison among seven nations. Eur Sociol Rev 6:103–124, 1990

Kim HS, Sherman DK, Taylor SE: Culture and social support. Am Psychol 63(6):518–526, 2008 18793039

Kleinman A: Anthropology and psychiatry. The role of culture in cross-cultural research on illness. Br J Psychiatry 151:447–454, 1987 3447661

Kogstad RE, Mönness E, Sörensen T: Social networks for mental health clients: resources and solution. Community Ment Health J 49(1):95–100, 2013 22290305

Lakey B, Orehek E: Relational regulation theory: a new approach to explain the link between perceived social support and mental health. Psychol Rev 118(3):482–495, 2011 21534704

Malchodi CS, Oncken C, Dornelas EA, et al: The effects of peer counseling on smoking cessation and reduction. Obstet Gynecol 101(3):504–510, 2003 12636954

Shalizi CR, Thomas AC: Homophily and contagion are generically confounded in observational social network studies. Sociol Methods Res 40(2):211–239, 2011 22523436

Smith K, Christakis N: Social networks and health. Annu Rev Sociol 34:405–429, 2008

Speck R, Attneave C: Family Networks: Retribalization and Healing. New York, Pantheon, 1973

Thoits PA: Mechanisms linking social ties and support to physical and mental health. J Health Soc Behav 52(2):145–161, 2011 21673143

Williams DR: Miles to go before we sleep: racial inequities in health. J Health Soc Behav 53(3):279–295, 2012 22940811

Windell D, Norman RM: A qualitative analysis of influences on recovery following a first episode of psychosis. Int J Soc Psychiatry 59(5):493–500, 2013 22532125

Suggested Readings

Kawachi I, Berkman L: Social ties and mental health. J Urban Health 78:458–467, 2001

Smith K, Christakis N: Social networks and health. Annu Rev Sociol 34:405–429, 2008

Supplementary Module 4: Psychosocial Stressors

Adil Qureshi, Ph.D.

Irene Falgàs, M.D.

Francisco Collazos, M.D.

Ladson Hinton, M.D.

Psychosocial stressors often play a central role in the genesis and course of psychiatric disorders and can be basic to how patients and families experience, understand, and express mental illness. For example, a Puerto Rican woman living in the United States who is the primary caregiver for her mother with Alzheimer's disease might understand her mother's illness as a consequence of the loneliness triggered by the erosion of family support and attention due to geographical fragmentation of the family and other factors (Hinton and Levkoff 1999). The meaning of the loss of family support for this caregiver and the central role it plays in her explanatory model of dementia may be understood in relation to *familismo*, a cultural construct that emphasizes the value of close interpersonal ties and reciprocal support among immediate and extended family members for health and well-being (Sabogal et al. 1987).

The core DSM-5 (American Psychiatric Association 2013) Cultural Formulation Interview (CFI; see Appendix A in this handbook) contains several questions about important psychosocial stressors influencing the patient's problems (especially questions 7 and 10, but also questions 4, 5, 9, and 13). In some situations, however, the clinician may want to inquire more deeply into the cultural aspects of psychosocial stressors affecting psychiatric diagnosis and treatment. The Psychosocial Stressors supplementary module was developed to assist clinicians in this endeavor. The objectives of this subchapter are to describe the role of culture in the process of stress activation, appraisal, and management, to review the structure and content of the Psychosocial Stressors module, and to provide guidelines on the use of the module in psychiatric assessment and care.

Culture and Psychosocial Stressors

What may be experienced as stressful can vary considerably across cultures (Chun et al. 2006). According to the transactional stress model of Lazarus (1993), stress occurs if the demands of an event, situation, or endeavor exceed those that the individual is able to manage. Stress can be said to occur if an individual appraises a situation as a threat to his or her well-being and believes that he or she does not have the resources to respond to it. Culture is essential to the process of stress activation, appraisal, and management in several fundamental ways: 1) cultural values and meanings are fundamental to the appraisal process; 2) the kinds of resources brought to bear for coping with stress may depend on cultural factors and the person's immigration status; and 3) the frequency and nature of stressors may vary depending on a person's history (e.g., being an immigrant or refugee), positioning within the host culture (e.g., as a member of a racial or ethnic minority group), and cultural background (Arbona et al. 2010; Berry et al. 1987; Lindencrona et al. 2008). An important aspect of the interpretation of events as stressful is the person's assessment of the adequacy of resources to cope with the event. The patient's cultural orientations and sociocultural context may influence the types and availability of social and local community resources to deal with stressful events.

One important example of how culture can shape the appraisal process comes from research on individualism and collectivism (Markus and Kitayama 2010). Cited frequently in the literature as foundational for selfhood, the dimension of individualism-collectivism (sometimes referred to by the term *independence-interdependence*) can help make sense of potential sources of stress and mitigating factors in the appraisal process. For a woman with a collectivistic (interdependent) orientation, for example, her very notion of selfhood is such that her group, however defined, is central to her experience of self and sense of well-being. In this case, the individual's role in life is more likely to be ascribed rather than chosen, and fulfilling the socially defined role may be central to her sense of well-being; conversely, not doing so can be a considerable source of stress (Chun et al. 2006). In contrast, individualism, or the independent self, is characterized by achievement and differentiation of self from others, in which each individual chooses his or her life path, and well-being is derived from individual accomplishments, be they personal, social, or professional. In this respect, not living up to one's own expectations for individual achievement can be a considerable source of stress.

The following examples illustrate the difference: An individual characterized by a collectivistic mind-set may migrate to a new country to earn a sufficiently high income to help the rest of the family; not finding a job that allows him or her to send money home would be a source of stress, because the well-being of the family is paramount. Conversely, for an individual who migrates with the individualistic goal of "making it big" to fulfill his or her own sense of success, not doing well in this respect would be stressful because of the associated personal feelings of failure rather than because of any impact on his or her family's well-being.

Although the expectations of others still play an important role in the lives of many individualistically oriented persons, the pressure to conform to the wishes of family and community is considerably lower than in collectivistic cultures. It is important to keep in mind that individualism-collectivism can be understood as dimensional and cannot simply be reduced to geography; individualists can live in highly collectivistic cultures, and collectivists can live in cultures valuing individualism. Clinicians should be aware that their patients may experience stress because of their inability to fulfill their social role and that this stress is not simply a function of a lack of autonomy or individuation but may also be due to a very real threat to their well-being. The threat does not necessarily derive from a negative response from family (although it can) but rather stems from not fulfilling one's social role, which is, in and of itself, a source of stress given that a person's value derives, in large part, from doing his or her part within the group.

Culture influences not only the appraisal process but also the kinds and levels (i.e., frequency and severity) of psychosocial stressors to which people are exposed as well as the resources that people have at hand to manage those stressors. This is highly relevant for members of historically marginalized social groups, such as racial/ethnic and sexual minorities, immigrants, and refugees. Disadvantaged social status can reduce the individual's access to social, economic, and political resources and therefore magnify stressors that commonly appear to be of low concern to majority group members (Magaña and Hovey 2003; Revollo et al. 2011). Conversely, collectivism in general and strong family values in particular can serve as resources mitigating against mental health problems.

Acculturative stress is triggered by stressors generated through contact across cultures. There is some debate as to whether this is strictly a "cultural" process or includes any and all aspects specific to migration (Rudmin 2003). For the purposes of the CFI, what is important is that clinicians be aware of the different possible sources of stress. To that end, the literature has identified the following types of acculturative stress: *perceived discrimination, intercultural contact stress* (stemming from the person's adaptation to a new culture), *cultural bereavement,* and *bicultural identity stress* (Rudmin 2009; van Tilburg and Vingerhoets 2007).

The subjective experience of racism and/or other forms of discrimination (e.g., as a result of ethnicity or sexual orientation)—potential stressors that can negatively impact health and well-being (Agudelo-Suárez et al. 2011; Bhui et al. 2005; Carter 2007; Pachankis 2014)—is not solely the result of overtly hostile and active/explicit behaviors; more subtle, quite possibly unconscious or implicit behaviors of others also have an impact (Dovidio 2001).

Intercultural contact stress encompasses multiple aspects of distressing culture change that result from living in a new and different culture (Berry et al. 1987). It can be triggered by rather banal details (e.g., differences in shop hours and public transportation), more complex differences (e.g., unfamiliar language and norms for social interaction), and even more complex adaptations (e.g., cultural values such as individualism and collectivism).

Cultural bereavement involves the losses associated with migration, which become all the more salient in the face of intercultural contact stress (Bhugra and Becker 2005). These losses frequently include language, social status, housing, natural environment, relationships with friends and family, and the experience of "at-homeness"; all of these losses can constitute important sources of stress.

Bicultural identity stress derives from the push-pull experience that two cultures can exert on the individual (Benet-Martínez and Haritatos 2005). An immigrant or a member of an ethnic minority group may be subject to the expectations of the culture of origin to maintain cultural norms and practices and of the majority culture to integrate; this is especially difficult for adolescents and youth. The youngster may need to live two, separated, indeed mutually incompatible lives, resulting in acute stress. For example, a teenager whose Pakistani parents are strongly identified with their culture of origin may well hide from them that she has a "local" boyfriend, a tattoo or piercing, and the like.

All of these stressors can potentially exacerbate existing mental health problems and also represent important domains for psychosocial treatment. Working with patients' resources to reduce the psychosocial stressors described in this section can help decrease overall distress.

Overview of the Supplementary Module

The Psychosocial Stressors supplementary module (provided in Appendix C in this handbook) explores psychosocial stressors that may have a substantial impact on the mental health of the individual. Five main questions help guide a conversation with the patient about areas of stress that are not usually part of the diagnostic interview, such as perceived discrimination, lack of group support, and adaptation difficulties. For example, psychotherapists report that they do not usually address race-related issues in routine practice (Maxie et al. 2006).

Given the goal of the CFI to facilitate access to the patient's narrative about his or her situation, the supplementary module's instructions invite the interviewer to tailor the specific questions to the particular patient. Interviewers are also encouraged to match their language to that of the patient; thus, the specific wording used by the clinician—whether it is the term used by the patient to refer to the stressor, the word *problem*, or other wording—should be consonant with the patient's usage.

Questions 1 and 2 elicit specific stressors that are affecting the individual. Questions 3–5 focus on understanding as well as evoking possible means for managing the patient's difficulties, taking into account the patient's social and cultural context and origin.

Guidelines for Clinical Use of the Module

The Psychosocial Stressors module is most relevant when the core CFI questions concerning the problem definition and the causes identify prominent psychosocial contributors to the problem. Indeed, this module seeks to identify and explore what could be called exacerbating factors of the existing mental disorder or psychological distress. To that end, it is best viewed not as a separate module but rather as one that complements the other modules and can serve to get a better sense of multiple aspects of the patient's lived experience.

Because of the diversity of issues that can impact the incidence and experience of stress, the clinician should begin by taking into consideration the following questions:

- What cultural model best describes the patient's environment? Is it influenced by collectivistic/interdependent values, individualistic/independent ones, or a combination?

- What stressors are affecting the patient? Is his or her cultural group subject to discrimination? Might the patient be facing stigma for the presented problem?
- How does the patient perceive the stress and how does he or she express it?

The clinician needs to be self-aware. An empathic approach in which the clinician openly listens to the patient can help create the trust necessary for an accurate diagnosis. It is worth noting that patients may be reluctant to raise certain issues, for example, those related to prejudice and racism, out of concern that they may offend the clinician. It may be worthwhile for clinicians to raise these issues themselves, by saying, for instance, "Some people who are in a similar situation to yours find themselves exposed to racism or discrimination. Would this be something you have experienced?" or "For you, as a gay Muslim man here in the United States, what is life like?" The specific content of these questions can be taken from the patient's answers to the core CFI questions on cultural identity. It is important that each patient's interview be tailored to the stressors raised by the patient as well as those inferred as likely by the clinician, so that the questions are specific to each individual. Research suggests that some ethnic minority patients may not be comfortable raising issues of race and diversity with majority group clinicians (Chang and Yoon 2011), fearing that they may be misunderstood. To that end, the questions in the module provide clinicians with a way to broach these potentially important topics.

The following case illustrates the clinical use of the Psychosocial Stressors module.

Case Vignette

Camila, a 43-year-old woman from a rural area of Bolivia, migrated by herself to Germany and presented to a mental health clinic for anxiety symptoms (e.g., trembling, difficulty sleeping, sweating). She was living in a low-income neighborhood of Frankfurt, sharing an apartment with two other families, and working sporadically as an informal caregiver for elderly individuals. She was markedly affected by immigration-related stressors. Her four daughters, all under age 15 years, lived in Bolivia with her mother; her command of German was limited; she did not have residency papers; she had been stopped by the police on a few occasions to review her documents; and she reported that she felt that native Germans stared at her with disapproving expressions. The initial cultural assessment revealed that Camila understood her problem as *nervios* (nerves), which had gotten worse because of the constant stressors of her new environment and the migration process as a whole (Guarnaccia et al. 2003).

Because administration of the supplementary module should be tailored to each patient, in Camila's situation the clinician could phrase the first question of the module as follows: "You have told me about some things that have affected your *nervios,* such as your separation from your daughters. I would like to learn more about that: Are there things going on that have made your *nervios* worse, such as difficulties with being alone, finding a job, money, or something else? Tell me more about that."

The interviewer can then proceed to elicit more detail on stressors the patient has already mentioned, using the questions listed in the module. For example, the interviewer might ask, "Have you experienced discrimination or been treated badly as a result of your background or identity? Have these experiences had an impact on your *nervios*?" Subsequent questions can continue to weave in the information already provided by the patient with the topics raised in the supplementary module: impact on others (question 2), coping (question 3), suggestions from social network (question 4), and additional sources of help, support, and treatment (question 5).

In this case, questions from other supplementary modules might also be useful, such as from the Social Network module and the Immigrants and Refugees module. Together with the information obtained through the core CFI, these questions may lead to a deeper and more synthetic conversation with the patient, with the goal of accurate diagnosis and more effective treatment.

Figure 3–2 illustrates how a well-crafted CFI assessment can reveal the psychosocial stressors exacerbating this patient's presented problem and possible avenues for intervention.

Conclusion

The Psychosocial Stressors supplementary module provides clinicians with a method for exploring cultural aspects of stressors that may be exacerbating the problem the patient presents. Cultural influences on the perception and experience of stress are substantial. Compared to the majority population, immigrants, refugees, and members of cultural minorities may be subject to additional stressors and have access to fewer resources for coping with them. The CFI questions help clinicians to explore these important topics directly with all patients, contributing to the assessment of key stressors in routine psychiatric practice.

KEY CLINICAL POINTS

- Cultural values such as the individualism-collectivism continuum are central to what is experienced as stressful.
- Asking specific questions about culturally and biographically relevant stressors with the help of the Cultural Formulation Interview can facilitate a better understanding of the patient's overall situation and help formulate diagnosis and treatment plans.

Questions

1. How does culture impact the perception of stress?

2. What are some subtypes of acculturative stress?

3. How might a collectivistic cultural mind-set influence how a person experiences stress differently from someone with an individualistic mind-set?

4. How does disadvantaged social status impact the process of stress activation, appraisal, and management?

5. How does the clinician's own cultural background affect the assessment of acculturative stress with an immigrant from a cultural minority group?

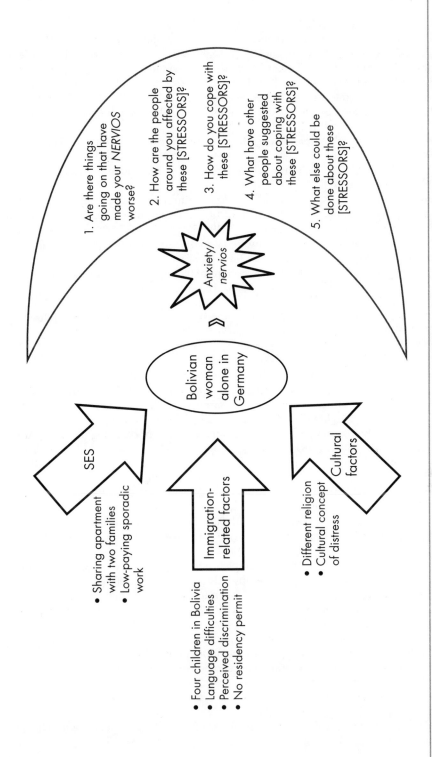

FIGURE 3–2.   **Types of psychosocial stressors affecting a patient's clinical presentation and possible CFI assessment questions.**

Note.   SES=socioeconomic status.

References

Agudelo-Suárez A, Ronda-Pérez E, Gil-González D, et al: The effect of perceived discrimination on the health of immigrant workers in Spain. BMC Public Health 11:652, 2011

American Psychiatric Association: Diagnostic and Statistical Manual of Mental Disorders, 5th Edition. Arlington, VA, American Psychiatric Association, 2013

Arbona C, Olvera N, Rodriguez N, et al: Acculturative stress among documented and undocumented Latino immigrants in the United States. Hisp J Behav Sci 32:362–384, 2010

Benet-Martínez V, Haritatos J: Bicultural identity integration (BII): components and psychosocial antecedents. J Pers 73(4):1015–1049, 2005 15958143

Berry J, Kim U, Minde T, et al: Comparative studies of acculturative stress. Int Migr Rev 21:491–511, 1987

Bhugra D, Becker MA: Migration, cultural bereavement and cultural identity. World Psychiatry 4(1):18–24, 2005 16633496

Bhui K, Stansfeld S, McKenzie K, et al: Racial/ethnic discrimination and common mental disorders among workers: findings from the EMPIRIC Study of Ethnic Minority Groups in the United Kingdom. Am J Public Health 95(3):496–501, 2005 15727983

Carter RT: Racism and psychological and emotional injury: recognizing and assessing race-based traumatic stress. Couns Psychol 35:13–105, 2007

Chang DF, Yoon P: Ethnic minority client's perceptions of the significance of race in cross-racial therapy relationships. Psychother Res 21(5):567–582 2011 21756191

Chun CA, Moos RH, Cronkite RC: Culture: a fundamental context for the stress and coping paradigm, in Handbook of Multicultural Perspectives on Stress and Coping. Edited by Wong PTP, Wong LCJ. New York, Springer, 2006, pp 29–53

Dovidio JF: On the nature of contemporary prejudice: the third wave. J Soc Issues 57(4):829–849, 2001

Guarnaccia PJ, Lewis-Fernández R, Marano MR: Toward a Puerto Rican popular nosology: nervios and ataque de nervios. Cult Med Psychiatry 27(3):339–366, 2003 14510098

Hinton WL, Levkoff S: Constructing Alzheimer's: narratives of lost identities, confusion and loneliness in old age. Cult Med Psychiatry 23(4):453–475 1999 10647944

Lazarus RS: From psychological stress to the emotions: a history of changing outlooks. Annu Rev Psychol 44:1–21, 1993 8434890

Lindencrona F, Ekblad S, Hauff E: Mental health of recently resettled refugees from the Middle East in Sweden: the impact of pre-resettlement trauma, resettlement stress and capacity to handle stress. Soc Psychiatry Psychiatr Epidemiol 43(2):121–131, 2008 18060523

Magaña CG, Hovey JD: Psychosocial stressors associated with Mexican migrant farmworkers in the midwest United States. J Immigr Health 5(2):75–86, 2003 14512761

Markus HR, Kitayama S: Cultures and selves: a cycle of mutual constitution. Perspect Psychol Sci 5:420–430, 2010

Maxie AC, Arnold DH, Stephenson M: Do therapists address ethnic and racial differences in cross-cultural psychotherapy? Psychotherapy (Chic) 43(1):85–98, 2006 22121961

Pachankis JE: Uncovering clinical principles and techniques to address minority stress, mental health, and related health risks among gay and bisexual men. Clin Psychol (New York) 21(4):313–330 2014 25554721

Revollo HW, Qureshi A, Collazos F, et al: Acculturative stress as a risk factor of depression and anxiety in the Latin American immigrant population. Int Rev Psychiatry 23:84–92, 2011

Rudmin F: Critical history of the acculturation psychology of assimilation, separation, integration, and marginalization. Rev Gen Psychol 7:3–37, 2003

Rudmin F: Constructs, measurements and models of acculturation and acculturative stress. Int J Intercult Relat 33:106–123, 2009

Sabogal F, Marín G, Otero-Sabogal R, et al: Hispanic familism and acculturation: what changes and what doesn't? Hisp J Behav Sci 9:397–412, 1987 van Tilburg M, Vingerhoets A (eds): Psychological Aspects of Geographical Moves: Homesickness and Acculturation Stress. Amsterdam, the Netherlands, Amsterdam University Press, 2007

Suggested Readings

Berry J, Kim U, Minde T, et al: Comparative studies of acculturative stress. Int Migr Rev 21:491–511, 1987

Chun CA, Moos RH, Cronkite RC: Culture: a fundamental context for the stress and coping paradigm, in Handbook of Multicultural Perspectives on Stress and Coping. Edited by Wong PTP, Wong LCJ. New York, Springer, 2006, pp 29–53

Lindencrona F, Ekblad S, Hauff E: Mental health of recently resettled refugees from the Middle East in Sweden: the impact of pre-resettlement trauma, resettlement stress and capacity to handle stress. Soc Psychiatry Psychiatr Epidemiol 43(2):121–131, 2008 18060523

Supplementary Module 5: Spirituality, Religion, and Moral Traditions

David M. Gellerman, M.D., Ph. D.

Devon E. Hinton, M.D., Ph.D.

Francis G. Lu, M.D.

A patient's relationship with spirituality, religion, and moral traditions is important to assess as part of a standard mental health evaluation for several reasons. This relationship often provides meaning and purpose to life, and religious faith, spiritual affiliations, and/or moral commitments can be essential components of a person's individual identity. Religious and spiritual belief systems and faith communities can play an important part in transmitting culturally held values, social behavior, and meaning even in early stages of psychological development (Shafranke 1992).

For the purposes of the DSM-5 (American Psychiatric Association 2013) Cultural Formulation Interview (CFI), *spirituality, religion, and moral traditions* are defined as systems of meaning and practice that help the individual and his or her community address the existential problems posed by suffering, morality, mortality, and the need for transcendence in the face of uncertainty. These systems can contribute a general understanding of reality in the context of human existence, similar to the concept of a "worldview" (Nicholi 2004). Spirituality and religion are related but distinct concepts. *Spirituality* can be defined as a personal experience or awareness of, or a relationship to, a nonmaterialistic or supernatural reality or life philosophy, whereas *religion* is usually considered to be a more formal and institutionalized set of beliefs, history, identities, and practices, often including guidance on how to achieve a spiritual experience (Josephson and Wiesner 2004; Lukoff et al. 2011). In addition, some individuals may subscribe to a system of moral reasoning and practice, also akin to a worldview, typically connected to principles of spiritual and religious traditions yet often experienced as a secular and philosophical guide for ethical behavior and a "good" life. These systems are referred to as *moral traditions* in the CFI; for example, it is debated whether systems such as Confucianism and Buddhism are "religions," because neither ascribes or promotes a theistic reality despite teachings on the nature

90

of existence and the promotion of behaviors meant to attune oneself to an underlying reality. These meaning systems include moral codes, values, systems of beliefs, and practices that guide individuals' everyday behavior, aspirations, and way of interpreting and giving meaning to illness, suffering, loss, and death—questions that are just as important to moral traditions as they are to religious and spiritual traditions. Exploring how these systems—whether spiritual, religious, or secular—inform an individual's identity, beliefs, faith, and practices is essential to understanding his or her views of illness and coping and his or her decisions about health care and help seeking. The effective negotiation by patients and clinicians of alternative and sometimes conflicting life commitments in the face of suffering to attain a joint decision-making process constitutes an essential part of a "values-based" clinical practice as an important complement to DSM-based diagnostics (Fulford 2005).

In the core CFI, several questions may elicit information about a patient's spiritual, religious, and moral traditions, including questions about supports that make the problem better (question 6), conflicting views that may make a problem worse (question 7), and self-coping and help seeking (questions 11–12 and 14–15). However, the only questions that inquire specifically about "faith or religion" are questions 8–10 regarding cultural identity, and then only as one of several aspects of the person's background. The Spirituality, Religion, and Moral Traditions supplementary module is devoted to these topics, especially as they relate to the patient's current problem and the role of these domains with respect to stressors and supports, cultural identity, coping, and help seeking (provided in Appendix C in this handbook). In this subchapter, we provide outline of the importance of assessing spirituality, religion, and moral traditions; discuss the supplementary module in depth, including its organization; and illustrate the value of assessing these domains with a case vignette.

Importance of Assessing Spirituality, Religion, and Moral Traditions

Koenig (2007) summarizes several tools to help obtain what has been called "a spiritual history." For example, FICA is a mnemonic reminding the clinician to inquire into or listen for patients' **F**aith and beliefs, the **I**mportance of their religious or spiritual lives in regard to patients' medical care, and an indication of involvement in a religious or spiritual **C**ommunity, and then to determine how to **A**ddress spiritual issues in the patients' care, if appropriate (Pulchalski 2006). Other tools include SPIRIT, which involves inquiring into **S**piritual beliefs, **P**ersonal spirituality, **I**ntegration with a spiritual community, **R**ituals, **I**mplications for medical care, and **T**erminal events planning (e.g., advance directives) (Maugans 1996), and HOPE, in which the clinician asks about sources of **H**ope, **O**rganized religion, **P**ersonal spirituality, and **E**ffects on medical care (Anandarajah and Hight 2001). A spiritual history allows a patient to discuss his or her religious, spiritual, and moral beliefs, values, and practices; the ways that these may influence or affect his or her medical decision-making process or treatment goals; and potential sources of religious or spiritual strength or concern (Pulchalski 2006).

Video 7 explores how the patient's religious beliefs influence his ideas about treatment.

 Video Illustration 7: Bridging the gap (3:57)

This video illustrates use of the core CFI to explore the patient's preferences for care, which include reflecting on the role of his faith in treatment. When asked what kinds of help would be most beneficial in addressing his anxiety, the patient discusses the frustrations of reconciling his faith and values with the types of interventions that have been recommended so far. Most salient for the patient is that he desires his recovery and treatment to include his religious faith. He states clearly a desire to find a therapist who might understand his religious values and background, asking the interviewer for recommendations.

The purpose of this video is to illustrate use of the CFI as a continuous interview. Therefore, the interviewer chose to postpone an answer to this direct question and to press on with the CFI. An alternative response would be to explore at that point the patient's preferences and expectations in working with a therapist, completing the core CFI afterward.

The patient responded to the next CFI question by highlighting the discrepancy between his mother's stated positive response to the suggestions of family and friends for managing her own illness and their actual lack of effectiveness. He says, "If anything, she just pretended like they worked outside of the home, and she would just be in bed all day." As a result, the patient indicates a reluctance to talk to his family and friends about his anxiety, although it is unclear whether this is because of perceived stigma and shame or because he expects similar unhelpful advice. This is very useful information for the clinician in helping the patient decide what treatments to pursue: the clinician could explore the nature of these unhelpful suggestions at that point or he could return to this issue after completing the core CFI. Likewise, considering the importance of the patient's faith in the patient's care and his previously stated preference for spiritual counseling, another reasonable follow-up question would be to explore whether the patient has discussed his anxiety with a leader in his faith and whether this helped or possibly exacerbated his anxiety. This approach could involve integrating questions from the supplementary module Spirituality, Religion, and Moral Traditions at this point in the core CFI.

The video concludes with the last question of the core CFI, regarding concerns about doctors and patients misunderstanding each other because of differing backgrounds. The patient resumes discussing his struggle between understanding and appreciating his therapist's recommendations to address his anxiety symptoms, on the one hand, and his preference to base his recovery on his religious faith and to avoid medications, on the other. He indicates feeling pressured by providers to take medications in contrast to his values, as well as having many questions and doubts regarding the use of medications in general. The patient concludes by expressing a preference to discuss his treatment options with someone who has had similar experiences and has made progress in his or her own recovery, consistent with the patient's early preference for a therapist who might share his religious values. A follow-up interview with the Spirituality, Religion, and Moral Traditions module and the Coping and Help Seeking module could be very useful at this point.

The role of religious, spiritual, and moral factors in assessing suicide may be especially important, because many religions discourage or prohibit self-harm (Gearing and Lizardi 2009). In a study of depressed patients in hospitals, those patients endorsing religious affiliation were less likely to have a history of suicide attempts and had lower suicidal ideation (Dervic et al. 2004). A similar finding was reported among inpatients diagnosed with depression who reported childhood abuse (Dervic et al. 2006). Depressed inpatients with lower scores on a scale of moral objections to suicide had more lifetime suicide attempts and endorsed religious affiliation less often than inpatients with higher scores on the scale of moral objections to suicide (Lizardi et al. 2008).

Asking whether patients' faith or their religious, spiritual, or moral affiliation has changed over time may reveal key experiences in their lives, such as suffering due to trauma exposure. Individuals with posttraumatic stress disorder (PTSD) were more likely than individuals without PTSD to report changes in spiritual or religious beliefs (Falsetti et al. 2003). Fontana and Rosenheck (2004) assessed changes in religiosity over time in over 1,000 combat veterans being evaluated for PTSD, many of whom had endorsed religion as a "source of comfort" prior to military service. Whereas 24% reported that religion had become a greater source of comfort over time, 29% indicated the opposite. Thus, religiosity or spirituality may help some veterans cope with trauma, but for others the experience of trauma and/or the development of PTSD may result instead in a reduction in their sense of themselves as religious, spiritual, or moral persons.

Overview of the Supplementary Module

The Spirituality, Religion, and Moral Traditions supplementary module assesses four domains:

- Spiritual, religious, and moral identity (questions 1–4)
- Role of spirituality, religion, and moral traditions in the individual's life (questions 5–8)
- Relationship to the current problem (questions 9–12)
- Potential stresses or conflicts related to spirituality, religion, and moral traditions (questions 13–16)

Each domain is described below. The first domain is also described in "Aspects of Cultural Identity Related to Spirituality, Religion, and Moral Traditions."

Spiritual, Religious, and Moral Identity

Question 1 asks patients whether their religion, spirituality, or moral tradition is an important aspect of their lives. Subsequent questions explore a patient's connection to a group associated with that particular tradition (question 2); the religious, spiritual, and moral tradition background of his or her family (question 3); and any other spiritual, religious, or moral traditions that the patient may identify with or participate in (question 4). These questions contribute to a basic spiritual history.

Role of Spirituality, Religion, and Moral Traditions in the Individual's Life

Questions 5–8 inquire about the role of these traditions in the patient's and his or her family's life, specifically in their activities. The United States is home to a diversity of religious faiths (Koenig 2007). Many Americans endorse belief in a God, pray, and regularly attend a church, temple, or other religious institution. Spiritual, religious, or moral practices may include limiting or prohibiting the eating of meat, drinking of alcohol, or use of particular drugs or medications, as well as encouraging fasting during specific times of the year. Numerous studies have found associations between religiosity and positive mental health outcomes, although the means of measuring religious behaviors and the strength of the association vary substantially (Koenig 2007). Individuals who follow the prohibitions with respect to alcohol and drugs are obviously at lower risk for substance use disorders. In one recent study, frequency of church attendance was associated with decreased incidence of depression onset, whereas frequency of prayer was associated with decreased severity of depression in older adults (Ronneberg et al. 2014).

Relationship of Spirituality, Religion, and Moral Traditions to the Problem

Questions 9–12 examine the degree to which one's faith, spirituality, moral tradition, and participation in a religious community are sources of strength or coping in regard to the problem presented. Pargament et al. (2000) examined various ways in which patients use religious or spiritual beliefs to find meaning in times of suffering or illness. Examples of helpful or positive coping strategies included perceptions of spiritual support and guidance, congregational support, and reframing of negative life events within the conception of a still benevolent God. Negative coping strategies related to poorer outcomes included spiritual discontent, either with the congregation or with God, and perceiving negative life events as God's punishment (Pargament and Brant 1998). In a related study, positive religious coping strategies predicted increases in stress-related growth, spiritual outcomes, and cognitive functioning at follow-up, whereas negative coping methods predicted declines in spiritual outcomes and quality of life, as well as increased depressed mood and decreased independence in daily activities (Pargament et al. 2004).

In the United States, clergy have been described as de facto mental health counselors for some individuals because they offer a substantial amount of pastoral counseling (Weaver 1998). A study of 99 African American pastors in New Haven, Connecticut, revealed that participants averaged over 6 hours a week in pastoral counseling, with about 20% of pastors spending over 8 hours a week in this activity

(Young et al. 2003). Similarly, a study of Muslim imams in the United States found that 50% devoted 5 hours a week to counseling, whereas 30% spent 6–10 hours a week in counseling (Ali et al. 2005). Asking the patient about past or current counseling with his or her religious or spiritual teacher, pastor, or leader may reveal resources and specific religious or spiritual practices that can be incorporated or negotiated as part of the patient's care.

The roles of religion and spirituality among African American women suffering domestic violence have been examined in several studies. Most African Americans identify themselves as Christian (Miller 2007; Potter 2007), and participation in worship serves not only as a means of religious experience and of establishing a sense of community, but also as a venue for speaking against oppression and seeking social justice and freedom (Miller 2007). In one study of 40 African American women who had experienced intimate partner violence (Potter 2007), relying on religious or spiritual faith to cope with or end the abusive relationship was a prevalent theme.

Meditation and other Buddhist spiritual practices are key ways in which populations attempt to recover from and cope with psychological distress such as trauma and PTSD (Nickerson and Hinton 2011). Ideally, the clinician can encourage the patient to use these resources in recovery, and certain aspects of these religious practices—from specific techniques to proverbs and imagery used in the tradition—may be integrated into the clinical therapies to make them more culturally sensitive. For example, among Buddhist patients, loving-kindness meditation and breath-focused meditation may be supported and taught in the clinic setting (Hinton et al. 2013). By assessing the patient's use of religious and related traditions in dealing with the problem, the clinician can optimize treatment and increase empathy.

Potential Stresses or Conflicts Related to Spirituality, Religion, and Moral Traditions

Questions 13–16 explore conflicts that may arise between one's spiritual, religious, or moral identity and the clinical problem or other aspects of one's cultural identity (e.g., sexual orientation and gender identity). Question 13 asks whether issues related to one's spirituality, religion, or moral tradition contribute to the clinical problem, whereas questions 14–16 ask more specifically about personal challenges, discrimination, and conflict with others as a result of spiritual, religious, or moral commitments.

Video 8 demonstrates the conflict between the patient's religious upbringing and his current suicidal thoughts.

 Video Illustration 8: Crisis of faith (3:54)

The video begins as an interviewer is asking the last questions of the Spirituality, Religion, and Moral Traditions supplementary module of a young man in the emergency department who is struggling with thoughts of suicide. When asked about practices related to his Catholic faith that might be helpful for his predicament, the patient indicates that while at one time he felt God listened to his prayers, this is no longer the case. At this point in the interview, it might have been useful to explore the patient's prior religious experiences in prayer and how and when he began not to feel heard by God. As the interviewer goes on to assess any potential stressors or conflicts related to his faith, the patient discusses the tension between his family and the Catholic Church, on the one hand, and his own suffering and thoughts of suicide, on the other. Instead of being a source of support, his family's Catholic faith is experienced as a further cause of his alienation from them; he feels the family would simply encourage him to pray instead of trying to understand his feelings of being "out of control." This alienation is highlighted in his response to the later question about being in conflict with others, when he reiterates that his suffering and his ambivalence about whether to continue living are creating emotional distance between him and his wife and family because he feels they cannot understand his experiences.

One central conflict described by the patient is the tension between living with intense suffering and taking his life and going to hell, which he believes is the consequence of a mortal sin such as suicide. His assertion that his family and church "won't accept what it is I'm feeling right now, what it is I'm thinking about," communicates his sense of isolation. We cannot assume that his Catholic faith will be a protective factor against suicide; it seems to be acting just as much as a significant source of stress and alienation.

Conflicts between aspects of a person's cultural identity do not necessarily lead to marked distress and impairment. For example, although many Western mainstream religions discourage, forbid, or even oppress homosexuality, Tan (2005) examined the "religious well-being" and "existential well-being" of 93 gay and lesbian individuals in the American Midwest and found that respondents endorsed high levels of both types of well-being. García et al. (2008) reviewed the challenges faced by gay, bisexual, and transgender (GBT) individuals in the United States whose sexual orientation conflicted with their religious upbringing and faith, especially among Latino men raised Catholic. Despite endorsing conflict between their sexual orientation and Catholicism, all GBT men described reconciling their religious faith and their sexuality to some degree, whether they remained Catholic, converted to another faith, or did not identify any formal religious or spiritual affiliations. Many who did not identify with a particular group described continuing to believe in God, pray, or read books on spiritual development.

Spiritual and religious factors in men diagnosed with HIV and AIDS have also been examined. HIV infection can exacerbate the sense of alienation from the church, and in Miller's (2005) sample of interviewees, many African American gay men with AIDS left their religious institutions as a result. Seegers (2007) noted that the gay men infected with HIV in her study endorsed an active and valued spiritual life and religious practices and expressed their spirituality through church-related activities; however, none had openly revealed their homosexuality or shared their HIV status with their clergy or church community. Thus, when evaluating gay, lesbian, bisexual, and transgender patients, clinicians also need to ask about how their religious, spiritual, and moral beliefs affect their feelings about their sexuality and their participation in a spiritual community.

Guidelines for Clinical Use of the Module

Case Vignette

Matthew is a 27-year-old non-Latino white man who presented to the local Veterans Affairs hospital for treatment of PTSD and chronic pain. He had been deployed to Iraq during Operation Iraqi Freedom, engaged in combat, and been discharged after suffering injuries from an improvised explosive device. In his spiritual history, Matthew identified as Roman Catholic (question 1), having been raised primarily by his Catholic grandmother and attending mass with her until he joined the U.S. Army at the end of high school (questions 2–3). Since returning from Iraq, he had not returned to church or participated in services (questions 5–6). Although he wanted to attend mass with his wife, he could not tolerate being among large groups of people, and therefore he was concerned about missing out on an important practice of his faith (question 8). He endorsed praying regularly at home (question 7) and reading the Bible (question 11) but felt unsure that God heard his prayers (question 12). When asked if his Catholic faith was a source of comfort or strength for him, he replied that despite his frequent wish to be dead and thoughts of killing himself, his belief that suicide is a sin kept him from acting on these thoughts (question 9). However, he also believed he was likely to go to hell after he died anyway, having "destroyed families" by killing enemy combatants.

In discussing this last point, Matthew's therapist asked whether forgiveness was an important concept in the Catholic faith, and the patient responded that it was. The patient then met with his local bishop (question 10), who emphasized to him God's forgiving nature. Although somewhat comforted, the patient noted that ultimately even if God forgave him for having to kill people as a soldier, he was unable to forgive himself. The dissonance between being assured of God's forgiveness and being unable to forgive himself remained a constant challenging theme in his mental health care (questions 13–14). Matthew subsequently engaged in group psychotherapy with another therapist, who was a Protestant and who at one point commented, "God is not in the Catholic Church." The patient was very offended by this remark (questions 15–16) and dropped out of group therapy. Although the patient was able to restart individual therapy with a new therapist, the insensitive comment by the former therapist precipitated a serious setback in the patient's mental health care.

This case illustrates several issues related to spirituality, religion, and moral traditions. It is important to highlight that although Matthew did not belong to a U.S. racial or ethnic minority group, a culturally sensitive approach to his care was very valuable in understanding his perception of the problem and his coping and help-seeking choices because his religious affiliation was a central component of his cultural identity. Obtaining a spiritual history and trying to understand a person's faith and the role this may play in care can identify possible areas of dissonance, distress, and cognitive distortions related to spirituality, religion, or moral commitments. Although Matthew considered his faith an important aspect of his identity and a guide to understanding the world, his experiences of trauma reduced his ability to practice his faith, to be part of his religious community, and to feel close to God. In this case, consultation with a local religious leader was an appropriate help-seeking choice for the patient, although it ultimately did not provide the reassurance that he hoped for. Finally, the group therapist's lack of empathy and insensitive remark highlight the importance of culturally competent care and the risk of harm when a person's spiritual, religious, or moral traditions are ignored or, in this case, insulted.

Conclusion

Given the prominent role of spirituality, religion, and moral traditions in the values, attitudes, and beliefs of different cultural groups, the supplementary module on these domains can help clinicians obtain a useful spiritual history. Routinely assessing this kind of information provides insight into the patient's personal coping and social resources and allows the patient to express beliefs about existential meaning that may contribute to his or her perception of the problem presented. With practice, care, and respect, clinicians can become increasingly comfortable with obtaining spiritual histories. This evaluation adds minimal time to the session and can greatly enhance the clinician-patient relationship and increase therapeutic impact. Clinicians may choose to administer the supplementary module as a separate element of the evaluation to systematically assess these key domains. Alternatively, clinicians may weave questions about spirituality, religion, and moral traditions into their assessment of patients' illness representations, developmental history, and cultural identity. Clinicians may also find it useful to discuss patients' level of comfort with the clinician's stated or divined religious beliefs, including as part of the evaluation of the patient-clinician relationship. Attention to the role of spirituality, religion, and moral traditions in the patient's life is an important component of a comprehensive clinical evaluation.

KEY CLINICAL POINTS

- The routine assessment of a spiritual history allows a patient to discuss his or her religious, spiritual, and moral beliefs, values, and practices; the ways in which these may influence or affect his or her medical decision-making process or treatment goals, personal coping, and social resources; and potential sources of religious or spiritual strength or concern.

- The Spirituality, Religion, and Moral Traditions supplementary module provides a framework for exploring a patient's identity; the role of spirituality, religion, and moral traditions in the patient's life; possible relationships between these traditions and the clinical problem; and any potential stressors or conflicts related to spirituality, religion, and moral traditions.

Questions

1. How does a clinician initially assess a patient's religious, spiritual, and moral traditions?

2. In what ways do spiritual, religious, and moral traditions influence decisions about health care and other forms of help seeking?

3. How do spiritual, religious, and moral traditions contribute both adaptive and possibly maladaptive strategies for coping with uncertainty and illness?

4. What are two spiritual or religious coping strategies that have been associated with positive health care outcomes?

5. How can leaders or teachers of spiritual, religious, or moral traditions contribute to the patient's level of resiliency or stress in facing a clinical problem?

References

Ali OM, Milstein G, Marzuk PM: The imam's role in meeting the counseling needs of Muslim communities in the United States. Psychiatr Serv 56(2):202–205, 2005 15703349

American Psychiatric Association: Diagnostic and Statistical Manual of Mental Disorders, 5th Edition. Arlington, VA, American Psychiatric Association, 2013

Anandarajah G, Hight E: Spirituality and medical practice: using the HOPE questions as a practical tool for spiritual assessment. Am Fam Physician 63(1):81–89, 2001 11195773

Dervic K, Oquendo MA, Grunebaum MF, et al: Religious affiliation and suicide attempt. Am J Psychiatry 161(12):2303–2308, 2004 15569904

Dervic K, Grunebaum MF, Burke AK, et al: Protective factors against suicidal behavior in depressed adults reporting childhood abuse. J Nerv Ment Dis 194(12):971–974, 2006 17164639

Falsetti SA, Resick PA, Davis JL: Changes in religious beliefs following trauma. J Trauma Stress 16(4):391–398, 2003 12895022

Fontana A, Rosenheck R: Trauma, change in strength of religious faith, and mental health service use among veterans treated for PTSD. J Nerv Ment Dis 192(9):579–584, 2004 15348973

Fulford KWM: Values in psychiatric diagnosis: developments in policy, training and research. Psychopathology 38(4):171–176, 2005 16145268

García DI, Gray-Stanley J, Ramirez-Valles J: "The priest obviously doesn't know that I'm gay": the religious and spiritual journeys of Latino gay men. J Homosex 55(3):411–436, 2008 19042279

Gearing RE, Lizardi D: Religion and suicide. J Relig Health 48(3):332–341, 2009 19639421

Hinton DE, Pich V, Hofmann SG, et al: Mindfulness and acceptance techniques as applied to refugee and ethnic minority populations: examples from culturally adapted CBT (CA-CBT). Cogn Behav Pract 20:33–46, 2013

Josephson AM, Wiesner IS: Worldview in psychiatric assessment, in Handbook of Spirituality and Worldview in Clinical Practice. Edited by Josephson AM, Peteet JR. Washington, DC, American Psychiatric Publishing, 2004, pp 15–30

Koenig HG: Spirituality in Patient Care: Why, How, When and What, 2nd Edition. Philadelphia, PA, Templeton Foundation Press, 2007

Lizardi D, Dervic K, Grunebaum MF, et al: The role of moral objections to suicide in the assessment of suicidal patients. J Psychiatr Res 42(10):815–821, 2008 18035375

Lukoff D, Lu FG, Yang CP: DSM-IV religious and spiritual problems, in Religious and Spiritual Issues in Psychiatric Diagnosis. Edited by Peteet JR, Lu FG, Narrow WE. Washington, DC, American Psychiatric Publishing, 2011, pp 171–198

Maugans TA: The SPIRITual history. Arch Fam Med 5(1):11–16, 1996 8542049

Miller RL Jr: An appointment with God: AIDS, place, and spirituality. J Sex Res 42(1):35–45, 2005 15795803

Miller RL Jr: Legacy denied: African American gay men, AIDS, and the black church. Soc Work 52(1):51–61, 2007 17388083

Nicholi AM: Introduction: definition and significance of a worldview, in Handbook of Spirituality and Worldview in Clinical Practice. Edited by Josephson AM, Peteet JR. Washington DC, American Psychiatric Publishing, 2004, pp 3–12

Nickerson A, Hinton DE: Anger regulation in traumatized Cambodian refugees: the perspectives of Buddhist monks. Cult Med Psychiatry 35(3):396–416, 2011 21630119

Pargament KI, Brant CR: Religion and coping, in Handbook of Religion and Mental Health. Edited by Koenig HG. San Diego, CA, Academic Press, 1998, pp 111–128

Pargament KI, Koenig HG, Perez LM: The many methods of religious coping: development and initial validation of the RCOPE. J Clin Psychol 56(4):519–543, 2000 10775045

Pargament KI, Koenig HG, Tarakeshwar N, et al: Religious coping methods as predictors of psychological, physical and spiritual outcomes among medically ill elderly patients: a two-year longitudinal study. J Health Psychol 9(6):713–730, 2004 15367751

Potter H: Battered black women's use of religious services and spirituality for assistance in leaving abusive relationships. Violence Against Women 13(3):262–284, 2007 17322271

Pulchalski C: Spiritual assessment in clinical practice. Psychiatr Ann 36:150–155, 2006

Ronneberg CR, Miller EA, Dugan E, Porell F: The protective effects of religiosity on depression: a 2-year prospective study. Gerontologist July 25, 2014 [Epub ahead of print] 25063937

Seegers DL: Spiritual and religious experiences of gay men with HIV illness. J Assoc Nurses AIDS Care 18(3):5–12, 2007 17570295

Shafranke EP: Religion and mental health in early life, in Religion and Mental Health. Edited by Schumaker JF. New York, Oxford University Press, 1992, pp 163–176

Tan PP: The importance of spirituality among gay and lesbian individuals. J Homosex 49(2):135–144, 2005 16048898

Weaver AJ: Mental health professionals working with religious leaders, in Handbook of Religion and Mental Health. Edited by Koenig HG. San Diego, CA, Academic Press, 1998, pp 349–364

Young JL, Griffith EE, Williams DR: The integral role of pastoral counseling by African-American clergy in community mental health. Psychiatr Serv 54(5):688–692, 2003 12719499

Suggested Readings

George Washington Institute for Spirituality and Health: http://smhs.gwu.edu/gwish/

Koenig HG: Spirituality in Patient Care: Why, How, When and What, 2nd Edition. Philadelphia, PA, Templeton Foundation Press, 2007

Pulchalski C: Spiritual assessment in clinical practice. Psychiatr Ann 36:150–155, 2006

Supplementary Module 6: Cultural Identity

Neil Krishan Aggarwal, M.D., M.B.A., M.A.

This subchapter focuses on the rationale and utility of the Cultural Identity supplementary module of the Cultural Formulation Interview (CFI) and the module's relationship to the identity-related questions of the core CFI. The Cultural Identity module has 34 questions presented in multiple sections (see Appendix C in this handbook), which are grouped in this discussion as follows: 1) national, ethnic, racial, linguistic, and migration factors; 2) spirituality, religion, and moral traditions; and 3) gender identity and sexual orientation identity. This introductory section offers a common definition for cultural identity, discusses the need for clarifying cultural identity in relation to clinical practice as presented in DSM-IV and then in DSM-5 (American Psychiatric Association 1994, 2013), and explains the core CFI and the supplementary module on cultural identity.

Monroe et al. (2000) define *identity* as "the idea of a sense, developed early in childhood, of oneself as both an agent and an object that is seen, thought about, and liked or disliked by others" (p. 420). This definition emphasizes that identity is a sense of self that is inherent to each individual emerging in relation to others. The CFI invites clinicians to discover which aspects of the self are most important for the patient, whom the patient names as close associates, and how aspects of the self are given meaning in relation to these associates.

The Cultural Identity module focuses on three key aspects of identity that routinely present clinicians with difficulties during clinical evaluation. In a literature review of publications on the DSM-IV Outline for Cultural Formulation (OCF), Lewis-Fernández et al. (2014) found that these three specific areas related to cultural identity would benefit from greater clinical attention. These three different aspects of cultural identity are explored subsequently in this volume; the authors present the latest relevant theories for each aspect and illustrate practical assessments through use of the CFI.

Historical Background: From the DSM-IV OCF to the DSM-5 CFI

The core CFI differs markedly from the OCF in two significant ways. First, the CFI differs in its *placement* of cultural identity exploration. Clinicians were encouraged to begin the OCF with questions about the cultural identity of the individual. Supporting text for the OCF clarified that clinicians should note "the individual's ethnic or cultural reference groups," "the degree of involvement with both the culture of origin and the host culture" for immigrants and ethnic minorities, and "language abilities, use, and preference" (American Psychiatric Association 1994, p. 843). However, clinicians struggled to formulate questions using these instructions (Lewis-Fernández 2009). Psychiatric trainees have also felt uncomfortable exploring patient identities without feeling intrusive or concerned that patients would find such questions irrelevant to experiences with care (Aggarwal and Rohrbaugh 2011). Therefore, members of the DSM-5 Cross-Cultural Issues Subgroup decided to introduce questions on cultural identity after the section on the cultural definition of the problem, enabling clinicians to cultivate the patient trust necessary to discuss such a personal topic and to address the most relevant and immediate patient concerns first.

Second, the CFI differs from the OCF in its *treatment* of cultural identity. The CFI questions have been revised in response to theoretical innovations on culture in the social and behavioral sciences. Cultural competence initiatives in the U.S. mental health system have historically paralleled the rise of the civil rights movements in the 1960s that emphasized race ("African American," "Asian," "Native American") and ethnicity ("Hispanic/Latino") as the most important markers of identity (Jenks 2011; Shaw and Armin 2011). However, experience with such initiatives has revealed that clinicians risk offering irrelevant recommendations on the basis of group-level racial and ethnic stereotypes (Aggarwal 2011; Kleinman and Benson 2006). For this reason, contemporary cultural competence initiatives emphasize that all people, not only racial and ethnic minorities, create distinct cultures in an ongoing and dynamic process of meaning-making based on their social affiliations (Aggarwal 2010; Carpenter-Song et al. 2007).

Cultural theorists have called attention to the notion of *hybridity*—that is, the idea that all people belong to multiple subcultures at any given time—challenging the notion that identities are only inherited, static in time, and group based rather than acquired, adaptable, multifaceted, and individualized (Bhabha 1994). For example, different situations may determine whether language, ethnicity, gender, or any other social affiliation is important at any given time. The task for a clinician is to help a patient explore which affiliation is essential to the experience of health care at a particular point in time. Moreover, a patient and clinician relate to each other's hybrid identities in any number of ways, often without awareness at the start of the clinical encounter, and these relationships influence how the patient shares his or her cultural identity (Aggarwal 2012). An open inquiry into cultural identity is all the more important in this era of information technology and globalization in which patients and clinicians can accumulate cultural affiliations through unprecedented travel to new societies both in person and over the Internet (Kirmayer 2006). This stance is not intended to suggest that group identities are unimportant but instead it intended to promote direct inquiry by clinicians about which group identities are most meaningful for patients rather than making assumptions.

Overview of the Supplementary Module

The CFI is a patient-centered approach; it encourages clinicians not to make any assumptions about patient identities. The core CFI's approach to cultural identity has already been introduced in Chapter 2, "The Core and Informant Cultural Formulation Interviews in DSM-5." Therefore, the focus in this subchapter is on the Cultural Identity supplementary module. The Guide to Interviewer for the Cultural Identity module (see Appendix C) notes the following:

> We use the word *culture* broadly to refer to all the ways the individual understands his or her identity and experience in terms of groups, communities or other collectivities, including national or geographic origin, ethnic community, racialized categories, gender, sexual orientation, social class, religion/spirituality, and language.

The CFI encourages clinicians to expand their understandings of identity beyond race, ethnicity, and language preferences to include the communities to which patients belong. The introduction to the "Role of Cultural Identity" in the core CFI for the individual being interviewed follows a similar format to the Guide to Interviewer in adopting a patient-centered approach to identity that makes no prior assumptions:

> Sometimes, aspects of people's background or identity can make their [PROBLEM] better or worse. By *background* or *identity,* I mean, for example, the communities you belong to, the languages you speak, where you or your family are from, your race or ethnic background, your gender or sexual orientation, or your faith or religion. (American Psychiatric Association 2013, p. 753)

The Cultural Identity supplementary module includes 34 questions that cover different aspects of identity. Clinicians may not need to use all questions with every patient but may find these sample questions helpful for investigating specific aspects of identity that may serve as a clinical focus. There are three main sections on cultural identity and a final section on how this information relates to the problem presented by the patient.

National, Ethnic, and Racial Background; Language; and Migration

The first seven questions of the module focus on an individual's national, ethnic, and racial background. National, ethnic, and racial identities are forms of social affiliation that have long been rooted in geography, with the understanding that a particular cultural group resides in a territorially constrained area (Gumperz and Cook-Gumperz 2008). These questions explore the birth locations of the patient and family, definitions of cultural community, the contexts in which these definitions arise, and the extent of any current health or life problems due to identity. These questions may be clinically useful when national, ethnic, and racial issues are defining features of the patient's presentation, as detailed subsequently in "Aspects of Cultural Identity Related to National, Ethnic, and Racial Background; Language; and Migration."

Questions 8–13 in the module uncover information about language, including fluency, situations in which certain languages are preferred, and preferences for language use in health care settings. Anthropologists have increasingly shown that language is not constrained within geographical borders (Urciuoli 1995); therefore, a clinician should not assume that all patients speak his or her language without first inquiring into their preferences. Clinicians may find these language questions helpful when the patient seems to express difficulties in speaking the dominant language of the clinic and would prefer interpreters.

Questions 14–22 on migration explore the circumstances of leaving a birth country, challenges of acculturation, and the impact of these factors on a patient's current presentation. Clinicians who treat immigrant and refugee populations may find these questions especially pertinent, especially because legal status may affect the extent to which patients decide to access health services.

Spirituality, Religion, and Moral Traditions

Questions 23–25 pertain to spirituality, religion, and moral traditions. They are posed to obtain information on specific beliefs and practices that inform the current illness and life in general, as discussed in "Aspects of Cultural Identity Related to Spirituality, Religion, and Moral Traditions." Clinicians may find that answers to these questions illuminate existential concerns raised by the current episode of sickness and indicate how patients continually derive meaning from their suffering throughout the experiences of illness and healing.

Gender and Sexual Orientation Identity

Questions 26–28 on gender identity and questions 29–32 on sexual orientation identity inform clinicians about the patient's identifications and their impact on the illness experience and general access to services. As explained in "Aspects of Cultural Identity Related to Gender Identity and Sexual Orientation Identity," stigma and discrimination have long acted as barriers to care for populations with gender and sexual orientation identity issues, and the CFI Cultural Identity module can inform clinicians about such potential barriers in formulating better alternatives for the current clinical encounter.

Summary

The supplementary module ends with two open-ended summary questions (questions 33 and 34). They seek information about other aspects of identity that might help the clinician better understand the patient's health care needs and about which aspects of identity are most important in relation to the current problem.

Conclusion

The questions on cultural identity in the core CFI and the supplementary module are intended to help clinicians develop practical, patient-centered approaches for diagnostic assessment and treatment planning. The DSM-5 field trials have demonstrated the need to translate theories from the social sciences for practical clinical care (Aggarwal et al. 2013). Case reports, controlled studies, and the experiences of clinicians, researchers, patients, and administrators can provide valuable information about how the developers of the CFI and its supplementary modules have succeeded and where revisions are needed for future editions of DSM. For example, experience with these supplementary modules may point to aspects of identity that seem most relevant to clinical situations. By the same token, clinicians may find that the supplementary modules include too much information for practical use. Because virtually no information is available on what patients deem important to ask regarding cultural identity, various stakeholders are invited to treat these supplementary modules as works in progress that elucidate how cultural identity relates to sickness and health.

KEY CLINICAL POINTS

- People adopt different identities based on social relationships, suggesting that clinicians need to ask patients how they identify rather than making general assumptions.
- The core Cultural Formulation Interview and its supplementary modules contain practical questions to address the relevance of a patient's identity to the problem he or she presents.

Questions

1. How is culture defined in DSM-5?

2. How does culture affect the care of patients in clinical practice?

3. What types of barriers to care do immigrants and refugees experience?

4. What types of barriers to care do people with gender and sexual orientation identity issues experience?

5. Why should patients be asked about their spiritual, religious, or moral traditions?

References

Aggarwal NK: Reassessing cultural evaluations in geriatrics: insights from cultural psychiatry. J Am Geriatr Soc 58(11):2191–2196, 2010 20977437

Aggarwal NK: Intersubjectivity, transference, and the cultural third. Contemp Psychoanal 47:204–223, 2011

Aggarwal NK: Hybridity and intersubjectivity in the clinical encounter: impact on the cultural formulation. Transcult Psychiatry 49(1):121–139, 2012 22218399

Aggarwal NK, Rohrbaugh RM: Teaching cultural competency through an experiential seminar on anthropology and psychiatry. Acad Psychiatry 35(5):331–334, 2011 22007094

Aggarwal NK, Nicasio AV, DeSilva R, et al: Barriers to implementing the DSM-5 Cultural Formulation Interview: a qualitative study. Cult Med Psychiatry 37(3):505–533, 2013 23836098

American Psychiatric Association: Diagnostic and Statistical Manual of Mental Disorders, 4th Edition. Washington, DC, American Psychiatric Association, 1994

American Psychiatric Association: Diagnostic and Statistical Manual of Mental Disorders, 5th Edition. Arlington, VA, American Psychiatric Association, 2013

Bhabha H: The Location of Culture. New York, Routledge, 1994

Carpenter-Song EA, Nordquest Schwallie M, Longhofer J: Cultural competence reexamined: critique and directions for the future. Psychiatr Serv 58(10):1362–1365, 2007 17914018

Gumperz JJ, Cook-Gumperz J: Studying language, culture, and society: sociolinguistics or linguistic anthropology? Journal of Sociolinguistics 12:532–545, 2008

Jenks AC: From "lists of traits" to "open-mindedness": emerging issues in cultural competence education. Cult Med Psychiatry 35(2):209–235, 2011 21560030

Kirmayer LJ: Beyond the 'new cross-cultural psychiatry': cultural biology, discursive psychology and the ironies of globalization. Transcult Psychiatry 43(1):126–144, 2006 16671396

Kleinman A, Benson P: Anthropology in the clinic: the problem of cultural competency and how to fix it. PLoS Med 3(10):e294, 2006 17076546

Lewis-Fernández R: The cultural formulation. Transcult Psychiatry 46(3):379–382, 2009 19837777

Lewis-Fernández R, Aggarwal NK, Bäärnhielm S, et al: Culture and psychiatric evaluation: operationalizing cultural formulation for DSM-5. Psychiatry 77(2):130–154, 2014 24865197

Monroe KR, Hankin J, van Vechten RB: The psychological foundations of identity politics. Annual Review of Political Science 3:419–447, 2000

Shaw SJ, Armin J: The ethical self-fashioning of physicians and health care systems in culturally appropriate health care. Cult Med Psychiatry 35(2):236–261, 2011 21553151

Urciuoli B: Language and borders. Annu Rev Anthropol 24:525–546, 1995

Suggested Readings

Cerulo KA: Identity construction: new issues, new directions. Annu Rev Sociol 23:385–409, 1997. A good review of how social scientists such as anthropologists and sociologists think about cultural identity.

Mezzich JE, Caracci G, Fabrega H Jr, et al: Cultural formulation guidelines. Transcult Psychiatry 46:383–405, 2009. Explanation of how social science theories can be used to explore cultural identity through the cultural formulation.

Aspects of Cultural Identity Related to National, Ethnic, and Racial Background; Language; and Migration

Simon Groen, M.A.

Hans Rohlof, M.D.

Sushrut Jadhav, M.B.B.S., M.D., MRCPsych, Ph.D.

Ton and Lim (2006) define *cultural identity* as follows:

> a multifaceted core set of identities that contributes to how an individual understands his or her environment. Ethnic identity is often a crucial facet of an individual's overall cultural identity, but many other facets may contribute to it as well. The greater the amount of detail a clinician is able to ascertain about the individual's cultural identity, the better understanding he or she will have of the individual's perspectives on health, illness, and the mental health system. (p. 10)

The Cultural Identity supplementary module (provided in Appendix C in this handbook) of the Cultural Formulation Interview (CFI) offers an opportunity for clinicians to explore the complexity of patients' cultural identity by unpacking its various elements. Here, in addition to evaluating the problem presented, we examine the first three parts of the module in an attempt to explore clinical relevance with respect to identity: national, ethnic, and racial background; language; and migration. Finally, we provide suggestions on how to use this portion of the module.

National, Ethnic, and Racial Background

Questions 1–7 of the Cultural Identity module ask about the patient's national, ethnic, and racial background.

National Identity

National identity expresses the feeling of difference one person has from another based on the conceptualization that they belong to different nations or to distinct national groups within a multicultural setting (Smith 1993). When clinicians elicit the national identity of individuals with mental health problems during diagnosis and treatment, they may need to be aware of the patient's sense of belongingness, which could include the patient's relationship to national symbols, language(s), the nation's history, national values, politics, religions, national media, music, food habits, and so on. The awareness of difference is addressed by the question "Who are we?" as opposed to "Who are they?" Anderson (1983) introduced the concept of *nation* as a socially constructed imagined community as conceived by the persons who believe themselves to be a part of that community. The community is "imagined" because "the members of even the smallest nation will never know most of their fellow members, meet them, or even hear of them, yet in the minds of each lives the image of their communion" (Anderson 1983, p. 49). It is important to bear in mind that national, geographical, and cultural boundaries are not coterminous.

For the clinician, it is useful to explore the individual's notion of that imagined community. A nation's history and the everyday values prized by the group have developed over time, and this history plays a major role in the sociocultural construction of the national identity of its community members. Cases in point are the dramatic sociohistorical changes after the independence of formally colonized nations in Africa and Asia in the 1960s, the Islamic Revolution in Iran in the 1980s, and national development of former Soviet satellite states in the 1990s. There are also more distant events, such as the origin of the United States as a nation in the struggle against the British and the historical development of Latin American countries opposed to Spanish rule. In psychoanalytical literature, this is known as *large-group identity,* which is based on chosen victories and chosen traumas (Volkan 1999). A clinician does not have to be aware of the entire historical development of a patient's nation or community. However, when the clinician is eliciting a patient's national background (questions 1–6), understanding the historical context is helpful for eliciting his or her life story in a culturally sensitive manner.

Place of birth is an important aspect of identity (question 1). Cultural differences based on regional distinctions are common. For instance, if a patient is born in Iraq, it matters whether he or she is from Baghdad, Kirkuk, or Basra. Baghdad has a multiethnic population that is mainly divided into Sunni and Shiite districts. In the current moment, Baghdad is a city with frequent ethnic conflicts, car bombings, and other forms of violence. Kirkuk, a city in northern Iraq, is economically one of the most important municipalities in the autonomous region of Kurdistan, mostly populated by Iraqi Kurds. Basra is the most important city in the Shiite-dominated southeastern part of Iraq that was heavily involved in the Iran-Iraq War from 1980 to 1988. The differences between these various localities may be more important to the patient at times than their commonalities as part of the more recent nation-state of Iraq.

In Europe, many immigrants were born in the former Yugoslavia, the Punjab, or Bengal before geopolitical partitions, and these places of origin have evolved over time both politically and culturally. As another example, if someone is from the southern Indian state of Tamil Nadu, it may be relevant to establish whether the patient is of Tamil or Sinhalese origin from Sri Lanka, because this fact may provide clues to social exclusion or experiences of military trauma and genocide. In many countries, urban and rural areas differ in important ways. This is the case in many African nations: rural areas have less access to mental health care; different knowledge of psychopathology; and variation in adherence to indigenous belief systems, secret societies, witchcraft, ideas about ghost or spirit possession, and other supernatural concepts.

In many countries, especially those populated by diaspora cultures, identity is shaped by parental place of birth (question 2). If one or both parents were born in another nation or culturally distinct area, this often influences a person's identity. A Chinese American man whose parents were born in China and who himself was born in California may see himself more as Chinese at times or more as American at times, depending on the context. If the parentage is mixed, especially if parents are from areas in conflict with each other, such as individuals of Bosnian-Serbian or Azeri-Armenian heritage, this can pose substantial challenges: these individuals run the risk of being rejected, threatened, or even chased and murdered by those whose parentage is not mixed.

As these examples show, identity is an active process of representing oneself to others. Someone's place of birth (question 1), parentage (question 2), and national, ethnic, and/or racial background (question 3) play important roles in self-representation in everyday life—that is, how that person describes himself or herself to others (question 4).

Ethnic Identity

Ethnicity refers to the classification of people as belonging to a group that claims a common descent, frequently attributed to a specific geographical region; usually a common language and other cultural characteristics; and possibly a common religion (Eriksen 1993). Such group identities are always defined in relation to nonmembers of that group (Barth 1969). Ethnic groups within a nation may differ from each other in terms of primary language, religion, rituals, values, symbols, clothing, and food. Of course, within ethnic groups, subgroups also vary in terms of these characteristics, but the point of the concept of ethnicity is that it minimizes these particular differences in the name of the postulated group similarities. For example, Puerto Ricans may speak English or Spanish as their primary language, depending on the extent and duration of their U.S. migration experience, but this difference is minimized in the name of a common Puerto Rican ethnicity. A nation may contain multiple ethnic groups; for instance, Ethiopia has more than 80 such groups. Alternatively, an ethnic group may span more than one currently defined nation-state; the Kurds, for example, live in parts of Iraq, Turkey, Iran, and Syria. In most African countries, the word *tribe* is more common than *ethnic group* in everyday speech. In Somalia, there is a complicated *clan* genealogy with major clans and many subclans. Somalis may recognize each other's lineage by their double last names. The clan or subclan to which a Somali belongs can influence educational and work opportunities as well as experiences of protection and discrimination (Groen 2009). The U.S. Census distinguishes only one *ethnicity*, Hispanic/Latino, and five *races*, white/Caucasian, black/African American, Asian, American Indian and Alaskan Native, and Native Hawaiian and Pacific Islander. The distinction of Latino-ness as an ethnicity is a recent development, stemming from political recognition of the diversity of characteristics usually considered racial that characterize the Latino group; Latinos can be of European, African, Native, or Asian descent but are supposedly unified by their cultural similarities, including language and Latin American geographical background. Obviously, Latinos also differ markedly from each other, underlining the primarily political aspect of the definition of ethnicity.

In some nations, there are violent conflicts between ethnic groups. For example, there were large-scale warlike conflicts between Hutu and Tutsi in the late 1980s in Rwanda; between Azeri and Armenians (the Nagorno-Karabakh conflict) also starting in the late 1980s; and among Bosnians, Croatians, and Serbs in the former Yugoslavia during the 1990s. There may also be less intense conflicts between mainstream and minority ethnic groups regarding whether or not the latter belong to the larger national group. The Pashtun claim the Hazara are not real Afghans; other Angolans claim the Bakongo are not real Angolans; many Congolese claim the Banyamulenge belong to Rwanda. The position of ethnic groups varies across different states and time periods; currently, Kurds are relatively safe in the autonomous region of Kurdistan in northern Iraq, but they are sometimes persecuted in Iran, Syria, and Turkey. Canadians may define their ethnic identities in terms of the complexities of their colonial past; also, as a result of a common history of colonialism and foreign domination, the Irish may see themselves as a separate ethnic group but define themselves as politically aligned with the black population in the United Kingdom.

Racial and "Racialized" Identity

The term *race* has no scientific or biological basis; it is instead a social construct that acquired its modern form in the eighteenth to nineteenth centuries. *Racialized identity* is an alternate social construct that highlights the point that the experience of race is based on the *perception* of having a common heritage with a particular group defined in racial terms (Helms 1993). A commonly defined racialized identity is that of skin color. This popular folk notion often clumps people into blacks, whites, reds, or yellows. Responses and attitudes toward skin color vary across and within countries. In the United States, being part of a racialized community, such as white Americans, American Indians, or African Americans, may play a crucial role in defining one's cultural identity, particularly if viewed by others as a "true" characteristic of a person. Therefore, it is important to ask patients how they locate themselves with respect to racialized identities prevailing within their community or culture. Many patients of African, Asian, and Afro-Caribbean background in the United Kingdom may think their mental health problems are misunderstood by local white British clinicians. They may feel that they have been wrongly diagnosed or have been treated in a culturally insensitive manner, which may result in poor adherence to care (Littlewood and Lipsedge 1997). The reverse may also apply to clinicians in other countries providing consultations to local white British or white U.S. patients. In many regions, such as in India, the term *race* or *racial identity* may not resonate with local ideas of identity. Instead, *caste* (*jāti*) or social class may constitute the core of a person's or community's cultural identity. In such contexts, caste and class identity of both patient and clinician may hinder or facilitate access to care and engagement with treatment. Therefore, clinicians eliciting a person's "racial background" need to be sensitive to locally prevalent notions of "racial identity" and the manner in which these terms are expressed and understood in different contexts and cultures (Jadhav and Jain 2012).

Videos 9 and 10 illustrate the use of the National, Ethnic, and Racial Background section of the Cultural Identity supplementary module.

 Video Illustration 9: A small town, which is why I'm here (4:39)

In the video "A small town, which is why I'm here," a psychiatrist conducts an interview with a middle-aged Puerto Rican man who suffers from anxiety symptoms at work after his mother, who lives in Puerto Rico, has a stroke. The aim of the National, Ethnic, and Racial Background portion of the Cultural Identity supplementary module is to assess how a person's national, ethnic, and racial background affects his or her sense of self and his or her place in society and how these aspects of identity influence behavior. In this video, the clinician frames the purpose of the interview. This is an important part of any supplementary module, because it clarifies for the patient how the subsequent questions relate to the patient's reason for seeking help. In this case, the interviewer emphasizes that he wants to understand whether the patient's cultural identity influences his mental health problems and his expectations of care. The initial questions immediately reveal the reason for seeking help. The patient is experiencing substantial anxiety because his mother is in Puerto Rico in a town with limited access to the tertiary medical care she needs for her stroke. He feels pressure to return to the island to provide the care she needs, as seems to be expected of any good Puerto Rican son. In fact, if he does not go, his family might think less of him and perhaps even repudiate him to some extent. The conflict stems from the fact that his sense of himself is connected to being the kind of person who takes risks to become successful, including migrating to the United States for a better future. To complicate matters further, he fears that he could lose his job if he responds to what he and his community in Puerto Rico interpret as his filial duty. He appears puzzled by the reaction of his employers, who are unwilling to grant him leave from work to travel. He says, "At work they…kinda don't get this thing with family. I don't quite understand how it works over here, but it's almost like family isn't important, like you're supposed to go working anyway, you can't take any time off." His current predicament highlights the cultural differences between his new environment and key aspects of his identity, and this conflict appears to be heightening his anxiety.

Information on a patient's cultural identity can help clarify perspective on health, illness, and the mental health system. The way an individual represents himself to others, how he feels about his position in society, and how this relates to his mental health problems is useful information for the clinician. Starting from the information obtained in the video, the interviewer can proceed to elicit additional details. For example, the interviewer could obtain more information on the patient's role in his family. The clinician could ask if the patient is the eldest son, who is thought to have a special responsibility for his mother, or how his family reacted to his migration and to his drive to succeed, which may put extra pressure on him that could contribute to his symptoms. To help with the current situation at work, the clinician could inquire whether he has felt misunderstood there in other situations, whether there are other Puerto Rican coworkers, whether they have experienced the same kind of misunderstandings, and whether he is afraid to be discriminated against as a result of his ethnicity if he asks for unpaid leave.

 Video Illustration 10: It gets kind of confusing (2:41)

In the video "It gets kind of confusing," the interviewer explores the cultural identity of a young woman of mixed Panamanian–U.S. descent who is being evaluated for apparently having auditory hallucinations of her grandmother's voice (see the video "Full CFI" for longer segments from the complete CFI assessment). The goal of this section of the Cultural Identity supplementary module is to assess how a person's national, ethnic, and racial background affects his or her sense of self and his or her place in society and how these aspects of identity influence behavior. The patient calls herself "American" but is exposed to "traditions and culture that I carry with me from the Panamanian side of my family." Her juxtaposing of these aspects of her background as in some sense opposed to each other carries through the rest of the interview. Her father is "from America" and "white," while her mother and her relatives are from Panama. Her mother "is a citizen now," apparently somewhat recently. The patient tends to resolve the conflict by telling people she is "Hispanic," but in general "I try to not even enter the topic." She feels people "get confused" about ethnicity and race in general, given that people "can be a mix of anything, can be a mix of black, or white, or Native American, everything." She feels "like any other like American person growing up in my hometown," but she also feels closest to the Panamanian side of the family. This is partly because of the cultural traditions that endure in her nuclear family and also because of her close, loving relationship with a grandmother in Panama. The interview illustrates some of the complexities of identity that may be affecting her clinical presentation, resulting in a deep-set conflict expressed via hallucinatory experiences. Information on her cultural identity would be essential for her treatment going forward, for example, in certain types of psychotherapy.

The interview illustrates some of the complexities of identity that may be affecting her clinical presentation, resulting in a deep-set conflict expressed via hallucinatory experiences. Information on her cultural identity would be essential for her treatment going forward, for example, in certain types of psychotherapy. The clinician could obtain more information on each of the points raised by the patient—for example, regarding the role of cultural traditions in her household and whether these led her to feel "different" from her peers growing up. These questions are likely to elicit useful material for the process of psychotherapy.

Language

Questions 8–13 of the Cultural Identity module evaluate language with respect to identity. Language is a key component of identity and serves as a marker of belonging to a certain cultural group. Consider the following statement by an Iranian woman from Tabriz in the province of East Azerbaijan in northeastern Iran, which is populated by Turkish, Turkmen, and Bulgarian Iranians:

> As long as I know, my family has been in Tabriz. Because my parents did not have many opportunities to go to school, they hardly spoke Farsi. We spoke Azeri at home. In primary school, until fifth grade, the books were in Farsi, but the teachers taught in Azeri. From fifth grade on, they started to teach in Farsi. I felt I was different from others, because I was fluent in Azeri but not in Farsi. (Azeri patient from Iran seen in a Dutch clinic)

This example shows how language influences the sense of belonging. For this woman, speaking a certain language marks her sense of being different from others. The language a person uses can vary across situations: at home, on the street, in school, or in official documents. In some places during certain time periods, the languages of particular national subgroups have been forbidden in public space, such as the Kurdish language Kurmanji in Turkey or Catalan in Franco's Spain. People may refrain from speaking their mother tongue in public if they are afraid to be recognized as a member of a particular group.

After people migrate, the languages they speak at home often vary depending on speaking partner (question 10). For instance, parents may feel most comfortable speaking their native language with each other but may mix their language with the language of the host country when speaking to their children. Sometimes, the children do not learn the language of the host country until they go to school. Frequently, the children are more fluent than the previous generation in the language of the host nation and may have to help their parents read letters or official documents. At times, children may forget their native language. This may pose communication problems with their parents and also contribute to intergenerational conflicts. Parents may find it upsetting that their children are no longer able to speak with family members left behind in their home country and may feel that they have lost touch with their culture of origin.

Some migrants are proud of their fluency in the host language. This may become clear during their interaction with clinicians in mental health care (question 12). Using an interpreter in such a situation could be regarded as an insult and as a refutation both of their progress and of their acculturation to the host country. However, when expressing intense emotions, these patients may well be more fluent in their native language. In such instances, a clinician could point out the benefit of speaking in the native language but express respect for their language acquisition in the host country. Some patients refuse an interpreter because, despite confidentiality regulations, they do not trust other members from their cultural group, particularly when the migrant community is composed of diverse subgroups, some of whom were in conflict in the culture of origin. Some patients from tightly knit communities may refuse interpreters because of concern over the risk of disclosure leading to stigmatizing consequences for their family, including decreased marriage prospects for their children. Alternatively, interpreter refusal may be the result of the realistic or imagined fear of being identified and thus persecuted after escaping from their countries of origin for cultural and political reasons. The clinician should respect and address all of these concerns during treatment.

Language literacy may also be an important aspect of identity. For example, whether a person can read and write in his or her native language may indicate a certain sociocultural status in the home country (question 13). For instance, many Afghan women, particularly those in rural areas, are forbidden to go to school and therefore are usually illiterate. This situation can become a major obstacle to their efforts to integrate within the host country.

Migration

Questions 14–22 of the Cultural Identity module evaluate migration in relation to identity and the problem presented. For immigrants, a major stressor is leaving loved ones and a familiar sociocultural context and having to develop a new life in the host country. Migration may be forced or due to personal choice. Both types result in cultural displacement and dislocation. However, migration may not always be detrimental to the person's health because his or her experiences are also shaped by responses from members of the host society. Migration and postmigration living problems—for example, those problems due to experiences in transit to the host nation or events in the host nation such as the asylum procedure—may be the most important causes of distress (Laban et al. 2005). The clinician needs to know how long the patient has lived in the host country, what was the reason for leaving the country of origin, and how his or her life has changed as a result of the migration process (questions 14–16). For example, for individuals originating from a collectivistic society, adapting to a more individualistic culture might add new dimensions to their mental health problems. Having been accustomed to the group taking care of its members' problems, they may feel alienated in the new setting because they are responsible for their own individual health care–seeking choices. Equally, there may be intracultural variations among individuals from a collectivistic society, in that some might be primarily *allocentric* (other focused) and others may be egocentric (self-focused) (Bhugra 2005). For clinicians, it is important to use the Cultural Identity module to distinguish a patient's individual characteristics and not to fall into the trap of stereotyping on the basis of fragmented knowledge about the person's country of origin.

Guidelines for Clinical Use of the Module

Using this supplementary module in clinical practice is best illustrated by a clinical vignette. The vignette does not address all of the questions in the module but touches on its key components.

Case Vignette

Amir, a 39-year-old Iraqi man who had worked as an interpreter for Western allied forces in Iraq, was referred to mental health care in a European country for severe depressed mood and nightmares after suffering a traumatic exposure. His most pressing concern was that he felt his problems were not acknowledged by the government of the country where he found refuge. He mentioned that he worked quite hard for the army of occupation. He thought it would bring him great respect. But over time, he came to feel like a traitor to his country and had great difficulty proceeding with his life as usual. During the early phase of treatment, the clinician and patient elaborated on what Amir meant exactly by this statement. He explained that he hoped that by becoming an army interpreter he would bring prosperity and freedom for his people. This idealistic view of his activities eroded over time, as he felt increasingly that he was exploited and trapped in a power dynamic in which he could not participate any longer. He came to feel that he was used as a tool for the suppression of his own people. Moreover, when Amir made a return trip to Iraq from his host country, he was regarded as a traitor by his fellow countrymen.

He told the clinician that his family in Iraq was in great danger because of his interpreter work and was viewed as an enemy by the Iraqis opposing the Western occupation. When asked what he would do if they attacked his family, Amir turned very pale and said, "I would kill myself, because it would be my fault and I would not be able to cope with my guilt." He stated that in his culture, family meant everything. On another occasion, he said that he was proud to be an inhabitant of his "new" country; now he felt that if asked to choose, he would want to remain there. This was because in Iraq he felt physically unsafe and he would also feel controlled by his family. Amir appreciated the possibility for further educational development and other opportunities to advance his life because of the support he had received in his "new" country. As a result of his conflicting feelings, his cultural, national, and ethnic identity had become intensely mixed and chaotic.

This vignette demonstrates how national and migration issues are intertwined with multiple aspects of cultural identity. A person's cultural identities mutually influence and shape each other. In addition, different aspects of identity may come to the fore depending on the context in question. This man is an Iraqi by national identity, but his work and experiences in the host country after migration changed his attitude toward his country of origin and his fellow countrymen. The case illustrates the dynamic aspect of identity. What is crucial for the clinician to explore is the value a patient attaches to the various dimensions of identity and how these dimensions influence his or her sense of belonging, self-esteem, and other elements of self-experience that are important clinically. The Cultural Identity supplementary module can help the clinician perform a relatively thorough evaluation of identity if the clinician approaches the assessment with an inquisitive and respectful attitude in an atmosphere of open exchange. When conducting a cultural assessment, the clinician elicits the cultural aspects of the person's identity but also should not forget the position of the individual in the culture.

Conclusion

The Cultural Identity supplementary model assesses the impact of national, ethnic, and racial background; language; and migration because eliciting a patient's multifaceted cultural identities helps the clinician better understand the individual's perspectives on his or her mental health problems. This subchapter focuses on these issues, how they relate to mental health problems, and how they can be addressed by clinicians.

KEY CLINICAL POINTS

- Aspects of a patient's cultural identity related to national, ethnic, racial, and linguistic background as well as migration status can affect the type and severity of risk factors for mental health problems, the patient's interpretation of illness causation and symptomatology, and help-seeking expectations.

- Exploration of these aspects of cultural identity with the Cultural Formulation Interview may improve patient engagement and clinician understanding of the person's mental health problems, especially among cultural minorities, including migrant populations.

Questions

1. What are some of the aspects of cultural identity that can affect the onset, interpretation, and care of mental health problems?

2. How can cultural identity affect the causes of mental health problems and the person's help-seeking choices?

3. How can language differences and migration experiences influence diagnosis and treatment?

References

Anderson B: Imagined Communities: Reflections on the Origin and Spread of Nationalism. London, Verso, 1983

Barth F: Introduction, in Ethnic Groups and Boundaries: The Social Organization of Cultural Difference. Edited by Barth F. Boston, Little, Brown, 1969, pp 9–38

Bhugra D: Cultural identities and cultural congruency: a new model for evaluating mental distress in immigrants. Acta Psychiatr Scand 111(2):84–93, 2005 15667427

Eriksen TH: Ethnicity and Nationalism: Anthropological Perspectives. London, Pluto Press, 1993

Groen S: Recognizing cultural identity in mental health care: rethinking the cultural formulation of a Somali patient. Transcult Psychiatry 46(3):451–462, 2009 19837781

Helms JE: Introduction: review of racial identity terminology, in Black and White Racial Identity: Theory, Research and Practice. Edited by Helms JE. Westport, CT, Praeger, 1993, pp 3–8

Jadhav S, Jain S: Clinical appeal of cultural formulations in community rural mental health, in Comprehensive Textbook on Community Psychiatry in India. Edited by Chavan BS, Gupta N, Arun P, et al. New Delhi, Jaypee Brothers, 2012, pp 560–565

Laban CJ, Gernaat HBPE, Komproe IH, et al: Postmigration living problems and common psychiatric disorders in Iraqi asylum seekers in the Netherlands. J Nerv Ment Dis 193(12):825–832, 2005 16319706

Littlewood R, Lipsedge M: Aliens and Alienists: Ethnic Minorities and Psychiatry, 3rd Edition. London, Routledge, 1997

Smith AD: National Identity: Ethnonationalism in Comparative Perspective. New York, Penguin Books, 1993

Ton H, Lim RF: The assessment of culturally diverse individuals, in Clinical Manual of Cultural Psychiatry. Edited by Lim RF. Washington, DC, American Psychiatric Publishing, 2006, pp 3–31

Volkan VD: Psychoanalysis and diplomacy: part I. Individual and large group identity. J Appl Psychoanal Stud 1:29–55, 1999

Suggested Readings

Berry JW, Poortinga YH, Segal MH, et al: Cross-Cultural Psychology: Research and Application. Cambridge, UK, Cambridge University Press, 2002

Groen S: Recognizing cultural identity in mental health care: rethinking the cultural formulation of a Somali patient. Transcult Psychiatry 46(3):451–462, 2009 19837781

Multicultural Mental Health Resource Centre: http://www.multiculturalmentalhealth.ca/clinical-tools/cultural-formulation/

Ton H, Lim RF: The assessment of culturally diverse individuals, in Clinical Manual of Cultural Psychiatry. Edited by Lim RF. Washington, DC, American Psychiatric Publishing, 2006, pp 3–31

UCL Cultural Consultation Service: http://www.ucl.ac.uk/ccs/specialist-services

van de Vijver FJR, van Hemert DA, Poortinga YH: Multilevel Analysis of Individuals and Cultures. New York, Erlbaum, 2008

Aspects of Cultural Identity Related to Spirituality, Religion, and Moral Traditions

David M. Gellerman, M.D., Ph.D.

Francis G. Lu, M.D.

Spirituality, religion, and moral traditions often offer meaning and purpose to an individual's life, and religious faith, spiritual affiliations, and/or moral commitments can be essential components of a person's cultural identity. Religious and spiritual belief systems and faith communities can play an important part in transmitting culturally held values, social behavior, and meaning even in the early stages of psychological development (Shafranke 1992). Such beliefs and values may be challenged when one's perceived identity is threatened or distorted at times of crisis or transition (Peteet 2004b), further contributing to a person's distress. All of these components of identity can influence a patient's views and behaviors, including how the patient understands his or her psychiatric illness and how the patient chooses to navigate among available mental health care choices (Peteet 2004a).

Assessment of Cultural Identity in the Core Cultural Formulation Interview and Supplementary Modules

The core Cultural Formulation Interview (CFI) has three questions on the patient's cultural identity (questions 8–10); "faith or religion" is indicated as a component of this identity. These basic questions on general cultural identity are supplemented with three additional questions in the Cultural Identity supplementary module that focus specifically on the spiritual, religious, and moral aspects of identity (question 23); the importance of these issues in patients' everyday lives (question 24); and the contribution of the patient's family to this aspect of identity (question 25). If the clinician wants to follow up the answers to these questions, a separate module on the overall role in the person's life of spirituality, religion, and moral traditions lists domains and specific questions for further exploration (for more information see subchapter "Supplementary Module 5: Spirituality, Religion, and Moral Traditions" and Appendix C in this handbook).

In the Cultural Identity module, question 23 opens a dialogue with the patient about the aspect of his or her identity that has to do with religious, moral, or spiritual traditions. Even though the question refers to the present time, the patient may respond in terms of past affiliations or even aspirational ones. If the patient describes a change in affiliations over time, use of the Spirituality, Religion, and Moral Traditions supplementary module may be advised because these changes and the reasons for them can be important markers of identity development, community engagement, and/or attempts at coping with a clinical problem. Question 24 asks the patient about the significance of spiritual, religious, and moral traditions in everyday life as a way of evaluating his or her level of identification with that tradition and its importance as a support or even potentially a stressor. The extent to which one or more traditions affect everyday life likely correlates with the level of the person's identification and its impact on cultural identity. Question 25 asks the patient whether family members share his or her traditions. If the answer is more toward the affirmative, this may clarify the cultural context that supports the patient's identification with the tradition. Also, the patient's identification might be preliminarily assessed to be normative for the patient as an outgrowth of the family's traditions. If the answer is more toward the negative, the clinician would need to understand how this came to be and how much of a stressor this discrepancy with family norms might be for the patient. Question 25 has a built-in follow-up question to ask for more details in either case.

Video 11 delves into the interconnectedness of spirituality, religion, and moral traditions with cultural identity.

 Video Illustration 11: You still show up on Sunday (3:26)

This video illustrates the use of the cultural identity questions (8–10) from the core CFI. The patient's answers reveal important values as well as conflicts about his sense of himself that stem from the role of spirituality and religion in his life. While attending church and Sunday school is a central aspect of his background, and a source of his value system, he also indicates learning to "put up a front." He says this behavior was influenced by his mother, who had "multiple nervous breakdowns" and "wouldn't leave her bed" during the week but would take pains to appear well enough in church on Sunday despite being severely impaired at home. Not only does this comment provide important family psychiatric history, but it also suggests an early conflict in the patient's social development, in the sense of endorsing versus behaving consistently with one's values.

In response to the next question of the core CFI, on aspects of cultural identity that make a difference to his anxiety, the patient describes the challenges of reconciling his faith with his studies in cognitive science and his need for treatment. On the one hand, the patient suggests that his anxiety, as "part of God's creation," has value and is "beautiful in that way"; on the other hand, he also says that he does not wish, or even need, to suffer as his mother did, suggesting that she avoided treatment in part because of her religious values. While acknowledging his need for anxiety treatment, he also states his preference to not take medications, a preference guided by his religious values. The video concludes with the third and final core CFI question on cultural identity, inquiring whether aspects of his background or identity cause these concerns or difficulties. The patient responds that living in New York challenges him to keep living up to his religious values, suggesting that this tension contributes to his anxiety symptoms.

Additional probes could elicit more information on these conflicts related to the patient's faith. Questions from the Spirituality, Religion, and Moral Traditions supplementary module might be helpful in this regard. For example, it would be useful to know more about the patient's specific faith tradition and moral values, including the role of the religious community in faith members' lives and their attitudes about mental health services. It could be useful to treatment planning to explore the potential role of religious practices such as reading or studying religious materials or prayer and the patient's past experience of the usefulness of these practices for coping with his anxiety symptoms. Finally, in response to the last question of the video, exploring specific "temptations" faced by the patient could identify stressors, conflicts, and coping strategies in relation to his anxiety symptoms and whether he has found a church in New York that can expand his social network in a supportive way.

Relationship to Gender Identity and Sexual Orientation Identity

One specific aspect of the impact of spirituality, religion, and moral traditions bears mentioning. Conflicts may arise between the patient's spiritual, religious, or moral identity in the context of his or her sexual orientation and gender identities. These latter aspects of identity are explored in Cultural Identity supplementary module questions 26–32, discussed next in this chapter. They may be particularly important in clarifying how the patient negotiates his or her sexual orientation and gender identity in the context of his or her religious, spiritual, or moral life. For example, although many Western mainstream religions may discourage, forbid, or even oppress homosexuality, several studies suggest that gay and lesbian individuals can identify themselves as having rich spiritual and religious lives (García et al. 2008; Tan 2005). In García et al.'s (2008) study, gay, bisexual, and transgender men described reconciling their religious faith and their sexuality to some degree, whether they remained Catholic, converted to another faith, or did not identify any formal religious or spiritual affiliations. Many who did not identify with a particular group described continuing to believe in God, pray, and read books on spiritual development. Although this study included transgender individuals, few if any studies explore religious or spiritual identity specifically in transgender populations. HIV infection can exacerbate the sense of alienation from the church, and in Miller's (2005) sample of interviewees with AIDS, many left their religious institutions as a result. Seegers (2007) noted that the gay men infected with HIV in her study endorsed an active and valued spiritual life and religious practices and expressed their spirituality through practices at church; however, none had openly revealed their homosexuality or shared their HIV status with their clergy or church community.

Conclusion

Because the impact of spiritual, religious, and moral traditions on a person's life is important to explore among people presenting with psychiatric difficulties, these issues are included as topics of assessment in the core CFI, in a separate supplementary module, and as part of the Cultural Identity module. Here we focused on how clinicians should assess this domain through the Cultural Identity module.

KEY CLINICAL POINT

- Religious faith, spiritual affiliations, and/or moral commitments constitute important components of a person's cultural identity that can be explored with the Cultural Formulation Interview as part of a cultural assessment focusing on the person's illness interpretations and coping and help-seeking options.

Questions

1. How does a clinician assess the religious, spiritual, and moral components of a person's cultural identity?

2. In what ways do spiritual, religious, and moral traditions influence decisions about health care and other forms of help seeking?

3. In what ways might a person's engagement with spiritual, religious, or moral traditions contribute to increased emotional distress?

References

García DI, Gray-Stanley J, Ramirez-Valles J: "The priest obviously doesn't know that I'm gay": the religious and spiritual journeys of Latino gay men. J Homosex 55(3):411–436, 2008 19042279

Miller RL Jr: An appointment with God: AIDS, place, and spirituality. J Sex Res 42(1):35–45, 2005 15795803

Peteet JR: Doing the Right Thing: An Approach to Moral Issues in Mental Health Treatment. Washington, DC, American Psychiatric Publishing, 2004a

Peteet JR: Therapeutic implications of worldview, in Handbook of Spirituality and Worldview in Clinical Practice. Edited by Josephson AM, Peteet JR. Washington, DC, American Psychiatric Publishing, 2004b pp. 47–59

Seegers DL: Spiritual and religious experiences of gay men with HIV illness. J Assoc Nurses AIDS Care 18(3):5–12, 2007 17570295

Shafranke EP: Religion and mental health in early life, in Religion and Mental Health. Edited by Schumaker JF. New York, Oxford University Press, 1992

Tan PP: The importance of spirituality among gay and lesbian individuals. J Homosex 49(2):135–144, 2005 16048898

Suggested Readings

Anandarajah G, Hight E: Spirituality and medical practice: using the HOPE questions as a practical tool for spiritual assessment. Am Fam Physician 63(1):81–89, 2001 11195773
George Washington Institute for Spirituality and Health: http://smhs.gwu.edu/gwish/
Koenig HG: Spirituality in Patient Care: Why, How, When and What, 3rd Edition. Philadelphia, PA, Templeton Foundation Press, 2013
Maugans TA: The SPIRITual history. Arch Fam Med 5(1):11–16, 1996 8542049
Pulchalski C: Spiritual assessment in clinical practice. Psychiatr Ann 36:150–155, 2006

Aspects of Cultural Identity Related to Gender Identity and Sexual Orientation Identity

John E. Pachankis, Ph.D.

Mark L. Hatzenbuehler, Ph.D.

Sexual orientation and gender identity form important aspects of cultural diversity for lesbian, gay, bisexual, and transgender (LGBT) individuals. Unfortunately, until recently, the cultural relevance of these identities was obscured from mainstream mental health practice, or sexual orientation and gender identities were treated with censure and moral disapprobation, as evidenced by the inclusion of sexual orientation as a mental illness in DSM until 1973. In recent decades, however, LGBT individuals have made rapid social progress toward recognition and respect from mainstream institutions, including psychiatric ones. Recent evidence suggests that LGBT individuals are more likely than heterosexuals to seek mental health treatment (Cochran et al. 2003). Consequently, it is essential that mental health professionals are competent in assessing and treating individuals with diverse sexual orientations and gender identities.

The Cultural Formulation Interview (CFI), including the supplementary modules, advances clinicians' cultural competence by providing straightforward prompts for assessing the relevance of a patient's sexual orientation and/or gender identity to the mental health concerns presented by the patient. Here we review empirical research on five domains that are most relevant to the assessment of the impact of sexual and gender identity on mental health to provide guidance to clinicians on how to assess these clinically meaningful areas. We first discuss the assessment of sexual and gender identity as outlined in the Cultural Identity supplementary module (provided in Appendix C of this handbook), followed by brief summaries of the importance of these aspects of identity for all the domains assessed in the core CFI and further elaborated in the supplementary modules.

Gender and Sexual Orientation Identity

Gender refers to a socially constructed notion of masculinity or femininity that describes the roles, behaviors, activities, or attributes that society considers appropriate for men and women. Gender is not always aligned with biological sex and does not always describe a purely dichotomous phenomenon; that is, gender can be fluid. For transgender individuals, gender identity does not conform to conventional, dichotomous notions of male or female or the biological sex to which one was assigned at birth. *Sexual orientation,* in contrast, typically refers to the way in which an individual identifies his or her sexual orientation in relation to the gender or sex to which he or she is attracted.

Although it can be argued that LGBT individuals belong to a distinct culture (Duberman et al. 2002), the meaning of that culture and any LGBT individual's degree of identification with it vary widely and likely will continue to change in the face of rapid social progress and the greater possibility of assimilation into mainstream cultures. Therefore, the CFI prompts providers to broadly assess all patients' sexual orientation and gender identities and the developmental trajectories of these identities.

The Cultural Identity supplementary module prompts mental health practitioners to systematically assess these aspects of identity using matter-of-fact, open-ended questions. By assessing all patients' sexual orientation and gender identities, providers avoid making assumptions about those identities and their relevance to any given patient. By asking, for example, "How would you describe your sexual orientation?" (question 29) or "What label do you prefer for your gender identity?" clinicians pave the way for open sharing of many possible identities. Clinicians can expect a variety of responses to these questions, especially among younger generations of sexual and gender minority individuals (e.g., those who identify as LGBT, who engage in same-sex sexual behavior, who are gender nonconforming, or who otherwise do not identify their sexual orientation as heterosexual or their gender identity in binary terms), who are especially likely to identify their sexual orientations and gender identities using a range of options (e.g., queer, pansexual) rather than more traditional labels (e.g., lesbian, transgender) (Pantalone et al. 2014). Clinicians should use the term(s) that the client prefers and explore the meaning of these terms for the individual. Furthermore, clinicians should avoid assuming binary gender conceptualizations (i.e., male and female), because some patients identify themselves and their partners in nonbinary terms. Therefore, rather than asking, "Do you have sex with men, women, or both?" clinicians can pose more open-ended prompts, such as "Tell me about your recent sexual partners," to capture the full range of genders with which patients and their partners might identify.

LGBT individuals do not uniformly follow a single trajectory of identity-related development (Floyd and Bakeman 2006). However, certain aspects of sexual and gender identity development are common and therefore warrant consideration when conducting the CFI. Although many LGBT people become aware of their sexual or gender identity early in life—even in childhood—sexual and gender identity milestones can occur at any point in the life course. For sexual minority individuals, awareness of a nonheterosexual identity typically precedes self-identification as lesbian, gay, or bisexual, which typically precedes one's first same-sex sexual encounter. The first same-sex sexual encounter, in turn, typically precedes initial disclosure of one's sexual identity to another person (Calzo et al. 2011). Similarly, for transgender individuals, awareness typically precedes disclosure, which precedes considerations of transitioning gender identities, which may or may not be sought (Bockting and

Coleman 2007). However, because this sequence of identity-related milestones is not guaranteed across LGBT people, nuanced assessment is necessary. The attainment and sequence of these milestones represent important determinants of LGBT individuals' mental health. For example, early achievement of identity-related milestones may expose some LGBT people to greater lifetime victimization, such as from peers at school (Kosciw et al. 2010); conversely, later achievement of milestones, such as first disclosure, can lead to mental health challenges associated with exiting heterosexual life or prolonged exposure to living and publicly identifying as one gender before transitioning to another. Providers ought to be aware of age cohort influences on these milestone effects, because older cohorts may have attained identity-related milestones at a later age because of the greater stigma toward LGBT people in more distant decades than at present. Furthermore, compared to young LGBT individuals, older LGBT individuals who attained these milestones at an earlier age may have been subjected to more stigma and thus more threats to mental health (D'Augelli 2002). Supplemental prompts to the CFI for assessing identity-related milestones might include "When did you first know that you were [gender identity or sexual orientation]?" and "Tell me about your early sexual experiences."

Unlike some cultural identities, sexual orientation and gender identity are relatively concealable. After a period of initial awareness of one's sexual or gender identity, most LGBT individuals choose to disclose their sexual orientation or gender identity to others. When, how, and to whom LGBT individuals disclose depend on personal and situational contexts and can be both voluntary and involuntary. Disclosing one's sexual or gender identity—a process known as *coming out*—represents an important, and sometimes ongoing, task for most LGBT individuals and one that can have important implications for mental health. Coming out alleviates the mental burden of concealment (Pachankis 2007) but also invites the stress of navigating a new public identity (JE Pachankis, SD Cochran, VM Mays, "Mental health correlates of concealment and disclosure among sexual minority adults: a population-based study," Yale School of Public Health, Yale University, New Haven, Connecticut, 2014). Disclosure can usher in a period of exploration of LGBT communities, friendships, and romantic and sexual partners. LGBT individuals vary widely in their degree of affiliation with LGBT communities, and such affiliations can be associated with both risk and resilience (Lelutiu-Weinberger et al. 2013). Therefore, understanding a patient's experience of disclosure and concealment, as well as the factors motivating continued concealment, can help direct culturally sensitive case formulation. Recommended questions to facilitate an exploration of developmental experiences include these: "Whom have you told about your sexual orientation or gender identity? How did they react? Whom have you not told? How connected do you feel to an LGBT community?"

Conceptualizations of Distress Among LGBT Patients

The Cultural Identity module instructs providers to assess the relevance of gender identity and sexual orientation identity to LGBT patients' distress by asking, "Do you feel that your [gender identity or sexual orientation] has influenced your [PROBLEM] or your health more generally?" (questions 26 and 30). In asking this question, providers should be familiar with the vast amount of research suggesting that LGBT individuals experience more mental (Hatzenbuehler 2009; Meyer 2003) and physical (Lick et al. 2013) health problems than heterosexual individuals. Sexual minority individuals are disproportionately likely to experience mood, anxiety, and substance use disorders compared to heterosexuals (Cochran et al. 2003). Preliminary evidence also suggests that transgender individuals experience numerous mental health and psychosocial burdens, including high rates of incarceration, homelessness, and unemployment (Herbst et al. 2008). LGBT individuals are also disproportionately at risk for suicide ideation and attempts (Eisenberg and Resnick 2006). The preponderance of evidence suggests that these sexual and gender identity disparities in mental health and psychosocial risk are a function of stigma-related stress (i.e., the stress resulting from LGBT individuals' disadvantaged social status) (e.g., Meyer 2003).

In addition to being at disproportionate risk for experiencing these mental health problems compared to the general population, LGBT individuals are significantly more likely to meet criteria for more than one psychiatric disorder, including combined mental health and substance abuse disorders (Cochran et al. 2003). Providers ought to consider the possible impact of comorbidity on symptom presentation of LGBT patients and the severity of their distress and functional impairment. Comorbidity can complicate both diagnosis and treatment. Additionally, some evidence suggests that mental health problems arise earlier among LGBT individuals than in the general population (Gilman et al. 2001). Therefore, compared to other patients, LGBT patients might present for treatment at an earlier age or with more severe impairment after a potentially prolonged symptom course.

Mental health providers should carefully consider that although epidemiological evidence shows that social stigma affects mental illness etiology, presentation of symptoms, and course among LGBT individuals, LGBT patients themselves might not readily perceive the adverse impact of stigma on their mental health. Throughout history, narratives of LGBT identity often emphasized the burden of stigma-related stress, although more recent narratives of LGBT identity also emphasize the resilience and creativity displayed by sexual and gender minority individuals (Cohler and Hammack 2007). Therefore, providers ought to consider these narrative influences on their patients' responses to the identity-impact prompt in the CFI. Upon asking the query "Do you feel that your [gender identity or sexual orientation] has influenced your [PROBLEM] or your health more generally?" providers should also be aware that the influence of identity-related stress on LGBT individuals' health is often insidious and invisible.

Psychosocial Stressors and Cultural Features of Vulnerability in LGBT Patients

As mentioned in the section "Conceptualizations of Distress Among LGBT Patients," research convincingly links the substantial mental health disparities due to gender and sexual identity to LGBT individuals' disproportionate exposure to stigma-related stress. Therefore, providers should familiarize themselves with the specific forms of stress experienced by LGBT individuals, because these stressors can impact symptom presentation, inform treatment planning, and complicate diagnosis. These stressors include stigmatizing social contexts, which operate through concealment, expectations of rejection, internalized homophobia, and elevations in general vulnerability factors to heighten the risk for psychiatric disorder among LGBT individuals (Hatzenbuehler 2009; Meyer 2003).

Stigmatizing social contexts can include parents, peers, religious communities, school environments, and workplaces that perpetuate stereotypes, generate distance, and deny LGBT individuals the same rights and opportunities afforded heterosexual and *cisgender* individuals (i.e., individuals whose gender identity matches their assigned sex at birth) (Meyer 2003). LGBT youth experience significantly more parental and peer rejection than heterosexual youth (Balsam et al. 2005). For LGBT individuals, parental rejection is associated with adverse mental health outcomes (Ryan et al. 2009), whereas parental support is protective against the development of mental health problems (e.g., Goldfried and Goldfried 2001). Similarly, religious communities, schools, and workplaces can serve as sources of either stress or support depending on the degree of acceptance they communicate toward LGBT individuals (e.g., Russell et al. 2009). Furthermore, laws and policies that deny LGBT individuals the same rights as heterosexuals, as well as community-level attitudes that communicate mistrust or dislike of an LGBT identity, are associated with elevated risk for psychiatric disorders and suicide attempts among LGBT individuals (e.g., Hatzenbuehler 2011; Hatzenbuehler et al. 2010). Therefore, clinicians should assess the degree of LGBT-related stigma or support in the current and past contexts in which LGBT patients live. Provider assessments of social-contextual factors surrounding LGBT patients might include the following, for example: "How supportive are your parents, school, and religious community of your sexual orientation?" "In what situations do you feel most comfortable being LGBT?"

An LGBT identity for some individuals is central and salient to their overall identity, whereas an LGBT identity is secondary for others. The influence of stigmatizing contexts on LGBT individuals' mental health likewise varies as a function of LGBT identity centrality and salience. A central and salient LGBT identity is more likely than a less central and salient identity to be associated with distress in stigmatizing social contexts (Quinn and Chaudoir 2009). Thus, in addition to the contextual assessment described in the previous paragraphs, providers ought to consider assessing the interaction of contexts with identity centrality and salience. For example, the core CFI suggests the question "For you, what are the most important aspects of your background or identity?" (question 8), which can be supplemented with questions such as "How important is your sexual orientation or gender identity to you?"

Stigma operates through several stress mechanisms to elevate risk for psychiatric disorders (Hatzenbuehler 2009). LGBT-specific stress mechanisms through which stigma impairs mental health include concealment, chronic expectations of rejection, and internalized stigma (Meyer 2003). Although many LGBT individuals may have disclosed their gender identity or sexual orientation to many people in many situations, coming out is an ongoing process, because new situations have to be assessed for safety and a decision has to be made regarding the benefits versus costs of disclosure in each new context. LGBT individuals who choose to conceal their sexual or gender identity may experience well-documented cognitive, affective, and interpersonal strains that elevate the risk for mood, anxiety, and substance use disorders (Pachankis 2007). LGBT individuals who experience early or ongoing rejection directed toward their sexual or gender identity might be particularly likely to expect ongoing rejection, especially in ambiguous situations (Pachankis et al. 2008), which can also elevate risk for psychiatric disorder (Feinstein et al. 2012). Finally, LGBT individuals who live in stigmatizing locales or experience more frequent prejudice and discrimination are more likely to direct stigmatizing attitudes toward themselves (Berg et al. 2013), with adverse implications for mental health (Newcomb and Mustanski 2010).

Evidence also suggests that because of their disproportionate exposure to stigma-related stressors, LGBT individuals have elevations compared to the general population in general psychiatric vulnerability factors, including emotion regulation difficulties, negative cognitive biases, and interpersonal problems. Elevations in these processes can begin early for LGBT individuals (Hatzenbuehler 2009). In addition to assessing stigma-related stressors and mechanisms, mental health providers should also closely assess elevations in general vulnerability factors among LGBT patients, even when full diagnostic criteria for psychiatric disorders are absent.

Psychiatric diagnosis of LGBT individuals is often complicated by the fact that some symptoms of psychiatric disorders represent functional adaptations to stigma rather than forms of psychopathology. For example, social anxiety and concomitant fears of negative evaluation are common among individuals who possess a concealable stigma (Pachankis 2007). Social anxiety disorder would be an inappropriate diagnosis among LGBT individuals whose fears of rejection or negative evaluation are grounded in accurate expectations of rejection or negative evaluation in LGBT-hostile social climates. Similarly, identity confusion is built into developmental models of LGBT identity formation (e.g., Cass 1984) and is normative in social contexts that stigmatize LGBT identities. Fears of disease are normative among gay and bisexual men (Odets 1995) given the very high rates of HIV infection in the gay and transgender communities. Finally, substance use norms are more permissive within LGBT communities, which at least partially explains LGBT individuals' greater use of substances compared to the general population (Cochran et al. 2012; Green and Feinstein 2012). These cultural features of distress influence diagnostic decision making and therefore underscore the paramount importance of assessing the relevance of LGBT stigma to psychiatric symptoms. This assessment can be complemented by a review of LGBT patients' own attributions for their distress as well as the developmental and contextual influences discussed above. The CFI can help providers formulate the relevance of LGBT stigma to diagnosis and includes questions such as "Why do you think this is happening to you? What do you think are the causes of your [PROBLEM]?" (core CFI question 4) and "Do you feel that your [gender identity or sexual orientation] has influenced your [PROBLEM] or your health more generally?" (Cultural Identity module questions 26 and 30). Asking these questions can help providers recognize cultural features of vulnerability among LGBT patients in order to make culturally informed diagnoses.

Video 12 deals with anger and impulsive behavior issues that stem from sexual orientation identification.

 Video Illustration 12: Ties that bind (3:35)

In this video, the clinician illustrates the use of the core CFI with a young Pakistani woman who is being evaluated in the emergency department for anger issues and impulsive behavior in the context of a tumultuous relationship with her family, exacerbated by her parents' discovery that she has been involved in a romantic relationship with another woman. In response to the clinician's general prompts about the nature of the problem, the patient describes her social isolation and feelings of not fitting in at home or school as causing her to adopt an angry, defensive stance. Hewing closely to the CFI, the provider then asks the patient to describe the most important aspects of her identity among several options, including gender and sexual identity. In response, the patient describes the strict, religious household in which she was raised. She then confides that her present problems stem from her family's discovery of her romantic relationship with another woman, which led her family to view the patient as a disappointment and to contact the other woman's family to discuss the situation. The provider then continues using the CFI to explore how the patient's background shapes her coping skills and help-seeking needs. The patient focuses her answers to these questions on her strict upbringing.

The provider's use of the CFI yields a strong picture of the patient's cultural background. The provider's open questioning regarding important aspects of identity likely paved the road for the patient to disclose her recent romantic relationship with a woman and the ensuing stress caused by her parents' discovery of this relationship. The supplementary guidance provided in this chapter suggests further areas of questioning to specifically ascertain the relevant features of the patient's sexual orientation. Given that many patients might have difficulty discussing their gender or sexual identity and given the sometimes invisible impact of these identities on mental health, we suggest that providers ask several specific follow-up questions beyond the core CFI to capture these aspects of identity. For instance, in this assessment, the provider might have gained a deeper understanding of the patient's sexual identity had he asked how she describes her sexual identity (e.g., lesbian, bisexual, queer), about the importance she ascribes to this identity, and when she first became aware of this identity. By pointedly asking, "Do you feel that your sexual orientation has influenced your current problems or your health more generally?" the provider might have gained insight into how the patient conceptualizes her current distress in light of her sexual orientation and the stress it poses to her family relationship. Given this patient's strained relationship with her family, it would also be important to assess her other sources of support, including from friends, romantic or sexual partners, and the LGBT community. Assessing the resilience that she has displayed in establishing a minority sexual identity might have introduced a relatively positive perspective on this presently stressful situation.

Cultural Features of Coping and Help Seeking Among LGBT Patients

The CFI instructs providers to assess factors related to coping and help seeking. Specifically, the core CFI suggests that providers ask, "Sometimes people have various ways of dealing with problems like [PROBLEM]. What have you done on your own to cope with your [PROBLEM]?" (question 11) and "Often, people look for help from many different sources, including different kinds of doctors, helpers, or healers. In the past, what kinds of treatment, help, advice, or healing have you sought for your [PROBLEM]?" (question 12). LGBT individuals are significantly more likely to seek help for mental health problems than the general population (Cochran et al. 2003). This greater treatment seeking may be a result of the significant mental and physical health disparities that exist for sexual orientation and gender identity or a function of the self-exploration and personal growth that might be embedded within LGBT communities because of the LGBT identity development process (Balsam et al. 2006). This greater use of treatment among LGBT individuals compared to the general population is all the more striking given the structural barriers (e.g., fewer financial resources, greater lack of health insurance) and history of ineffective and unethical mental health treatments (e.g., sexual orientation conversion therapy) faced by this population (Cochran 2001). To facilitate an understanding of the treatment-seeking barriers that LGBT patients may face, the Cultural Identity module instructs providers to ask, "Do you feel that your [gender identity or sexual orientation] influences your ability to get the kind of health care you need for your [PROBLEM]?" (questions 27 and 31).

In addition to their higher use of professional mental health services, LGBT individuals may be more likely to seek and receive social support from families of choice than from families of origin (Oswald 2002), given that they often do not share the same sexual or gender identity as their parents and often experience rejection from families. Relatedly, social networks may be more fluid among LGBT individuals, who may embrace the opportunity to redefine traditional connections and relationships to create a support network. For example, LGBT individuals' social networks might be more likely to include former romantic or sexual partners than might be usual for heterosexual or cisgender individuals. Additionally, LGBT role models are an important source of resilience and support for LGBT individuals (Bird et al. 2012), but role models are also not easily accessible in all contexts, especially for young LGBT individuals, for whom a generation of potential role models was decimated by the early HIV/AIDS epidemic and because of stereotypes surrounding bonds between older and younger LGBT individuals (Bird et al. 2012). Finally, the coming-out process, given its potential challenges, provides LGBT individuals a mastery experience that can be drawn on to overcome subsequent challenges. In addition to asking the standard core CFI questions about coping and help seeking, providers can ask additional questions to assess the coping and social support resources available to their LGBT patients, such as "What role do your friends and partners play in your life? Who are your role models? What strengths do you possess because of your gender identity [or sexual orientation]?"

Cultural Features of the Relationship Between LGBT Individuals and Clinicians

Given that gender identity and sexual orientation represent important components of cultural identity for many LGBT individuals, providers ought to become familiar with LGBT cultures and apply models of multicultural competence to the treatment of LGBT patients (e.g., Pachankis 2014; Pachankis and Goldfried 2004). To this end, providers should familiarize themselves with the unique issues and social norms among this group. For example, the term *homosexual* has pathological and medicalizing undertones given its historical usage. The term fails to describe individuals who possess bisexual identities as well as lesbian and gay men who identity as lesbian or gay without engaging in same-sex sexual behavior. Furthermore, different cultures and societies use terms other than *lesbian, gay, bisexual,* or *transgender* to refer to their sexual and gender minority populations. Providers should become familiar with these terms as well as the intersection of sexual orientation and gender identity with other forms of cultural diversity (e.g., race, ethnicity, nationality). Additionally, given that there is no single LGBT culture, providers should become familiar with the heterogeneity within the various LGBT cultures and assess the nature of the LGBT cultures with which their patients identify.

The CFI suggests assessing patient concerns about provider discrimination and cultural misunderstanding because such concerns act as barriers to receiving help. Specifically, the Cultural Identity module suggests asking, "Do you feel that health care providers have certain assumptions or attitudes about you or your [PROBLEM] that are related to your [gender identity or sexual orientation]?" (questions 28 and 32). In fact, LGBT individuals may experience shame and embarrassment about disclosing relatively normative features of LGBT life that may be nonnormative among heterosexuals. For example, relationship arrangements for same-sex partners are often more flexible and open than they are in heterosexual relationships (e.g., multiple partners concurrently; Parsons et al. 2013). Some bisexual individuals are married to an opposite-sex partner and therefore may have difficulty finding support for their bisexual identity. Furthermore, some transgender individuals may seek mental health services related to the gender transition process and therefore require that their provider possess sufficient understanding of that process (Bockting et al. 2006). Without direct examination of patients' potential expectations of provider bias and the provider's explicit demonstration of LGBT cultural competence, these features of some LGBT patients' lives might remain undisclosed, despite potential relevance to the issues presented by patients.

Although providers should assess the relevance of LGBT patients' sexual and gender identity to the presented problem, providers should also be careful not to overemphasize sexual orientation or gender identity, especially when these identities are irrelevant to the patient's presented problem. Some patients' problems will be closely related to their experience of being LGBT (e.g., fear of coming out to others); for other patients, however, sexual orientation and gender identity may form part of the general background but not be directly related to the presented problem (e.g., general social isolation, including from LGBT peers) (Safren and Rogers 2001). The CFI directs providers to assess the relevance of this feature of cultural diversity to ensure optimal service delivery.

Conclusion

The CFI provides straightforward guidance for assessing the relevance of patients' sexual orientation and gender identities to the mental health concerns presented. The CFI supplementary modules regarding psychosocial stressors, identities, and coping and help-seeking tendencies will likely be particularly relevant for assessing the cultural context of LGBT patients' current mental status. Assessment of sexual orientation and gender identities, the mental health concerns particularly relevant to LGBT patients, the cultural conceptualizations of distress and coping among LGBT individuals, and the relevance of LGBT identities to the provider-patient relationship should form a core part of culturally competent psychiatric care. The questions contained in the core CFI and the supplementary modules can assist providers in conducting such an assessment.

KEY CLINICAL POINTS

- A patient's gender and sexual identities can affect his or her conceptualizations of distress, generate insidious psychosocial stressors, and yield distinct forms of coping and help seeking, all of which form essential components of a culturally sensitive case formulation.
- Because gender and sexual identities occur in a distinct and changing social context characterized by both stigma and social progress, systematically eliciting the meaning and experience of gender and sexual identity for each patient against a backdrop of familiarity with LGBT culture will yield an LGBT-sensitive case formulation.

Questions

1. What features of LGBT identities are relevant to a culturally sensitive case formulation?

2. How do gender identity and sexual orientation identity affect distress for LGBT clients?

3. How does LGBT stigma complicate psychiatric diagnosis?

References

Balsam KF, Rothblum ED, Beauchaine TP: Victimization over the life span: a comparison of lesbian, gay, bisexual, and heterosexual siblings. J Consult Clin Psychol 73(3):477–487, 2005 15982145

Balsam KF, Martell CR, Safren SA: Affirmative cognitive-behavioral therapy with lesbian, gay, and bisexual people, in Culturally Responsive Cognitive-Behavioral Therapy: Assessment, Practice, and Supervision. Edited by Hays PA, Iwamasa GY. Washington, DC, American Psychological Association, 2006, pp 223–243

Berg RC, Ross MW, Weatherburn P, et al: Structural and environmental factors are associated with internalised homonegativity in men who have sex with men: findings from the European MSM Internet Survey (EMIS) in 38 countries. Soc Sci Med 78:61–69, 2013 23261257

Bird JD, Kuhns L, Garofalo R: The impact of role models on health outcomes for lesbian, gay, bisexual, and transgender youth. J Adolesc Health 50(4):353–357, 2012 22443838

Bockting WO, Coleman E: Developmental stages of the transgender coming out process: toward an integrated identity, in Principles of Transgender Medicine and Surgery. Edited by Ettner R, Monstrey S, Eyler E. New York, Haworth Press, 2007, pp 185–208

Bockting WO, Knudson G, Goldberg JM: Counseling and mental health care for transgender adults and loved ones. International Journal of Transgenderism 9:35–82, 2006

Calzo JP, Antonucci TC, Mays VM, et al: Retrospective recall of sexual orientation identity development among gay, lesbian, and bisexual adults. Dev Psychol 47(6):1658–1673, 2011 21942662

Cass VC: Homosexual identity formation: Testing a theoretical model. Journal of Sex Research 20(2):143–167, 1984

Cochran SD: Emerging issues in research on lesbians' and gay men's mental health: does sexual orientation really matter? Am Psychol 56(11):931–947, 2001 11785169

Cochran SD, Mays VM, Sullivan JG: Prevalence of mental disorders, psychological distress, and mental health services use among lesbian, gay, and bisexual adults in the United States. J Consult Clin Psychol 71(1):53–61, 2003 12602425

Cochran SD, Grella CE, Mays VM: Do substance use norms and perceived drug availability mediate sexual orientation differences in patterns of substance use? Results from the California Quality of Life Survey II. J Stud Alcohol Drugs 73(4):675–685, 2012 22630806

Cohler BJ, Hammack PL: The psychological world of the gay teenager: social change, narrative, and "normality." J Youth Adolesc 36:47–59, 2007

D'Augelli AR: Mental health problems among lesbian, gay, and bisexual youths ages 14 to 21. Clin Child Psychol Psychiatry 7:433–456, 2002

Duberman M, Vicinus M, Chauncey G: Hidden from History: Reclaiming the Gay and Lesbian Past. New York, New American Library, 2002

Eisenberg ME, Resnick MD: Suicidality among gay, lesbian and bisexual youth: the role of protective factors. J Adolesc Health 39(5):662–668, 2006 17046502

Feinstein BA, Goldfried MR, Davila J: The relationship between experiences of discrimination and mental health among lesbians and gay men: an examination of internalized homonegativity and rejection sensitivity as potential mechanisms. J Consult Clin Psychol 80(5):917–927, 2012 22823860

Floyd FJ, Bakeman R: Coming-out across the life course: implications of age and historical context. Arch Sex Behav 35(3):287–296, 2006 16804747

Gilman SE, Cochran SD, Mays VM, et al: Risk of psychiatric disorders among individuals reporting same-sex sexual partners in the National Comorbidity Survey. Am J Public Health 91(6):933–939, 2001 11392937

Goldfried MR, Goldfried AP: The importance of parental support in the lives of gay, lesbian, and bisexual individuals. J Clin Psychol 57(5):681–693, 2001 11304707

Green KE, Feinstein BA: Substance use in lesbian, gay, and bisexual populations: an update on empirical research and implications for treatment. Psychol Addict Behav 26(2):265–278, 2012 22061339

Hatzenbuehler ML: How does sexual minority stigma "get under the skin"? A psychological mediation framework. Psychol Bull 135(5):707–730, 2009 19702379

Hatzenbuehler ML: The social environment and suicide attempts in lesbian, gay, and bisexual youth. Pediatrics 127(5):896–903, 2011 21502225

Hatzenbuehler ML, McLaughlin KA, Keyes KM, et al: The impact of institutional discrimination on psychiatric disorders in lesbian, gay, and bisexual populations: a prospective study. Am J Public Health 100(3):452–459, 2010 20075314

Herbst JH, Jacobs ED, Finlayson TJ, et al: Estimating HIV prevalence and risk behaviors of transgender persons in the United States: a systematic review. AIDS Behav 12(1):1–17, 2008 17694429

Kosciw JG, Greytak EA, Diaz EM, et al: The 2009 National School Climate Survey. New York, Gay, Lesbian, and Straight Education Network, 2010

Lelutiu-Weinberger C, Pachankis JE, Golub SA, et al: Age cohort differences in the effects of gay-related stigma, anxiety and identification with the gay community on sexual risk and substance use. AIDS Behav 17(1):340–349, 2013 22038078

Lick DJ, Durso LE, Johnson KL: Minority stress and physical health among sexual minorities. Perspect Psychol Sci 8:521–548, 2013

Meyer IH: Prejudice, social stress, and mental health in lesbian, gay, and bisexual populations: conceptual issues and research evidence. Psychol Bull 129(5):674–697, 2003 12956539

Newcomb ME, Mustanski B: Internalized homophobia and internalizing mental health problems: a meta-analytic review. Clin Psychol Rev 30(8):1019–1029, 2010 20708315

Odets W: In the Shadow of the Epidemic: Being HIV-Negative in the Age of AIDS. Durham, NC, Duke University Press, 1995

Oswald RF: Resilience within the family networks of lesbians and gay men: intentionality and redefinition. J Marriage Fam 64:374–383, 2002

Pachankis JE: The psychological implications of concealing a stigma: a cognitive-affective-behavioral model. Psychol Bull 133(2):328–345, 2007 17338603

Pachankis JE: Uncovering clinical principles and techniques to address minority stress, mental health, and related health risks among gay and bisexual men. Clin Psychol (New York) 21(4):313–330, 2014 25554721

Pachankis JE, Goldfried MR: Clinical issues in working with lesbian, gay, and bisexual clients. Psychotherapy 41:227–246, 2004

Pachankis JE, Goldfried MR, Ramrattan ME: Extension of the rejection sensitivity construct to the interpersonal functioning of gay men. J Consult Clin Psychol 76(2):306–317, 2008 18377126

Pantalone DW, Pachankis JE, Bankoff SM, et al: The health and wellness of sexual and gender minorities, in Multicultural Approaches to Health and Wellness in America. Edited by Gurung RAR. New York, Praeger, 2014, pp 195–224

Parsons JT, Starks TJ, DuBois S, et al: Alternatives to monogamy among gay male couples in a community survey: implications for mental health and sexual risk. Arch Sex Behav 42(2):303–312, 2013 22187028

Quinn DM, Chaudoir SR: Living with a concealable stigmatized identity: the impact of anticipated stigma, centrality, salience, and cultural stigma on psychological distress and health. J Pers Soc Psychol 97(4):634–651, 2009 19785483

Russell ST, Muraco A, Subramaniam A, et al: Youth empowerment and high school Gay-Straight Alliances. J Youth Adolesc 38(7):891–903, 2009 19636734

Ryan C, Huebner D, Diaz RM, et al: Family rejection as a predictor of negative health outcomes in white and Latino lesbian, gay, and bisexual young adults. Pediatrics 123(1):346–352, 2009 19117902

Safren SA, Rogers T: Cognitive-behavioral therapy with gay, lesbian, and bisexual clients. J Clin Psychol 57(5):629–643, 2001 11304703

Suggested Readings

Eubanks-Carter C, Burckell LA, Goldfried MR: Enhancing therapeutic effectiveness with lesbian, gay, and bisexual clients. Clinical Psychology: Science and Practice 12:1–18, 2006

Pachankis JE, Goldfried MR: Clinical issues in working with lesbian, gay, and bisexual clients. Psychotherapy 41:227–246, 2004

Pantalone DW, Pachankis JE, Bankoff SM, et al: The health and wellness of sexual and gender minorities, in Multicultural Approaches to Health and Wellness in America. Edited by Gurung RAR. New York, Praeger, 2014, pp 195–224

Supplementary Module 7: Coping and Help Seeking

Martin La Roche, Ph.D.
Devon E. Hinton, M.D., Ph.D.

The DSM-5 (American Psychiatric Association 2013) Cultural Formulation Interview (CFI) is a powerful clinical tool for assessing cultural factors using a person-centered approach. Two areas critical to a person-centered assessment are coping and help seeking. *Coping* refers to the techniques an individual employs to redress a problem, whereas *help seeking* refers to the specific ways the person seeks assistance for the problem from others (Hwang et al. 2008). Coping can target emotional and/or somatic aspects of distress. For example, a veteran of the Iraq War may use prayer to relieve combat-related distress, focusing on the psychological aspects of anxiety and guilt, whereas a Cambodian refugee may use "coining" to relieve panic symptoms, focusing on the somatic aspects of anxiety. (In coining, a coin dipped in a camphor-containing substance such as tiger balm is rubbed vigorously against the body to provide a path for the "bad wind" to be released from the body [Hinton et al. 2010].) Help-seeking behavior is often classified into two general types: *formal* and *informal*. *Formal help seeking* involves assistance from clinicians (e.g., psychologists) who are regulated by government agencies, whereas *informal help seeking* recruits the support of individuals not scrutinized by government officials (e.g., nontraditional healers, priests, friends) (Hwang et al. 2008). Questions about both formal and informal help seeking are included in the CFI assessment.

The core CFI prioritizes the assessment of coping and help seeking, featuring them prominently in two domains: 1) "Cultural Factors Affecting Self-Coping and Past Help Seeking" and 2) "Cultural Factors Affecting Current Help Seeking." In addition, clinicians may choose to further investigate these areas using the supplementary module Coping and Help Seeking, which is the topic of this subchapter. We briefly review the literature that underscores the importance of assessing coping and help-seeking behavior, give a description of the supplementary module, and illustrate the module's use with a case example that highlights the importance of obtaining this information to maximize treatment efficacy and adherence.

Why Assessing Coping and Help-Seeking Behavior Is Important

Assessing coping and help seeking can provide useful information as to what the patient hopes for from the current treatment and what he or she wants to avoid. An account of past choices can reveal what the patient found to be more or less useful in dealing with the problem. For example, the patient may have previously found psychiatric treatment not to be helpful, and exploring past treatment experiences should provide invaluable information, particularly when the clinician is a psychiatrist. Information on the patient's practices and help-seeking choices can also help the clinician reconcile proposed therapeutic approaches with the patient's expectations, including potentially how to amplify the clinical therapies by pairing them in some way with the patient's own behavior. For example, coping techniques such as Buddhist meditation or other forms of spiritual practice may be valuable healing modalities that can be encouraged and amplified in treatment, for instance, by incorporating them into cognitive-behavioral therapy interventions (Hinton et al. 2012). To obtain more detail on spiritual practices, the clinician can administer the Spirituality, Religion, and Moral Traditions supplementary module, which may be useful in conjunction with the module Coping and Help Seeking because many coping and help-seeking behaviors involve spiritual traditions. The module Coping and Help Seeking also explores the current presentation to treatment as the most recent instance of help seeking. Useful information for engagement and treatment planning can be obtained by determining who suggested that the patient present for care at this time and what treatments the patient currently expects to receive. To increase positive expectancy and adherence, treatment may be presented in terms of the patient's current means of self-coping.

Another reason why information about past coping and help seeking is valuable to clinical care is that it constitutes a window into how the patient conceptualizes the problem, including his or her explanatory model (or models) of the disorder. For example, if a Latino patient has sought help for the problem from a Santeria priestess, it is important to find out what problem the patient presented to the healer, how the healer explained the problem, what treatments were suggested, and whether the patient found them helpful. The clinician would also like to know whether such treatments are ongoing, because this may reveal the patient's current views on the illness and potentially the patient's expectations about the treatment being sought from the clinical provider.

Video 13 uncovers the patient's coping mechanisms.

 Video Illustration 13: I don't have a problem (3:00)

The video entitled "I don't have a problem" illustrates how a patient may employ various strategies to cope with her condition. Initially, the patient denies any difficulties: "First of all, I don't have a problem.... I think I'm fine." As the

CFI interview proceeds, however, asking what is most troubling about her situation reveals some of her coping strategies, which include overeating and oversleeping. These help her feel a little better but then exacerbate her depressive symptoms—which the patient labels "a little down" or "moody"—and also lead to distressing weight gain. In response to core CFI question 5, another important coping strategy emerges. The patient speaks to her sister Rachel "every day," who knows "everything that is going on in my life." Rachel believes that the patient is depressed because "all of my friends are getting married" and "I don't have [a relationship] of my own." Rachel also fears that the patient has the same depressive illness that affected their aunt.

Talking with her sister is a help-seeking strategy in which the patient seeks assistance from her social network. The Coping and Help Seeking supplementary module could help the clinician explore these issues further, particularly the two social network items (questions 6 and 7). It would be beneficial to explore whether talking about "feeling down" with her sister helps her and in what way. Given the patient's reluctance about treatment, this material may be particularly useful to engage her in therapy. This information can also help the clinician reconcile the proposed therapeutic approaches with the patient's expectations, including potentially how to amplify the clinical therapies by pairing them in some way with the patient's own behavior.

Overeating and oversleeping constitute other important coping strategies for the patient. She feels ambivalent about these, because she dislikes the ensuing weight gain; this could be an avenue for assessing their effectiveness as behaviors. The Coping and Help Seeking supplementary module could be useful on this point, particularly the five questions (1–5) on self-coping. Enhanced awareness of the connection between eating and sleeping and feeling down may help her change her eating and sleeping habits as treatment progresses and may also guide her choices of alternative and more productive coping strategies. This kind of information is crucial for a person-centered approach to care that takes into consideration the meaning patients ascribe to symptoms and behaviors.

Video 14 addresses the patient's perception of how to cope and what treatment would best suit her.

 Video Illustration 14: Planning for something better (1:59)

In the video "Planning for something better," the core CFI questions (14–16) on help seeking and the clinician-patient relationship allow the patient to discuss directly what her coping and treatment preferences are. She believes that if she had a safe place to live and someone to talk to she would be doing better. Using the CFI, the interviewer explores her expectations and perceived barriers to treatment, and the patient explains that a female clinician could help her more effectively. At this point, the supplementary module on coping and help seeking, particularly the self-coping questions (1–5), might help further identify her resources and strengths and refine an effective treatment plan according to her needs and goals.

Arthur Kleinman (1978) introduced the concept of explanatory models of illness into psychiatry to emphasize that patients' interpretation and actual experience of an illness are embedded within specific social contexts. Individuals from different cultural backgrounds tend to categorize, label, and interpret their experiences differently. Furthermore, the ways in which they make sense of their problems affect how they cope with them and/or seek help from others (Hinton and Good 2009; Kleinman 1978, 1988; La Roche 2013). Patients' cultural views influence the selection of specific coping strategies and help-seeking behaviors. For example, those who believe their problems are psychological tend to seek help from mental health professionals, whereas those who believe their problems are somatic seek help from a primary care physician (Hwang et al. 2006). Demonstrating such a somatization perspective, 69% of Chinese Americans meeting screening criteria for depression in the waiting room of a primary care clinic had previously sought help for the depression from outpatient medical services, whereas only 3.5% had sought care from a mental health professional (Yeung et al. 2004). The CFI identifies patients' coping and help-seeking choices so that more effective and culturally consistent strategies can be designed to respond to their goals and characteristics, thereby enhancing treatment efficacy and adherence (La Roche 2013).

Informal healing services are popular in the United States generally (Eisenberg et al. 1998), but racial or ethnic minority groups may be more likely to turn to indigenous or complementary treatments for physical and mental health care (Barnes et al. 2004; Koss-Chioino 2000). For many racial or ethnic minority group members, religion can be a frequent source of coping strategies (e.g., prayers) and of help-seeking options, such as obtaining the assistance of priests or pastors (George et al. 2000). For example, African Americans may engage in more religious coping to deal with adversity than non-Latino white Americans (Conway 1985–1986). Similarly, many Latinos endorse Christian beliefs and prayer as a means to cope with adversity (La Roche 2013). Many racial or ethnic minorities report greater satisfaction with their religious coping efforts than whites and tend to feel that these efforts result in a greater personal connection with God (Myers and Hwang 2004).

Structural factors also influence patients away from the formal health care sector, and these factors reveal key areas that need to be addressed to ensure entry into and adherence to care. For example, the selection of formal or informal help may be related to economic barriers that are more prevalent among racial or ethnic minorities; these barriers include lack of insurance, limited job flexibility, and lower socioeconomic status (U.S. Department of Health and Human Services 2001). Lack of insurance in particular is a key predictor of lower formal help-seeking behaviors among racial or ethnic minorities (U.S. Department of Health and Human Services 2001). A contextually sound evaluation approach needs to elicit this information, as included in core CFI question 13.

In addition, accessing mental health services becomes even more difficult for many racial or ethnic minority groups because they tend to have negative attitudes toward mental health services. For example, because of historical experiences with racism and discrimination, many African Americans fear the mental health system (Keating and Robertson 2004); they lack confidence in it and feel that they have been mistreated and discriminated against by providers and the system as a whole (Smedley et al. 2003; U.S. Department of Health and Human Services 2001). Stigmatization can also limit access to mental health services (U.S. Department of Health and Human Services 1999). Stigma toward mental illnesses is a worldwide phenomenon and operates by motivating the general public to reject, avoid, fear, and discriminate against those with mental illness (Corrigan 2004). As a result, persons with mental illness become ashamed, conceal their problems, and delay or avoid seeking help owing to fear of being stigmatized and negatively labeled. Stigma may be more severe among some racial or ethnic minority communities and may have a more detrimental impact on help-seeking behavior, partly as a result of lower health literacy (U.S. Department of Health and Human Services 1999). In some Asian cultures, stigma may reflect badly on the patient but also may diminish the economic and marriage value for that person as well as his or her family (Ng 1997).

Overview of the Supplementary Module

The Coping and Help Seeking module has four sections and 13 questions (see Appendix C in this handbook). The questions are linked to the presented problem, and the first three sections emphasize the perceived helpfulness of self-coping and help seeking, whereas the fourth section, which is on the current treatment episode, explores treatment expectations rather than helpfulness.

Self-Coping

Questions 1–5 assess general self-coping. The first question examines the way in which an individual is currently addressing his or her problem and the level of helpfulness of this coping strategy. The second question broadens the question to similar problems in the past rather than the present. The next three questions ask about specific coping strategies—including use of the Internet and other media, spiritual practices, natural remedies, and over-the-counter medications—and inquire about the level of helpfulness of each.

Social Network

Questions 6 and 7 assess the patient's perception of the social network's ability to help him or her cope with the problem (e.g., by providing moral or other types of support) and the social network's influence on the method of coping and help seeking (e.g., a family member's etiological views of the problem often lead to certain suggestions about how to deal with it). Question 6 inquires whether the individual has informed a family member about the problem, whether the family member was helpful, and what suggestions were offered. Question 7 assesses the same topics with respect to a coworker or friend instead of a family member.

Help- and Treatment-Seeking Beyond Social Network

Questions 8–11 ask about helpers beyond the usual social network. The module taps the following sectors: spiritual, religious, and moral helpers; general doctors; mental health providers; and any other healers (e.g., acupuncturists, chiropractors). The questions inquire about the care received from each and its helpfulness.

Current Treatment Episode

The final two questions focus on the circumstances that led the individual to seek current treatment. Question 12 investigates who suggested accessing care now and why this type of treatment was suggested. Question 13 examines the patient's treatment expectations for the problem that brings him or her into care.

Clinical Use of the Module

The following case illustrates the clinical value of information about a patient's coping and help seeking. In this case, the information elicited by the supplementary module helped to prevent the patient from discontinuing treatment prematurely, as she had done in the past with a different provider, and helped in the selection of interventions that matched her treatment goals. The relevant sections of the module are noted in parentheses and italics.

Case Vignette

Elena, a 55-year-old woman from the Dominican Republic, is an unemployed mother of three and grandmother of eight who sought psychotherapy for the first time because of severe symptoms of anxiety, particularly insomnia (*presented problem on the core CFI*). She explained that the spirit of her recently deceased mother was visiting her at night. When asked how she coped with these visits, Elena reported "ignoring them" (*self-coping*). Unfortunately, this was not useful; her insomnia continued. Thus, she consulted with a friend (*social network*), who advised her to talk with her priest (*help and treatment seeking beyond social network*) because the patient is a devout Catholic. The priest encouraged her to pray a "Hail Mary" and an "Our Father" (*self-coping*) before going to bed. Although praying was somewhat helpful, she still had difficulties falling asleep. In further discussing her difficulties with her cousin (*social network*), Elena was encouraged to seek mental health help. At the first mental health clinic she attended, she met with a "tall, white, American psychiatrist" (*help and treatment seeking beyond social network*), who explained in English that spirits do not exist and that she should take medications to cope with her fears and high anxiety levels. She felt misunderstood and never returned to this psychiatrist or considered taking medications. Subsequently, Elena tried another mental health clinic with a Latino-focused program (*current treatment episode*). She reported liking this psychologist, who was Latino and communicated with her in Spanish. During this evaluation, she was able to talk about her fear of the spirit visitations. Unlike with the psychiatrist, she felt understood and accepted by the psychologist; she felt that her goals were being met, which allowed her to be open and engaged in the psychotherapeutic process.

Elena remained in treatment for eight sessions. Over time, her initial complaint of insomnia and spirit involvement evolved into a description of her feelings of guilt for having "abandoned" her mother in Santo Domingo to come to the United States. With the help of her psychologist, she was able to reframe her migration as a necessary and adaptive solution to the problem of being left by her husband in the Dominican Republic with three children and no economic support (*current treatment episode*). The psychologist's reframing coincided with that of Elena's priest, who also explained that she had not sinned in leaving her mother but instead had tried to do her best under extremely adverse circumstances (*help and treatment seeking beyond social network*). The patient, however, continued to feel guilty and depressed, especially when she missed her mother. Her priest recommended that she pray for her mother's soul every night (*help and treatment seeking beyond social network*), a suggestion that her psychologist heartily endorsed. The patient started to feel very close to her mother during her prayers and soon started praying in other circumstances when she was anxious or depressed (*self-coping*). As her symptoms began to lift, Elena explained this as a sign that God was giving her strength to cope with her problems.

Conclusion

We have highlighted the importance of systematically identifying and understanding a patient's coping and help-seeking behaviors and have shown how to use the CFI Coping and Help Seeking module to achieve this. The ways a patient has sought help in the past for a problem reveals key information about how the patient conceptualizes the problem and about previous treatment failures, stigmatization, access to treatment, and expectations about current care. This information is invaluable clinically, giving insight into how to overcome treatment barriers and increase adherence, cultural consonance of treatment, efficacy, and therapeutic alliance.

We also indicate future areas of research. First, self-coping narratives may reveal key local sources of resilience (Hinton and Kirmayer 2013; La Roche 2013), such as prayer or meditation. Both of these are consonant with current cognitive-behavioral therapy theory and can be integrated into care in order to increase efficacy and cultural acceptability of treatment, as well as treatment adherence, as illustrated in the case vignette (Hinton et al. 2012; La Roche 2013). Second, self-coping and help seeking represent key areas for research on treatment dissemination and implementation more generally, particularly in low-resource settings where shifting to less expensive helpers is a priority (Jordans and Tol 2013). A person's self-coping and help seeking reveal how problems are locally managed outside the formal health care system, which yields useful information about how to increase utilization and efficacy of, as well as adherence to, psychological and biomedical treatment.

Assessing coping and help seeking provides insight into the patient's conceptualization of his or her problem, previous treatment failures, and expectations about current treatment. This kind of information is crucial for a person-centered approach to care that takes into consideration the local sociocultural matrix of meaning.

KEY CLINICAL POINTS

- Coping and help seeking are strategies that individuals use to address their problems (e.g., emotional, relational, or somatic). *Coping* refers to the person's own efforts to deal with the situation, whereas *help seeking* refers to the steps taken by the person to seek assistance from others.

- Information on coping and help-seeking behaviors from the Cultural Formulation Interview can reveal what patients have found to be more or less useful for their problem, which can inform clinicians about what patients desire from the current treatment and what they want to avoid.

Questions

1. What are some examples of coping and help-seeking behaviors?

2. What clinical information can be obtained by assessing coping and help seeking with the CFI?

3. What are the differences between coping and help-seeking behaviors?

4. What are some examples of coping and help-seeking behaviors that are strongly influenced by culture?

5. What are the four components of the Coping and Help Seeking module?

References

American Psychiatric Association: Diagnostic and Statistical Manual of Mental Disorders, 5th Edition. Arlington, VA, American Psychiatric Association, 2013

Barnes PM, Powell-Griner E, McFann K, et al: Complementary and alternative medicine use among adults: United States, 2002. Adv Data 343(343):1–19, 2004 15188733

Conway K: Coping with the stress of medical problems among black and white elderly. Int J Aging Hum Dev 21(1):39–48, 1985–1986 3830893

Corrigan P: How stigma interferes with mental health care. Am Psychol 59(7):614–625, 2004 15491256

Eisenberg DM, Davis RB, Ettner SL, et al: Trends in alternative medicine use in the United States, 1990–1997: results of a follow-up national survey. JAMA 280(18):1569–1575, 1998 9820257

George LK, Larson DB, Koenig HG, et al: Spirituality and health: what we know, what we need to know. J Soc Clin Psychol 19:102–116, 2000

Hinton D, Good B: Culture and Panic Disorder. Stanford, CA, Stanford University Press, 2009

Hinton DE, Kirmayer LJ: Local responses to trauma: symptom, affect, and healing. Transcult Psychiatry 50(5):607–621, 2013 24142932

Hinton DE, Pich V, Marques L, et al: Khyâl attacks: a key idiom of distress among traumatized Cambodia refugees. Cult Med Psychiatry 34(2):244–278, 2010 20407813

Hinton DE, Rivera EI, Hofmann SG, et al: Adapting CBT for traumatized refugees and ethnic minority patients: examples from culturally adapted CBT (CA-CBT). Transcult Psychiatry 49(2):340–365, 2012 22508639

Hwang W, Lin K, Cheung F, et al: Cognitive-behavioral therapy with Chinese Americans: research, theory, and clinical practice. Cogn Behav Pract 13:293–303, 2006

Hwang WC, Myers HF, Abe-Kim J, et al: A conceptual paradigm for understanding culture's impact on mental health: the cultural influences on mental health (CIMH) model. Clin Psychol Rev 28(2):211–227, 2008 17587473

Jordans MJ, Tol WA: Mental health in humanitarian settings: shifting focus to care systems. Int Health 5(1):9–10, 2013 24029839

Keating F, Robertson D: Fear, black people and mental illness: a vicious circle? Health Soc Care Community 12(5):439–447, 2004 15373823

Kleinman A: Clinical relevance of anthropological and cross-cultural research: concepts and strategies. Am J Psychiatry 135(4):427–431, 1978 637136

Kleinman A: Rethinking Psychiatry: From Cultural Category to Personal Experience. New York, Freeman Press, 1988

Koss-Chioino JD: Traditional and folk approaches among ethnic minorities, in Psychological Intervention and Cultural Diversity. Edited by Aponte JF. Needham Heights, MA, Allyn & Bacon, 2000, pp 149–166

La Roche M: Cultural Psychotherapy: Theory, Methods and Practice. Thousand Oaks, CA, Sage, 2013

Myers HF, Hwang W: Cumulative psychosocial risks and resilience: a conceptual perspective on ethnic health disparities in late life, in Critical Perspectives on Racial and Ethnic Disparities in Health in Later Life. Edited by Anderson NA, Bulatao RA, Cohen B. National Research Council Committee on Population, Division of Behavioral and Social Sciences and Education. Washington, DC, National Academies Press, 2004, pp 492–539

Ng CH: The stigma of mental illness in Asian cultures. Aust NZJ Psychiatry 31(3):382–390, 1997 9226084

Smedley BDS, Stith AY, Nelson AR: Unequal Treatment: Confronting Racial and Ethnic Disparities in Health Care. Washington, DC, National Academies Press, 2003

U.S. Department of Health and Human Services: Mental Health: A Report of the Surgeon General. Rockville, MD, U.S. Public Health Service, Substance Abuse and Mental Health Services Administration, Center for Mental Health Services, National Institutes of Health, National Institute of Mental Health, 1999

U.S. Department of Health and Human Services: Mental Health: Culture, Race, and Ethnicity—A Supplement to Mental Health: A Report of the Surgeon General. Rockville, MD, Substance Abuse and Mental Health Services Administration (US), 2001

Yeung A, Chang D, Gresham RL Jr, et al: Illness beliefs of depressed Chinese American patients in primary care. J Nerv Ment Dis 192(4):324–327, 2004 15060408

Suggested Readings

Hinton D, Good B: Culture and Panic Disorder. Stanford, CA, Stanford University Press, 2009

Hwang WC, Myers HF, Abe-Kim J, et al: A conceptual paradigm for understanding culture's impact on mental health: the cultural influences on mental health (CIMH) model. Clin Psychol Rev 28:211–227, 2006

Kleinman A: Rethinking Psychiatry: From Cultural Category to Personal Experience. New York, Freeman Press, 1988

La Roche M: Cultural Psychotherapy: Theory, Methods and Practice. Thousand Oaks, CA, Sage, 2013

Supplementary Module 8: Patient-Clinician Relationship

Hans Rohlof, M.D.

Rob van Dijk, M.Sc.

Sofie Bäärnhielm, M.D., Ph.D.

The core Cultural Formulation Interview (CFI) contains only one question on the patient-client relationship (question 16; see Appendix A in this handbook), but the Patient-Clinician Relationship supplementary module is devoted entirely to this topic (see Appendix C in this handbook). In this subchapter, we first describe why it is useful for clinicians to assess the cultural aspects of the patient-clinician relationship. We then describe the supplementary module and provide guidelines for its use.

Clinical Utility of Assessing the Patient-Clinician Relationship

In mental health care, a positive patient-clinician relationship is of immense value (Nussbaum 2013). Without a basic trusting relationship, patients will not be open and honest about their thoughts, feelings, and behaviors, and the accuracy of psychiatric diagnosis will be reduced. In addition, patients may choose not to follow the clinician's advice, not to alter their behaviors, not to adhere to medication, or not to engage in psychotherapy; this lack of trust may lead to elevated rates of appointment no-shows and premature discontinuation. As expressed by Franz Kafka's country doctor, "To write prescriptions is easy, but to relate to people in other ways is difficult" (Kafka 1919).

Creating a relationship with patients is more challenging if patients and clinicians differ culturally. Patients may report idioms of distress that are unfamiliar to the clinician and may have different expectations about the clinical encounter, the course of treatment, and potential treatment effects. Any of these differences may result in the patient's lack of trust in the clinician. A poor clinician-patient relationship may contribute to the finding that the outcome of psychiatric treatment is much better when patients and clinicians share a similar cultural background (Fassaert et al. 2010).

The patient-clinician relationship constitutes an ongoing area of research in transcultural psychiatry. Kleinman (1980) pointed out the need to develop strategies so that the expectations of the patient and the possible solutions offered by the clinician can overlap. If the explanatory models of the patient and the clinician are too far apart, treatment is more likely to fail. Moreover, Kortmann (2010) suggested that distinct phases of treatment require the clinician to maintain different therapeutic "distances" from the patient. He distinguished the following three stages:

1. An *elementary-sympathetic* stage, in which the clinician tries to establish a positive and confidential relationship with the patient that facilitates trust and treatment adherence
2. A *diagnostic-therapeutic* stage, in which the clinician has to make a diagnosis and treatment plan, according to his or her professional standards
3. A *personal* stage, in which the clinician tries to integrate his or her observations and analysis in a tailored treatment that makes sense for the patient

The clinician should be aware that a positive relationship with a patient will improve treatment course and outcome by promoting progression through the three stages above. A patient who remains too long in the first stage may feel trust, empathy, and understanding but will not receive the necessary interventions from the clinician. If the second phase is too extensive, the patient may admire the clinician in his or her professional role but will miss a personal connection that motivates the patient to adhere to treatment and change his or her behavior. The relationship built during the initial diagnostic and treatment planning sessions is of crucial importance for the final outcome.

Cultural Aspects of Every Clinical Encounter

As in other contexts of human interaction, patients and clinicians produce, reproduce, and transform culture in the process of receiving and providing mental health care, in making contact, and in diagnosis and treatment. In other words, medical knowledge is also cultural and mental health care can be seen as a product of culture (Taylor 2003). In addition, clinical interaction is influenced by differences in power between patient and clinician in the clinical encounter, and between the social and cultural groups to which they belong. Notably, health care professionals have the power to define patients' worries and complaints and label them using classification systems such as DSM-5 (American Psychiatric Association 2013) or ICD-10 (World Health Organization 1992) in ways that give the patient access to scarce social resources, such as illness-related benefits and specific modalities of care.

Attention is often focused on linguistic and cultural differences in the clinical dyad, which are generally seen as blocking communication and the health care process. However, in every clinical encounter, medical culture and lay culture interact, even when patient and clinician share the same cultural or ethnic backgrounds or speak the same language (Boutin-Foster et al. 2008). Meanings of distress, complaints, and symptoms are negotiated in a continuous process of interpreting, defining, communicating, and redefining, with the goal of a shared understanding of the patient's mental health condition and agreement about diagnosis and treatment.

Because of a lack of objective biomarkers of mental disorders, diagnosis and treatment depend on the clinician's *interpretation* of the patient's *interpretation* of bodily and mental sensations, and of the way they are expressed, in ways that are socially acceptable and understandable to the patient and his or her social network. This double interpretation is complicated in a dyadic therapeutic relationship but is even more complex when a third party is involved, especially in situations where relatives or professional interpreters are present (Bot 2005; Willen 2011).

Cultural attitudes are co-constructed in interaction between patients and clinicians. Lewis-Fernández and Kleinman (1995) located culture not in the minds of individuals but rather between people in the medium of intersubjective engagements. Patients' attitudes toward clinicians are affected not only by factors such as cultural norms, transference, countertransference, and patients' prior experiences with health care but also by other social and individual factors. This influences their views about what is seen as appropriate to communicate about, how to communicate and interact with the clinician, and what to expect from care.

Different Clinical Encounter Models

Globally, there are a great variety of models of clinical encounters within health care systems, but the essence of all the models is that one person is in need of help and another is in a helping position. Various factors, such as social and cultural traditions, history, economy, ideologies, politics, and local contexts, affect the organization of health care systems. In Western industrialized societies, clinical encounters have shifted over the last half century from fairly authoritarian relations between clinicians and patients toward a more egalitarian person-centered approach. The latter requires that the clinician be more of a medical consultant and guide, while the patient is given more decision-making power. In this model, the focus is shifted to self-management on the part of the patient, resulting in an increased set of responsibilities for him or her.

In both primary care and mental health care in Western industrialized societies, clinicians play several roles when carrying out a psychiatric assessment. They act as medical experts, as well as helpers, guides, potential pharmacologists and psychotherapists, and gatekeepers of health care. In multicultural environments, these clinicians encounter patients who are socialized in various physical and mental health care systems, which they use simultaneously. Migrants and refugees face special situations. Migrants' expectations of the role of clinicians are diverse, as are their levels of trust in health care generally and in providers specifically. Patients with a refugee background may have experienced the mental health system as a collaborator in a repressive state and may even have experienced health professionals as participants in torture.

Emotional Reactions Between Patients and Clinicians

Clinicians must remember that all kinds of emotions can occur during psychiatric treatment. Cultural aspects of transference and countertransference are extensive (Comas-Díaz and Jacobsen 1991). The clinician should be aware of his or her own ethnocentric bias and of potential feelings of discrimination or overidentification, which can hinder diagnostic evaluation and treatment. In the unequal relationship of the clinician and the patient, it is difficult to express these feelings, but denying them is worse still. As early as the first encounter, the clinician should try to identify his or her own emotional reactions.

Role of Reflection in Understanding Culture

Reflexive stance means trying to see oneself through the eyes of the other. Self-reflection, or *reflexivity,* is a prerequisite for a comparative anthropological study of culture and society (Hylland Eriksen 2004). It is a structured approach to trying, to some extent, to take a step back from one's own cultural framework. Reflexivity can also be a useful approach in clinical work in multicultural environments when trying to better understand the perspective of the other.

Maintaining an attitude of self-reflection during ongoing clinical encounters may prove difficult. Rudolph et al. (2001) address the value of reflecting after an event on one's thoughts, feelings, and actions to enhance one's capacity for effective action in complex social situations. They take the view that off-line reflection provides sufficient distance in time and space to analyze and reexperience feelings, thoughts, actions, and results that are confusing. This approach can be helpful for identifying blind spots in assessment, including possible misunderstandings, miscommunication, and neglect of alternative diagnostic interpretations. Self-reflection is also a way to identify reactions of transcultural countertransference and to raise cultural awareness.

Why and When to Use
the Supplementary Module

The CFI facilitates exploration of cultural aspects of the interaction between clinician and patient by examining their present relationship and context. The only core CFI question on the patient-clinician relationship is question 16: "Sometimes doctors and patients misunderstand each other because they come from different backgrounds or have different expectations. Have you been concerned about this and is there anything we can do to provide you with the care you need?" The Patient-Clinician Relationship supplementary module suggests additional questions for a more comprehensive exploration. Addressing cultural aspects of the clinical interaction enables both clinicians and patients to improve their communication. The goal of the supplementary module is to assess the role of culture in the therapeutic relationship. More specifically, the questions in the module focus on how patient *and* clinician experience, interpret, and shape their cultural tool kits or repertoires, and how the development of the relationship is influenced as a result (Gregg and Saha 2006). The module therefore focuses on the *individual* experience of culture (Lakes et al. 2006)—that is, culture as it is experienced and performed by its individual agents, in this case the patient and the clinician.

The supplementary module addresses the dual process of interpretation described in the subsection "Cultural Aspects of Every Clinical Encounter." The questions explore the thoughts and beliefs that frame interpretation and help the clinician reflect on both interpretational processes: how the patient understands the relationship with the clinician and how the clinician understands the relationship with the patient. The module consists of two separate sets of questions: one to be asked of the patient during the clinical encounter and the other to facilitate self-reflection by the clinician after the interview. The module can be used when core CFI question 16 indicates the need for further exploration (e.g., if the patient reports substantial concerns about the relationship). Use of the module is also recommended if referral sources report difficulty achieving a working alliance, if the patient specifically mentions his or her cultural differences with the clinician or relates conflictive clinical relationships in the past, or if the clinician finds the patient reluctant to engage. In addition, the clinician's own past experiences and assumptions can be powerful reasons to complete the module. The self-reflective section may be a useful adjunct to care during every phase of treatment.

Overview of the Supplementary Module

The supplementary module has 12 questions, organized as two sets: the first five are asked of the patient, and the last seven encourage the clinician to take a self-reflexive stance. The first set evaluates four domains in the clinician-patient relationship: experiences, expectations, communication, and collaboration. The questions aim to accomplish the following objectives:

- Probe the thoughts and beliefs of the patient about health care in general, and health care professionals in particular, that may influence the therapeutic process in a positive or negative way
- Reveal past experiences that may impede or facilitate establishing an effective therapeutic relationship
- Elicit the patient's thoughts about the clinician and their future relationship
- Strengthen the clinician's presentation as a thoughtful and open provider, who can express his or her willingness to respect the patient, listen to the patient's experiences and take them seriously, and underscore the relevance attached to the patient's point of view

Questions 1 and 2 in the first set explore the patient's previous experiences of health care. The presentation of current complaints is contextual, depending on prior clinical experience, present needs, and cultural traditions and expectations. Negative experiences in the past, for instance, may explain the patient's reluctance to inform the clinician in an open way. Patients' expectations that the clinician cannot meet—for instance, immediate recovery from a chronic psychiatric illness or guaranteeing scarce social resources or a good outcome in a legal matter—may be identified and addressed early in therapy. In turn, the clinician can take into account in the treatment plan what the patient experienced as helpful or difficult in the past and what the patient's culturally patterned expectations are; sometimes, the clinician may also discover in the patient unexpected cultural and contextual resources.

Video 2 demonstrates how a prior negative experience can influence the current patient-clinician relationship.

 Video Illustration 2: What does that have to do with my lungs? (4:26)

In this video (highlighted in subchapter "Supplementary Module 1: Explanatory Model"), a consultation-liaison psychiatrist begins his consultation interview with a woman hospitalized for pulmonary disease by using the core CFI. The second question of the core CFI (How would you describe your problem if you were not talking to a physician?) quickly reveals that the patient is unaware that her physicians have requested a consultation-liaison visit, apparently because she is refusing diagnostic lung tests. The psychiatrist chooses to expand the basic core CFI assessment with some questions from the Explanatory Model supplementary module to clarify how the patient understands her illness. He hopes that this will help him clarify the communication difficulties between the patient and her inpatient team, because it appears very likely that there are differences in the way that she and her physicians perceive her medical problems. Elicitation of her explanatory model shows that she refuses the tests because she is afraid that these will lead to her demise. Her husband was also hospitalized for his lung problems and died during the admission; the patient is afraid the two are related. It appears that she has not been able to resolve this concern with her inpatient treatment team, a situation that demonstrates the value of using the CFI to elicit more detailed information that can be used in a negotiation process to agree on the next steps of evaluation and treatment.

This scenario also demonstrates how questions from different supplementary modules can be combined seamlessly in a single interview, depending on the needs of the situation. At the point that this video ends, for example, the psychiatrist could choose next to pursue questions from the module on the patient-clinician relationship in order to clarify further the conflictive relationship with the treatment team. The patient's mistrust of her clinicians and frank fear of tests may be motivated by many past experiences, including not only her own loss of her husband in at least superficially similar circumstances, but may possibly also be a consequence of racist policies affecting medical testing and treatment in the African American community. By providing a safe venue for her to express these concerns and expectations, the psychiatrist could help the patient develop a more collaborative relationship with the treatment team.

Questions 3–5 focus on the present situation and identify impediments to an effective therapeutic relationship. Question 3 explores the patient's views about the type of clinician he or she would prefer. It is best not to assume that one knows the patient's preferences but instead to inform patients openly about choices. If an interpreter is present, the patient's preferences regarding the interpreter's characteristics and role should be accommodated. The influence of racial or ethnic differences in therapeutic relationships is well known, but differences in gender, age, and religion may also play a role.

Video 15 demonstrates how eliciting a patient's clinician preference can lead to a more effective patient-clinician relationship.

 Video Illustration 15: In my own language (0:42)

The video "In my own language" shows how the core CFI question (16) on the patient-clinician relationship can yield useful concrete information to guide treatment planning even during an intake visit. Despite obvious English fluency, this patient explains that conducting therapy in English is "harder, I have to reach for words, I have to struggle." This kind of information is best if elicited during the initial visit, when treatment assignments are being decided, and validates the inclusion of this item in the core CFI, despite its potential sensitivity during an initial assessment.

It is important to keep in mind that matching on these characteristics is not always obvious or preferred. Differences, furthermore, are not facts, set once and for all. The initial preferences and the initially experienced differences may diminish as the therapeutic relationship unfolds in a positive way. Question 4 opens a dialogue about the patient's doubts over being understood in the diagnostic phase. For example, talking about homosexuality may be blocked if the patient and clinician share a religious background that does not approve of a homosexual orientation. Question 5 aims to promote a discussion about further collaboration.

The second set of questions in the Patient-Clinician Relationship supplementary module offers guidelines for clinician self-reflection after the interview. These questions may help raise the clinician's cultural self-awareness, including consciousness about how his or her approach is framed by medical culture. The questions may also promote the clinician's awareness of potential stereotyping, of effects that the context of treatment may have on the patient's behavior, and of possible limitations of the routines that clinicians develop and use in clinical practice to conduct evaluations and plan treatment. The questions perform a dual purpose, guiding the clinician's own thoughts about the clinical encounter to be applied in future sessions and serving as discussion points for consultation with colleagues on the care of the patient.

Questions 1 and 2 of this second set promote the clinician's reflection on feelings that may occur in the patient-clinician relationship. Discrimination and social exclusion often play an important role in the narratives of patients from underserved minority groups. Being part of the dominant social group, and therefore not having personal experience with discrimination and social exclusion, may unintentionally hinder clinicians from adequately assessing their impact on the life of the patient. Furthermore, the clinician can easily misjudge a patient when guided only by appearance. For example, because of the clinician's own assumptions, he or she may be surprised to discover that a person wearing a religious head covering or what appears to be a "traditional" mode of dress may espouse a thoroughly "modern" worldview.

Question 3 explores the impact of an interpreter on clinical communication. The presence of an interpreter may cause the patient to be less open about thoughts and feelings or, conversely, may improve trust and understanding. The clinician should consider whether the patient worries that the interpreter may not be trustworthy or sufficiently careful with confidential information. In small communities, the fear of unwanted disclosure is often present. Occasionally, especially in the case of refugees, patients may wonder about the allegiance of the interpreter to conflicting parties in the country of origin.

Question 4 encourages the clinician to reflect more generally about how the patient's cultural background may affect the clinician's understanding of the problem and its diagnosis, such as potential uncertainties about the diagnostic interpretation of clinical signs and expressions of distress. Question 5 encourages a reflexive stance toward the clinician's own treatment recommendations and more general routines for arriving at care planning. For example, the clinician may consider whether his or her treatment plans usually take into consideration the patient's conceptualization of the problem and whether the clinician checks his or her assumptions about the patient and his or her own cultural orientations in evaluating therapeutic possibilities. Questions 6 and 7 promote reflection on the clinician's own prejudices and stereotyping biases and their potential role in the encounter with the patient.

Obstacles and Caveats When Using the Module

A first obstacle is that the patient may wonder why the clinician is asking questions that may at first glance seem to have little or nothing to do with his or her complaints. Patients may not be accustomed to this kind of questioning, because most clinical settings encourage a more passive stance by the patient in relation to the clinician. It is important to introduce the questions in an appropriate way, and using the introduction to question 16 in the core CFI may help. In addition, the introduction to the supplementary module suggests the following framing: "I would like to learn about how it has been for you to talk with me and other clinicians about your [PROBLEM] and your health more generally. I will ask some questions about your views, concerns, and expectations." If the patient still appears uncertain, the clinician may stress that a good working relationship is important in mental health care and that it merits some exploration with the patient.

A second obstacle is that patients may not understand the questions or may be unwilling to disclose their thoughts about treatment or about the clinician, viewing themselves as dependent on the clinician's goodwill to access care. Sometimes, the patient discloses thoughts more naturally when talking about past experiences than when discussing the actual therapy situation itself. The clinician can also present examples from his or her clinical practice to convey to the patient that the clinician is well acquainted with the patient's situation.

A caveat to consider is the *culture pitfall*. This phrase refers to the clinician's focus on the culture of the group instead of on the individual patient as an agent who appropriates "culture" in certain ways and is involved in specific social contexts (Kleinman and Benson 2006). It also refers to an operationalization of culture as a set of static properties of patients instead of as a fluid intersubjective system of meanings and practices (Kirmayer 2012). Above all, patients usually do not like to be treated as a representative of an ethnic group instead of as an individual (Feldmann et al. 2007).

Another caveat is that both patients and clinicians may refer to "culture" as a defense mechanism: the patient may do so to avoid talking about personal issues and to legitimate his or her choices, whereas the clinician may do so to argue that problems that occur in treatment are externally caused and not therapist related. It is important to avoid talking about culture in general terms or to use it as an argument. The clinician should focus instead on the actual behaviors and views of the patient and his or her social system in everyday life. As Kleinman (2005) stated, it is important to keep in mind this injunction: "First, do no harm by stereotyping."

Conclusion

In this subchapter, we have provided a theoretical background to the evaluation of the patient-clinician relationship. We have described the supplementary module on this topic, shown how to implement it, and ended by describing possible obstacles and caveats to its use. Even if the clinician does not ask the questions verbatim, he or she should keep the topics of the module in mind during every phase of mental health assessment and treatment to enhance his or her reflexivity and cultural awareness.

KEY CLINICAL POINTS

- In psychiatric practice, a good patient-clinician relationship is of immense importance, reducing treatment nonadherence and nonretention.
- Transference and countertransference are affected by culture, including cultural similarities and differences between patient and clinician.
- The Patient-Clinician Relationship supplementary module can help the clinician obtain a quick and relatively thorough evaluation of the relationship to forestall later problems.

Questions

1. What is reflexivity in intercultural mental health care?

2. What are the goals of each of the two sets of questions in the Patient-Clinician Relationship supplementary module?

3. When in the process of care is it appropriate to use the questions in the Patient-Clinician Relationship supplementary module?

4. What are some obstacles to the use of the module?

5. What are some caveats for the use of the module?

References

American Psychiatric Association: Diagnostic and Statistical Manual of Mental Disorders, 5th Edition. Arlington, VA, American Psychiatric Association, 2013

Bot H: Dialogue Interpreting in Mental Health. Amsterdam, The Netherlands, Rodopi Publishers, 2005

Boutin-Foster C, Foster JC, Konopasek L: Viewpoint: physician, know thyself: the professional culture of medicine as a framework for teaching cultural competence. Acad Med 83(1):106–111, 2008 18162762

Comas-Díaz L, Jacobsen FM: Ethnocultural transference and countertransference in the therapeutic dyad. Am J Orthopsychiatry 61(3):392–402, 1991 1951646

Fassaert T, Peen J, van Straten A, et al: Ethnic differences and similarities in outpatient treatment for depression in the Netherlands. Psychiatr Serv 61(7):690–697, 2010 20592004

Feldmann CT, Bensing JM, de Ruijter A: Worries are the mother of many diseases: general practitioners and refugees in the Netherlands on stress, being ill and prejudice. Patient Educ Couns 65(3):369–380, 2007 17116386

Gregg J, Saha S: Losing culture on the way to competence: the use and misuse of culture in medical education. Acad Med 81(6):542–547, 2006 16728802

Hylland Eriksen T: What Is Anthropology? London, Pluto Press, 2004

Kafka F: A country doctor [in German], in Ein Landarzt, Leipzig, Germany, Kurt Wolff, 1919

Kirmayer LJ: Cultural competence and evidence-based practice in mental health: epistemic communities and the politics of pluralism. Soc Sci Med 75(2):249–256, 2012 22575699

Kleinman A: Patients and Healers in the Context of Culture. Berkeley, University of California Press, 1980

Kleinman A: Culture and Psychiatric Diagnosis. What Are the Necessary Tools? Utrecht, The Netherlands, Trimbos Institute, 2005

Kleinman A, Benson P: Anthropology in the clinic: the problem of cultural competency and how to fix it. PLoS Med 3(10):e294, 2006 17076546

Kortmann F: Transcultural psychiatry: from practice to theory. Transcult Psychiatry 47(2):203–223, 2010 20603386

Lakes K, López SR, Garro LC: Cultural competence and psychotherapy: applying anthropologically informed conceptions of culture. Psychotherapy (Chic) 43(4):380–396, 2006 22122131

Lewis-Fernández R, Kleinman A: Cultural psychiatry: theoretical, clinical, and research issues. Psychiatr Clin North Am 18(3):433–448, 1995 8545260

Nussbaum AM: The Pocket Guide to the DSM-5 Diagnostic Exam. Washington, DC, American Psychiatric Publishing, 2013

Rudolph JW, Taylor SS, Foldy EG: Collaborative off-line reflection: a way to develop skill in action science and action inquiry, in Handbook of Action Research: Participative Inquiry and Practice. Edited by Reason P, Bradbury H. London, Sage Publications, 2001, pp 405–412

Taylor JS: Confronting "culture" in medicine's "culture of no culture." Acad Med 78(6):555–559, 2003 12805033

Willen SS: Pas de trois: medical interpreters, clinical dilemmas, and the patient-provider-interpreter triad, in Shattering Culture: American Medicine Responds to Cultural Diversity. Edited by DelVecchio Good M, Willen SS, Hannah SD, et al. New York, Russell Sage Foundation 2011 pp 70–94

World Health Organization: International Statistical Classification of Diseases and Related Health Problems, 10th Revision. Geneva, Switzerland, World Health Organization, 1992

Suggested Readings

Beach MC, Saha S, Cooper LA: The Role and Relationship of Cultural Competence and Patient-Centeredness in Health Care Quality. New York, The Commonwealth Fund, 2006. Available at: http://www.commonwealthfund.org/publications/fund-reports/2006/oct/the-role-and-relationship-of-cultural-competence-and-patient-centeredness-in-health-care-quality. Accessed February 15, 2015.

Bernstein DM: Therapist-patient relations and ethnic transference, in Culture and Psychotherapy. Edited by Tseng WS, Streltzer L. Washington, DC, American Psychiatric Publishing, 2001, pp 103–122

Flores G: Culture and the patient-physician relationship: achieving cultural competency in health care. J Pediatr 136(1):14–23, 2000. Available at: http://peds.stanford.edu/Rotations/humanism_small_groups/documents/9_CulturePatientPhysicianRelationship.pdf. Accessed February 15, 2015.

Suchman AL: Research on patient-clinician relationships. J Gen Intern Med 18(8):677–678, 2003. Available at: http://www.ncbi.nlm.nih.gov/pmc/articles/PMC1494900/. Accessed February 13, 2015.

Tseng WS: Therapist and patient: relations and communication, in Handbook of Cultural Psychiatry. Edited by Tseng WS. San Diego, Academic Press, 2001, pp 435–442

Supplementary Module 9: School-Age Children and Adolescents

Cécile Rousseau, M.D.

Jaswant Guzder, M.D.

In this subchapter, we examine the importance of integrating the DSM-5 (American Psychiatric Association 2013) Cultural Formulation Interview (CFI) into a developmental and systemic perspective in clinical practice with youth and describe the use of the School-Age Children and Adolescents supplementary module (see Appendix C in this handbook). Integrating a cultural formulation dimension into the usual biopsychosocial assessment of youth must rely on a multi-informant model of interviewing. The CFI supplementary modules—including Cultural Identity, Explanatory Model, Psychosocial Stressors, and Coping and Help Seeking, among others— are all important in child and adolescent psychiatry, because unpacking the complexity of family and systemic issues may clarify the diagnosis and inform the treatment plan. In this subchapter, we address three of the most common challenges clinicians are likely to face when using the CFI in child and adolescent psychiatry: 1) accessing the voices of school-age children, including perceptions or dissonances related to normality and problem definition, assigning of cultural meaning, code switching, acculturation, racism, and language issues; 2) uncovering the evolution of feelings of belonging and multiple identities in cultural minority youth, such as hybridity and creolization of identities and daily realities of immigrant and refugee or undocumented communities; and 3) negotiating the gaps and divergent frames of reference between youth and their multiple caretakers (e.g., family, schools, youth protection agencies, clinicians).

Cultural Formulation in Child and Adolescent Psychiatry

The literature on culturally competent clinical practice underlines the importance of taking into account cultural and contextual factors throughout assessment in child psychiatry (de Anstiss et al. 2009; Measham et al. 2014; Rousseau et al. 2013). Some specific changes are required in the process of assessment to address linguistic and cultural breaches, not only between the family and the clinician but also among family members and numerous caretakers or agencies involved, including school social service agencies and day care programs.

Working with interpreters in child psychiatry must take into account the developmental level of the child and his or her ability to participate in linguistic interpretation and to comprehend translated written material. In the clinical setting, clinicians must also examine the effect of intergenerational differences in the alliance between the interpreter, the parents, and the child (Rousseau et al. 2011). It has been well established in the literature that immigrant children may differ from their host country same-age peers in that they present either more or fewer emotional and behavioral symptoms (Stevens and Vollebergh 2008). This difference is particularly important in the case of refugee children, who are exposed to multiple sources of adversity in both the premigration and the postmigration periods (Fazel et al. 2012). Recently, the question of cultural identity in immigrant and refugee youth, which has always been a key element of the acculturation process, has been emphasized in research because of its importance in the context of the intercommunity tensions associated with international conflicts and fears (Britto 2008). All of these factors, and others that are operationalized in the CFI, have a key role in child psychiatry and often need to be elicited in the assessment process in order to reach the comprehensive understanding that is needed to formulate an integrated treatment plan relevant to the family and the rest of the child's network.

However, literature on the cultural formulation approach and its application in work with children and adolescents is scant. A few clinically oriented papers describe its utility and question some of the limitations of the DSM-IV (American Psychiatric Association 1994) Outline for Cultural Formulation (OCF) for this population (Aggarwal 2010; Novins et al. 1997; Rousseau et al. 2008; Takeuchi 2000).

Discussing the application of the OCF to American Indian children, Novins et al. (1997) emphasize the difficulty of assessing cultural identity in children both because of the complexity of identity construction at this stage of life and because of the numerous identity shifts that may occur during the adolescent period (Canino and Spurlock 2000). Takeuchi (2000) demonstrates how cultural formulation can inform the development of an alternative treatment plan that takes into account family dynamics, explanatory models of illness, and sense of community. He also emphasizes the importance of taking time to establish a strong alliance and to formulate a culturally appropriate treatment plan. These few publications highlight the usefulness of the OCF in child psychiatry but also demonstrate that it may not always be an easy tool to implement in practice.

The CFI supplementary modules represent an important step in supporting clinicians working with families by providing specific questions to facilitate the assessment of the cultural dimensions of child psychiatric problems. To inform the development of training programs and clinical guidelines, the dissemination of the School-Age Children and Adolescents supplementary module will need to be supported in the future by a rigorous evaluation process. Although the core CFI is relevant individually to each youth, the supplementary module amplifies the collateral information (e.g., from family, peers, and school personnel) necessary to formulate an understanding of the youth's crucial developmental influences. The supplementary module can help the interviewer identify cultural and contextual influences that may hinder or facilitate developmental mastery.

Three principles should govern the application of the School-Age Children and Adolescents module and, to some extent, the use of any other supplementary modules with youth. First, brevity is essential; the validity of the assessment and the quality of the alliance require that the youth not be overburdened by the length of the interview. Because the patient's attention span and concentration increase with age and developmental stage, the culturally sensitive clinician should resist the desire to verbalize or gather all historical data at one time. The clinician should consider using other modalities, such as observation, drawing, or play, as auxiliary tools during the session, selecting carefully which cultural dimensions to investigate first. Second, the questions need to be adapted to the child's or adolescent's cognitive and linguistic development, particularly because the questions do not always correspond to chronological age. Cultural and contextual factors, including the impact of language differences and the dislocation experiences of refugees or immigrants, influence the relative maturity (or delay) in specific cognitive domains. Third, as in any standard biopsychosocial child psychiatry assessment, it is pertinent to include the collateral information gained from the perspective of the significant adults in the various life environments of the child.

Use of CFI Supplementary Modules in Child and Adolescent Psychiatry

The School-Age Children and Adolescents supplementary module does not replace the other modules of the CFI, which can also be used in child psychiatric assessments, particularly when the parents have undergone complex trauma, periods of absence due to migration trajectories, or reunification issues. The module has been developed to help the clinician explore age-related cultural dimensions with the youth themselves. Special care has been taken to avoid assigning a specific cultural identity to the youth by the examiner or collateral informants. The questions are purposefully indirect to allow the child or adolescent to express his or her feeling of being special or different without the clinician imposing the idea that he or she is in any way different. In terms of content, the questions are designed to yield the youth's representations of normality at home, at school, and with friends and some of the challenges of growing up.

The supplementary module is composed of four sections. The first section (questions 1–7) addresses the youth's feelings of age appropriateness in different settings (i.e., at home, at school, among friends), the perception of being different or special (in the youth's own view or the view of the family), and the pride or validation eventually associated with awareness of these differences. The second section (questions 8–10) targets age-related stressors and supports. The third section (questions 11–14) seeks to elicit expectations various people have of the child or adolescent and to uncover potential contradictions among these divergent expectations (e.g., a migrant family may expect a child to spend a lot of time on chores, but a teacher may consider these expectations to be abusive). The last section (questions 15–20) addresses markers, rituals, or processes in transition to adulthood or maturity. This set of questions is usually only for *adolescents*—that is, youth experiencing puberty. This developmental period, puberty and the periods immediately before and after, is universally considered important, although the specific concept of adolescence is not necessarily as formulated or well accepted in some communities as it can be in the European–North American context. This transition is commonly marked by celebrations or rituals that may be gender specific (e.g., the *quinceañera* for Latin American girls or the bar mitzvah for Jewish boys). The clash between youth culture in the host society and immigrant families' ideas about the transition to adulthood is a common source of conflict or challenge during the acculturation process. Dating, sibling responsibilities, financial responsibility toward family expenses, and degrees of autonomy are some frequent sources of tension that emerge because of diverging cultural norms. These familial transitions call for respectful acknowledgment of cultural norms and cultural differences that leaves room for mediation.

The supplementary module has an Addendum for Parents' Interview that can be used to elicit information from the adult caretakers of infants and preschoolers. Inquiring about the child's name or play activities is usually an easy route to rapport and often a nonthreatening way to address culture. Many names have special meanings that convey information about family dynamics (e.g., authority, degree of adhesion to tradition, or transgression of family and community practices) and about parental and extended family expectations regarding the particular child. Classic developmental milestones, such as walking, sleep habits, and toilet training, may vary culturally. Markers of autonomy (e.g., eating and dressing alone), assessment of age-appropriate risk taking, and forms of disciplining are also culturally constructed. Without taking into account intercultural differences among clinician, society, and family in the evaluation of those aspects of development, clinicians may arrive at inaccurate diagnoses or unsuccessful intervention plans (Hassan et al. 2011). The complexity of multiple language exposures at home and at school should also be actively elicited (Toppelberg and Collins 2010).

The School-Age Children and Adolescents module can be integrated into the intake assessment or a subsequent interview, in conjunction with the core CFI and other supplementary modules. It should not be administered as if it were a semistructured interview, with a preordained, fixed order of questioning. The child and adolescent clinician should learn to weave the CFI questions and dimensions into his or her usual comprehensive assessment. For example, the evaluation with the parents regarding pregnancy and delivery represents an excellent opportunity to ask about the child-naming process and the eventual meaning of the name; similarly, documenting a patient's developmental milestones can easily include questions about autonomy and discipline in the culture of origin, and likewise with other components of the usual clinical evaluation. Training child and adolescent clinicians to use all the components of the CFI can be done either through modeling—by watching an interview integrating a CFI perspective—or through case discussions that emphasize the significance of the cultural material, identify any missing information, and help clinicians and trainees integrate all available information into a case formulation to guide treatment planning.

Interviewing School-Age Children

Early in development, children grow up apprehending a world where they may be exposed to various cultural frames of reference. From age 4 years, they are able to distinguish their own cultural group's features and characteristics, especially those related to language, ethnicity, and visible minority status (Aboud 1993). As they individuate, youth learn how to navigate the cultural differences between home and a complex and heterogeneous outside world, including day care programs and schools. However, their capacity to articulate the cultural dimensions of their experience evolves more slowly, as they master language, learn to abstract, and develop cognitively. To access the cultural dimensions of their experience, interviews of school-age children should aim to elicit some of the internalized cultural norms and expectations that structure their perceptions of themselves and their roles in different contexts with various caregivers. These perceptions and mental representations should be distinguished from cognitive distortions associated with psychopathology or neurodevelopmental disorders. Children's participation in the assessment process does not imply that they are expected to become key informants about their cultures or that they can be expected to interpret their cultures for the clinician. Each family and child narrative is unique and may vary depending on context and other influences. The supplementary module suggests key questions to explore youth's perceptions of themselves and their role in the different environments they navigate, including the similarities and differences between the family's response to the youth's vocational goals, athletic interests, or artistic pursuits and the youth's perceptions of the host culture's responses to these activities. The following case vignette illustrates how the supplementary module may help elicit these perceptions.

Case Vignette

Hussein is a 9-year-old Eritrean refugee who was referred to child psychiatry by his Canadian school, which had recently expelled him and refused to take him back unless he was evaluated by mental health services for possible violent outbursts and unpredictable oppositional behavior. Hussein's mother explained that he was the oldest of five children and that she had to raise the children alone because her husband had been killed in the Eritrean civil war. Because of the war, Hussein had not been educated, and he was experiencing severe academic difficulties and increasing behavior problems. He had recently bitten another child and had hit two teachers before he was expelled. During the family phase of the interview, Hussein was withdrawn and almost mute. However, he agreed to stay with the clinician and be interviewed with the help of an interpreter. A bit reluctantly, he agreed to work on a puzzle but refused to speak about the problems at school.

Interviewer: Do you feel you are like other children your age?
Hussein: (Shakes his head no)
Interviewer: Do you feel different from other children here in Canada or in Eritrea?
Hussein: Both. (Frowns)

Interviewer: What would an Eritrean mother think of a son like you?
Hussein: (No answer)
Interviewer: What would an Eritrean grandmother think of a son like you?
Hussein: (In a muffled voice, visibly anxious) She would slit my throat.

This response opened a window to explore Hussein's negative self-image. He felt irresponsible and very apprehensive that he had not been a good example for his siblings as the oldest son. His school difficulties had led to remedial measures and placement in a special class, which he experienced as a terrible humiliation. He was convinced that school personnel considered him "crazy" or "bad," and these projected identifications led to his enactments of both "crazy" and "bad" behavior, leading to an escalation in the conflict with the school.

After the interview with Hussein, his mother acknowledged that she felt the school had hurt her son's sense of dignity and that his anger explained the intensity of his acting out. She felt that she could not criticize the school for fear of retaliation against Hussein and her other children, so she had kept her understanding of the situation to herself. The management plan included a change of school, because the original school would not agree to change their view of Hussein as violent and dangerous and to reintegrate Hussein into a regular classroom with academic support. Although Hussein continued to struggle academically throughout his schooling and remained quite hyperactive, his violent behavior completely disappeared and he successfully graduated from high school.

Hussein was caught between two very painful representations of himself. For the school and the host society, he was "crazy," and referral to the child psychiatrist embodied the confirmation of this view, which explained his reluctance to engage in the assessment. For his family (and his culture of origin), he was a failure because he could not fulfill his duties as the oldest son, especially in the absence of his father, and was a terrible example for his siblings. Partially restoring his self-image in these two worlds was crucial to the therapeutic process.

Use of the CFI modules with parents (including the Addendum for Parents' Interview of the School-Age Children and Adolescents module) may complement the assessment of the youth and offer useful information on illness explanations, aspects of cultural identity, and other factors that are relevant to understanding family dynamics and child-parent differences in appraising the impact of the youth's symptoms or behaviors. The symptom presented by the child may be understood differently by the youth and the parents in spite of the fact that they share a common culture at home.

Interviewing Adolescents: Eliciting Identities and Affiliations

Because of rapid developmental changes and the resulting shifts in social positioning, adolescence is always a period of identity formation, which for many youth living in multicultural settings will also include a series of identity negotiations (Akhtar 1995; Song 2004; Ungar 2008). In a clinical encounter, it could be incorrect to presume that an adolescent will have the same identity as his or her parents and elders or that the adolescent will necessarily be more acculturated than they are. Youth identities and affiliations can be elicited using the Cultural Identity supplementary module. However, it is important to understand that adolescents are far more vulnerable than adults, because their identities are in formation and thus are more fluid. The interviewer must be aware that the identity endorsed by the youth may shift with the interview context and with social circumstances.

Cultural Formulation and Systemic Interactions

Every aspect of a youth's environment plays a key role in understanding the individual's problem and in formulating a treatment plan. This multiplicity of perspectives within the assessment process is a fundamental asset to understanding the cultural frames of reference, not only of child and family but also of institutions, professionals, and other significant caretakers, who also engage the situation through a cultural lens. Often in CFI assessments, it is important for the clinician to complete a genogram with parents, once an alliance is established, to understand whether there are extended family members who may be geographically distant yet have a substantial impact on decision making, attachment roles, and emotional support in a way that is integral to the intervention plan.

Addressing institutional racism is always delicate when the clinician wants the institution to be a protective place for the child and family as part of establishing cultural safety. It is important not to deny the distress of institutional racism or abuses caused by prejudice, because this form of complicity may harm the family and the therapeutic alliance (Fernando 1995; Stanley 2009). The CFI can help to identify these issues, delineating their role in the clinical presentation, by taking these tensions into account and clarifying the need for professional advocacy.

Conclusion

The core CFI and the supplementary modules are useful tools for working with children, adolescents, and families. As in working with adult patients, all of the CFI modules may be helpful at different points in diagnosis and treatment planning with children and adolescents. Most often these assessments should include input from family (including extended family and/or family in the country of origin as needed), the day care program or school, and occasionally other legal actors such as youth protection services or the police. The cultural formulation approach not only should apply to the family and the youth interviews but also should inform a broader attempt to document the diverse perspectives of all the caretakers involved, because all of them are embedded in cultural predicaments and perspectives.

KEY CLINICAL POINTS

- Because the perceptions of children and adolescents are influenced by the various cultures to which they belong (at home, at school, in their community, and among their social networks), eliciting a multiplicity of perspectives is necessary to understand the cultural aspects of the individuals' mental health problems.

- The School-Age Children and Adolescents supplementary module of the Cultural Formulation Interview helps the clinician to elicit, through simple age-appropriate questions, cultural elements contributing to the assessment and formulation of a treatment plan, such as the norms and expectations that structure a youth's perception of self and of his or her role.

Questions

1. Who should be considered as an informant to understand the cultural aspects of a youth's mental health problem?

2. What are some of the factors to keep in mind when interviewing a child?

3. What are some aspects of child development that may vary with culture?

4. To what extent is adolescence a universal concept?

5. What characterizes cultural identity during adolescence?

References

Aboud FE: The developmental psychology of racial prejudice. Transcult Psychiatry 30:229–242, 1993

Aggarwal NK: Cultural formulations in child and adolescent psychiatry. J Am Acad Child Adolesc Psychiatry 49(4):306–309, 2010 20410723

Akhtar S: A third individuation: immigration, identity, and the psychoanalytic process. J Am Psychoanal Assoc 43(4):1051–1084, 1995 8926325

American Psychiatric Association: Diagnostic and Statistical Manual of Mental Disorders, 4th Edition. Washington, DC, American Psychiatric Association, 1994

American Psychiatric Association: Diagnostic and Statistical Manual of Mental Disorders, 5th Edition. Arlington, VA, American Psychiatric Association, 2013

Britto PR: Who am I? Ethnic identity formation of Arab Muslim children in contemporary U.S. society. J Am Acad Child Adolesc Psychiatry 47(8):853–857, 2008 18645418

Canino IA, Spurlock J: Culturally Diverse Children and Adolescents: Assessment, Diagnosis, and Treatment. New York, Guilford, 2000, pp 237–250

de Anstiss H, Ziaian T, Procter N, et al: Help-seeking for mental health problems in young refugees: a review of the literature with implications for policy, practice, and research. Transcult Psychiatry 46(4):584–607, 2009 20028678

Fazel M, Reed RV, Panter-Brick C, et al: Mental health of displaced and refugee children resettled in high-income countries: risk and protective factors. Lancet 379(9812):266–282, 2012 21835459

Fernando S: Mental Health in a Multi-Ethnic Society: A Multidisciplinary Handbook. New York, Routledge, 1995

Hassan G, Thombs BD, Rousseau C, et al: Child maltreatment: evidence review for newly arriving immigrants and refugees. Can Med Assoc J 2011. Available at: http://www.cmaj.ca/content/suppl/2010/06/07/cmaj.090313.DC1/imm-childmal-12-at.pdf. Accessed November 14, 2011.

Measham T, Heidenreich-Dutray F, Rousseau C, et al: Cultural consultation in child psychiatry, in Cultural Consultation: Encountering the Other in Mental Health Care. Edited by Kirmayer L, Rousseau C, Guzder J. New York, Springer, 2014, pp 71–87

Novins DK, Bechtold DW, Sack WH, et al: The DSM-IV Outline for Cultural Formulation: a critical demonstration with American Indian children. J Am Acad Child Adolesc Psychiatry 36(9):1244–1251, 1997 9291726

Rousseau C, Measham T, Bathiche-Suidan M: DSM-IV, culture and child psychiatry. J Can Acad Child Adolesc Psychiatry 17(2):69–75, 2008 18516309

Rousseau C, Measham T, Moro MR: Working with interpreters in child mental health. Child Adolesc Ment Health 16:55–59, 2011

Rousseau C, Measham T, Nadeau L: Addressing trauma in collaborative mental health care for refugee children. Clin Child Psychol Psychiatry 18(1):121–136, 2013 22626671

Song M: Choosing ethnic identity. Australian Journal of Social Issues 39:478, 2004

Stanley J: African and Caribbean mental health services in Manchester, in Mental Health in a Multi-Ethnic Society. Edited by Fernando S. London, Routledge, 2009 pp 205–207

Stevens GWJM, Vollebergh WAM: Mental health in migrant children. J Child Psychol Psychiatry 49(3):276–294, 2008 18081765

Takeuchi J: Treatment of a biracial child with schizophreniform disorder: cultural formulation. Cultur Divers Ethnic Minor Psychol 6(1):93–101, 2000 10975171

Toppelberg CO, Collins BA: Language, culture, and adaptation in immigrant children. Child Adolesc Psychiatr Clin N Am 19(4):697–717, 2010 21056342

Ungar M: Resilience across cultures. Br J Soc Work 38:218–235, 2008

Suggested Readings

Measham T, Heidenreich-Dutray F, Rousseau C, et al: Cultural consultation in child psychiatry, in Cultural Consultation: Encountering the Other in Mental Health Care. Edited by Kirmayer L, Rousseau C, Guzder J. New York, Springer, 2014, pp 71–87

Rousseau C, Measham T, Bathiche-Suidan M: DSM-IV, culture and child psychiatry. J Can Acad Child Adolesc Psychiatry 17:69–75, 2008

Supplementary Module 10: Older Adults

Neil Krishan Aggarwal, M.D., M.B.A., M.A.

Ladson Hinton, M.D.

In this subchapter, we present theoretical foundations and practical strategies for the cross-cultural assessment of older adults using the DSM-5 (American Psychiatric Association 2013) Cultural Formulation Interview (CFI). This type of cultural assessment assumes clear public health significance in light of population trends worldwide with respect to the growth and increasing ethnic and cultural diversity of older adult populations. The Older Adults supplementary module (in Appendix C in this handbook), along with the Caregivers supplementary module (also in Appendix C) and the CFI–Informant Version (in Appendix B), can assist clinicians in adapting the core CFI (in Appendix A) to meet the needs and circumstances of older adults, thereby facilitating more effective cross-cultural mental health assessment and initial treatment planning for older adults. This subchapter addresses the rationale for the Older Adults module to supplement the CFI, describes the structure and content of the Older Adults module, and provides clinicians with guidelines on use of this module and the other CFI components.

Rationale for the Supplementary Module

The aging population has grown because of medical innovations that have increased life expectancies to unprecedented levels. According to the Institute of Medicine (2008), the population of Americans age 65 and older is expected to double to 20% of the total population by 2030. In the mid-twentieth century, only 14 million people age 80 and older lived on the entire planet, a number that will skyrocket to 400 million by 2050 (World Health Organization 2012). This increase in the elderly population is also expected to increase the burden of mental health disorders, particularly of memory-impairment illnesses such as dementia, as people live longer. For example, 35.6 million people in 2012 were living with dementia worldwide, and this number is expected to double by 2030 and more than triple by 2050 (World Health Organization and Alzheimer's Disease International 2012). The rise in life expectancies has led to widespread social transformations, such as reducing traditional kinship ties from the extended family to the nuclear household with a consequent reduction in the extent to which family members provide care to elderly relatives (Sokolovsky 2009). Meanwhile, the responsibility of caregiving has shifted to a health care system that cannot adequately supply geriatric psychiatrists: in 2011, only 43% of the 131 postdoctoral fellowship positions in geriatric psychiatry were filled, an insufficient number to treat the 14%–20% of the elderly population suffering from a mental disorder (Institute of Medicine 2012). This lack of specialist resources increases the likelihood that mental health clinicians from all disciplines will treat older adults. Therefore, mental health clinicians would benefit from a basic introduction to cultural issues relevant to the care of this population.

We believe that clinicians who work with elderly patients would benefit from keeping two types of cultural competence in mind. First, we recommend that clinicians explore the unique identities of their patients and how these identities relate to their clinical care (see subchapter "Supplementary Module 6: Cultural Identity"). Second, we recommend that clinicians formulate the care of elderly patients based on common needs and challenges of this developmental phase. Culture shapes the attitudes, beliefs, and expectations of all humans about developmental transitions, such as retirement from work (Luborsky and LeBlanc 2003), the process of aging (Goldstein and Griswold 1998; Schulz and Heckhausen 1999), and the meanings and rituals associated with death (Hallenbeck et al. 1996). For this reason, cross-cultural gerontologists have emphasized the need to disentangle universal processes of aging common to all people and specific aspects of aging that vary based on individual cultural characteristics (Cattell 1989). The experience of aging is formed not only through interactions with close associates such as family and friends but also by social, political, and economic structures in which aging is embedded (Edmonson 2013), including the structures of the health care system. For example, culture influences the way elderly patients access health services, and attitudes vary on what constitutes elder abuse based on familial role expectations (Simpson 2005), the perceived need for treatment of disorders, such as dementia, that are considered a natural response to aging (Sadavoy et al. 2004), expectations about whether medications are useful (Chia et al. 2006), and which family members can serve as health care proxies for decision making (Rubinstein 1995; Morrison et al. 1998). Culture also influences how the elderly adopt self-care practices to maintain essential activities of daily living, and clinicians can inquire about these practices as a window into body image, psychological resilience, and cross-generational social relationships (Dill et al. 1995). In addition, culture influences how providers diagnose patients with age-related disorders; for example, international medical graduates, compared to U.S. graduates, diagnose depression less frequently in elderly individuals based on their own cultural attitudes and biases, which clearly impact treatment provision (Kales et al. 2006).

We acknowledge that culture envelops all of us in the health care system, not only patients or their close associates. A thorough and comprehensive cultural assessment should therefore account for the distinct characteristics of all participants in health care, including clinicians. Because of these complex interactions, specialists in cultural mental health have highlighted the need for a systematic method to elicit the relationship between cultural conceptions of aging and multiple domains of illness experience. A recent survey of textbooks on geriatric medicine and geriatric psychiatry has shown that authors either omit any mention of the need for cross-cultural assessment or suggest it without offering clear guidelines or methods (Aggarwal 2010). This led to suggestions that the DSM-IV (American Psychiatric Association 1994) Outline for Cultural Formulation (OCF) could be adapted for use with the elderly population based on the significant evidence base of its use in younger patients (Aggarwal 2010, 2013). The OCF's revision into the core CFI with a supplementary module for older adults offers standardized instructions and questions for clinicians to simultaneously assess cultural needs based on individual identities and common challenges in this developmental phase.

Overview of the Supplementary Module

The overall goal of the Older Adults supplementary module is to assist clinicians in gathering information to assess the role of cultural conceptions of aging and aging-related transitions in the patient's illness experience. Fundamental to this assessment is the notion that cultural concepts of aging can be important sources of identity, illness meanings, and interpersonal processes and experiences that are of direct relevance to the core domains of the CFI. The Older Adults module fleshes out these connections, offering concrete examples of questions to assist the clinician. The module consists of 17 open-ended questions that fall into six broad categories of inquiry. As in other supplementary modules, the questions in this module amplify particular sections of the core CFI (which parallel those in the CFI–Informant Version). In this section, we discuss important sections of this module and their relationships to the core CFI.

The first and last sets of questions in the Older Adults module address issues of identity as they relate to aging, but in very different respects. The first set, conceptions of aging and cultural identity, includes three questions that explore how older adults draw on culturally constructed concepts of aging and stages of the life cycle to create their own identities. These questions parallel the core CFI section on cultural identity (i.e., questions 8–10). Understanding the vocabularies that a person uses to describe his or her positioning in the developmental cycle (e.g., "an old person") and their associated meanings can be useful when these terms are invoked in other parts of the interview (e.g., "I am this way because I am old"). The final set, positive and negative attitudes toward aging and the clinician-patient relationship, includes questions 15–17. These questions (especially question 16) might evoke, for example, the experience of discrimination or stereotyping that older adults experience based on perceptions of how others treat them.

Aging can influence illness meanings through two pathways that are highlighted in this module. First, aging can be a powerful source of explanations for illness-related changes (e.g., "this is just part of getting old"); the specific meanings of growing old and associated expectations may vary substantially across cultures. The module's second set of questions (4 and 5) addresses how conceptions of aging shape explanatory models of illness and related coping strategies, directly expanding the core CFI questions on causes of the illness episode (core CFI question 4) and self-coping (question

11). Being older is associated with challenges and transitions that impinge on the experience and meaning of mental health problems. Older adults, for example, are much more likely than younger individuals to experience comorbid medical illness and associated challenges, such as medical treatments, functional disability, and increased reliance on others for assistance in completing activities of daily living. These challenges, in turn, influence how patients understand their mental health problems (e.g., as a result of a medical condition) and their approaches to coping. The third set of questions (6–9) probes relationships between physical health and mental health and may assist clinicians in understanding frameworks of explanation that may be relevant to older adults' conceptions of their mental health problems (core CFI question 4) and self-coping (question 11).

Video 16 presents the perspective of an older patient on his injury and recovery.

 Video Illustration 16: After the fall (4:00)

The CFI draws upon a definition of culture that includes the background, developmental experiences, and current social contexts of an individual and their resulting effect on perspective. The video "After the fall" highlights developmental experiences around aging as a source of dynamic cultural meaning-making during an illness, using questions from the supplementary module Older Adults. The interviewer begins with a series of open-ended questions on how age has affected the individual's current problem of a broken leg and subsequent recovery. The interviewer also encourages speculation on how being younger could have made a difference. The individual responds that being younger would not have made a difference to the conditions leading him to fall but that the rehabilitative exercises might have been "easier or faster." He also states: "I didn't consciously think, 'Yes, my age is a problem for this, or yes, I am getting more help because I am older for this.'" However, when the interviewer probes beyond physical factors to "context and life" in investigating additional domains of culture, the individual answers, "I have an extraordinary wife and she was there with me through this whole thing." He also adds with a laugh, "I wouldn't have had her if I was younger." We get a glimpse of how this individual views aging as a life phase filled with companionship and views his wife as an "advantage" of his age. The CFI invites clinicians to consider how members of a social network act as sources of support or stress during an individual's illness, recognizing that culture is transmitted within social groups such as families: the man in this video names his wife as a clear support and connects their positive relationship to aging.

For a subset of older adults, particularly those with functional limitations and frailty, older age brings with it increasing reliance on others for support, such as family members, friends, and paid workers. These social networks can be important for practical assistance with mental health treatment and act as sources of either emotional support or strain and conflict. For example, a perceived lack of support from family caregivers can be stressful for patients if caregivers violate culturally calibrated expectations of familial support. Questions 10–12 of this supplementary module assess the quality and nature of social supports and caregiving from the patient's perspective. Answers can provide clinicians with an understanding of the social context of illness that is meaningful for cultural formulation.

Video 17 focuses on social support, both physical and psychological, and the experience of recovery.

 Video Illustration 17: Getting back on my feet (3:46)

In this video, the interviewer transitions to the domain of the supplementary module on the quality and nature of social supports and caregiving by asking how recovery has changed relationships with friends and family, including with his wife. The man says emphatically, "It would be hard to imagine better support from colleagues—I had people come to the house so that we could get some work done.... It made it pretty easy for me to do the things I had to do to get back on my feet." These answers illustrate that people in his social network banded together for his psychological support and to facilitate activities of daily living such as work and basic ambulation. These answers also disclose this individual's resilience in refusing to compromise his baseline functioning prior to the fall. We learn about illness severity through certain sentences from the discussion on recovery: "It's uphill.... Any little sign of improvement is a big deal." These statements reveal a sense of the difficulties he has endured. He also adds, "It's bizarre...being wheeled through an air terminal flat on your back, looking up and seeing people who could walk." The interviewer recognizes that the individual is expanding the conversation beyond physical pain to discuss the psychological effects of illness. The interview closes with the individual clarifying, "They have pills for the pain, but if you're alert—which I was—the situation is very, very strange." Such statements impart a perspective on what is at stake for the individual during illness beyond the biomedical information obtained in a typical clinical interview, which can often be focused on symptom elicitation to make a diagnosis.

Guidelines for Clinical Use of CFI Components

In adopting what we term "the CFI approach" with older adults, we believe that clinicians can avail themselves of all three CFI components: 1) the core CFI, 2) the Older Adults supplementary module, and 3) the CFI–Informant Version. Each tool varies in terms of audience, length, and type of information elicited. In this section, we suggest one possible strategy for using the CFI with older adults. We hope that clinicians regard these components as complementary and synergistic rather than conflicting or confusing.

Core CFI

We believe that the core CFI can be used to begin the initial assessment of all patients in any clinical encounter. As explained in Chapter 2, "The Core and Informant Cultural Formulation Interviews in DSM-5," the DSM-5 field trials actively recruited patients between ages 18 and 80 (American Psychiatric Association 2013). Patients of a wide range of ages were included to test the feasibility, acceptability, and clinical utility of the CFI among different patient groups. Analyses showed that clinicians can use the CFI with older adults during initial assessments just as with younger adults. Therefore, we recommend that general clinicians use the core CFI for all older adults.

Older Adults Supplementary Module

We believe that the Older Adults module can be used to complement content elicited with the core CFI. Questions and techniques from this supplementary module assume that clinicians will have a working understanding of the core CFI. For example, substitution of "[PROBLEM]" with a patient's term in the supplementary module is designed to increase patient satisfaction and build therapeutic alliance as in the core CFI. At the same time, this supplementary module includes material unique to the cultural concerns of older adults, and there may be clinical scenarios when this content would be especially important. Mental health clinicians who work closely with primary care providers or geriatricians may find the third set of questions, influence of comorbid medical problems and treatments on illness (questions 6–9), to be helpful. Similarly, clinicians such as social workers, physical therapists, and occupational therapists who routinely perform functional assessments may benefit from the questions on quality and nature of social supports and caregiving (questions 10–13).

Thus, depending on the clinical circumstances, clinicians may choose to use only some of the questions from the supplementary module in conjunction with the core CFI. In addition, the questions in the supplementary module may be used during the clinical visit when the core CFI is used or later, in follow-up visits. Clinicians working with older adults may find that items from other supplementary modules are useful as well. For example, a clinician working with a frail older adult who is accompanied by a family caregiver may find the Caregivers module particularly useful for eliciting a more thorough understanding of the caregiver's perspective as a way of building rapport and developing culturally informed strategies to support the patient.

CFI–Informant Version

When a patient may not be able or willing to provide a detailed account of his or her illness, the CFI–Informant Version may help clinicians understand relevant cultural concerns from the patient's close associates. Neuropsychiatric conditions such as Alzheimer's disease, Parkinson's disease, and other dementias may affect memory, cognition, and other executive functions that are necessary for patients to complete the medical interview. General medical conditions such as diabetes, stroke, chronic pain, osteoporosis, imbalance, and falling may also lead patients to depend on close associates. In these instances, collateral information from informants can provide a fuller, richer picture of the patient's lived illness experiences, assuming that informed consent has been obtained.

Conclusion

We encourage clinicians to share their experiences using the CFI Older Adults supplementary module. In revising the DSM-IV OCF into the DSM-5 CFI, the DSM-5

Cross-Cultural Issues Subgroup drew upon case studies underscoring clinician experiences that the OCF could not be applied to older adults without significant modifications. The CFI approach encompasses a set of resources that may be particularly useful to clinicians working with older adults, including the Older Adults supplementary module, the CFI–Informant Version, and the Caregivers supplementary module. We hope that clinicians continue to write reflectively on the costs and benefits of implementing the CFI within their service settings. Such publications can help us iteratively improve the cross-cultural mental health care of older patients.

KEY CLINICAL POINTS

- Cultural competence in work with older adults consists of exploring the unique identities of patients, the relationship of these identities to clinical care, and cultural attitudes in this developmental phase.
- Older adults may have medical conditions and neuropsychiatric disorders that suggest a need for collateral history to complete a thorough cultural assessment.
- The core Cultural Formulation Interview (CFI), the CFI–Informant Version, and supplementary modules can be used to conduct a thorough cultural assessment of older adults.

Questions

1. Why is it important to understand cultural attitudes of aging in the care of older adults?

2. How does the clinician's cultural background or identity affect his or her attitude toward aging and the needs of the older population?

3. What aspects of aging are addressed in the Older Adults supplementary module?

4. What are some ethical concerns in using informants and caregivers to assess the cultural needs of patients?

References

Aggarwal NK: Reassessing cultural evaluations in geriatrics: insights from cultural psychiatry. J Am Geriatr Soc 58(11):2191–2196, 2010 20977437

Aggarwal NK: Cross-cultural geriatric psychiatry, in Fundamentals of Geriatric Psychiatry. Edited by Tampi RR, Williamson D. New York, Nova Science Publishers, 2013, pp 321–328

American Psychiatric Association: Diagnostic and Statistical Manual of Mental Disorders, 4th Edition. Washington, DC, American Psychiatric Association, 1994

American Psychiatric Association: Diagnostic and Statistical Manual of Mental Disorders, 5th Edition. Arlington, VA, American Psychiatric Association, 2013

Cattell MG: Being comparative: methodological issues in cross-cultural gerontology. J Cross Cult Gerontol 4(1):75–81, 1989 24389953

Chia LR, Schlenk EA, Dunbar-Jacob J: Effect of personal and cultural beliefs on medication adherence in the elderly. Drugs Aging 23(3):191–202, 2006 16608375

Dill A, Brown P, Ciambrone D, et al: The meaning and practice of self-care by older adults: a qualitative assessment. Res Aging 17:8–41, 1995

Edmonson R: Cultural gerontology: valuing older people, in Old Age in Europe: A Textbook of Gerontology. Edited by Komp K, Aartsen M. Dordrecht, The Netherlands, Springer, 2013, pp 113–130

Goldstein MZ, Griswold K: Cultural sensitivity and aging. Psychiatr Serv 49(6):769–771, 1998 9634155

Hallenbeck J, Goldstein MK, Mebane EW: Cultural considerations of death and dying in the United States. Clin Geriatr Med 12(2):393–406, 1996 8799356

Institute of Medicine: Retooling for an Aging America: Building the Health Care Workforce. Washington, DC, National Academies Press, 2008

Institute of Medicine: The Mental Health and Substance Use Workforce for Older Adults: In Whose Hands? Washington, DC, National Academies Press, 2012

Kales HC, DiNardo AR, Blow FC, et al: International medical graduates and the diagnosis and treatment of late-life depression. Acad Med 81(2):171–175, 2006 16436580

Luborsky MR, LeBlanc IM: Cross-cultural perspectives on the concept of retirement: an analytic redefinition. J Cross Cult Gerontol 18(4):251–271, 2003 14654730

Morrison RS, Zayas LH, Mulvihill M, et al: Barriers to completion of health care proxies: an examination of ethnic differences. Arch Intern Med 158(22):2493–2497, 1998 9855388

Rubinstein RL: Narratives of elder parental death: a structural and cultural analysis. Med Anthropol Q 9(2):257–276, 1995 7671117

Sadavoy J, Meier R, Ong AYM: Barriers to access to mental health services for ethnic seniors: the Toronto study. Can J Psychiatry 49(3):192–199, 2004 15101502

Schulz R, Heckhausen J: Aging, culture and control: setting a new research agenda. J Gerontol B Psychol Sci Soc Sci 54B:P139–P145, 1999 10363034

Simpson AR: Cultural issues and elder mistreatment. Clin Geriatr Med 21(2):355–364, 2005 15804555

Sokolovsky J: Aging, center stage: new life course research in anthropology. Anthropology News 50:5–8, 2009

World Health Organization: Good Health Adds Life to Years: Global Brief for World Health Day 2012. Geneva, Switzerland, World Health Organization, 2012

World Health Organization, Alzheimer's Disease International: Dementia: A Public Health Priority. Geneva, Switzerland, World Health Organization, 2012

Suggested Readings

Aggarwal NK: Reassessing cultural evaluations in geriatrics: insights from cultural psychiatry. J Am Geriatr Soc 58:2191–2196, 2010. This article on revising the OCF for use with older adults helped to revise the CFI in focusing on the needs of older adults.

American Association for Geriatric Psychiatry: Geriatric Core Competencies. McLean, VA, American Association for Geriatric Psychiatry, 2011. Available at: http://www.aagponline.org/index.php?src=gendocs&ref=GeriatricCoreCompetencies&category=Education. Accessed September 15, 2014.

Supplementary Module 11: Immigrants and Refugees

James Boehnlein, M.D., M.Sc.

Joseph Westermeyer, M.D., Ph.D.

Monica Scalco, M.D., Ph.D.

Mental health and adjustment of world refugee populations fleeing war and persecution has been a core area of study and practice in cultural psychiatry over the past several decades. The effects of premigration and migration trauma have been well described (Hollifield et al. 2006), along with the challenges of postmigration adjustment and acculturation (Finch and Vega 2003). Clinicians need practical tools to assess the mental health and functioning in these families and communities. The Cultural Formulation Interview (CFI) Immigrants and Refugees supplementary module allows clinicians to optimize assessment and treatment of these populations. This supplementary module can guide clinicians to efficiently recognize factors that influence mental health, such as premigration difficulties, exposure to violence and persecution, the historical time frame of migration, migration-related losses and challenges, continued ties to the country of origin, resettlement and life in the new country, and future expectations. After a discussion of the module, we explore some of the challenges involved in the assessment of refugees and immigrants.

Overview of the Supplementary Module

The Immigrants and Refugees supplementary module consists of 18 questions divided into seven sections (see Appendix C in this handbook). We discuss each of the sections, describing how exploration of these domains can enhance the clinician's ability to perform an effective assessment.

Background Information

Questions 1–4 obtain information on the patient's background and that of his or her entourage, including the reasons for migrating. A *migrant* is a person who relocates from a familiar sociocultural environment to an unfamiliar one (Westermeyer 1989b). This relocation may involve minimal geographical distance but represent a major sociocultural separation from the past. Alternatively, an individual may migrate thousands of miles but settle in a highly familiar sociocultural setting. Migration can be intranational or international. *Refugees* make up a special subgroup of migrants. Typically, they have involuntarily fled their homeland because of political, religious, or ethnic prejudice, pogroms, imprisonment, or armed conflict against the group to which they belong.

The individual's age at migration sets the stage for the subsequent story. The clinician can then proceed with age-appropriate topics, from location and conditions of birth, to family constellation, to education and socialization in the culture of origin or in the culture of relocation. If migration was motivated by economics, the patient's motivations and expectations should receive attention. If war or revolution predated migration, trauma and loss should be covered. If political, religious, or ethnic pogroms precipitated flight, their nature and personal effects should be plumbed (De Jesús-Rentas et al. 2010).

Understanding the patient's personal motivation for and expectations of migration is critical. *Voluntary* and *involuntary* migration can present differing clinical problems (Berry et al. 1987). Voluntary migrants may include students, guest workers, vacationers, entrepreneurs, and others. Typically, they travel alone or in family groups, although they may also affiliate with an expatriate group from the same country or region. They can return to their original country or community if they wish. Involuntary migrants might have their land taken from them so that it can be used for some social purpose (e.g., creating a water reservoir, building a road); they might remain in the same country. Involuntary migrants who leave their country of origin tend to be refugees. Unlike voluntary migrants, they are likely to migrate in large groups, perhaps as large as thousands or hundreds of thousands of people, and they often cannot return to the country of origin. International adoptees can be considered involuntary migrants who relocate alone or in small groups. *Temporary* or *permanent* migrations may occur. Temporary purposes consist of vacations, training, education, or temporary work. Permanent migrations include relocating to become a citizen of a new country, to marry a citizen of another country, to be adopted, or to start a new career. From a mental health perspective, each of these age-related factors contains specific liabilities and advantages.

Differences between "life before" and "life after" migration can precipitate disorder or undermine adjustment. For example, a subservient wife may become the new family breadwinner; a member failing to acculturate in a family whose other members are acculturating may become marginalized within the family; a family accustomed to servants may not be able to afford them; and students trained for rote memorization may have trouble with problem solving, group formats, informatics, statistics, or writing skills. Unfamiliar climate, food, dress, housing, laws, and language may be welcome to one migrant but anathema to another.

Premigration Difficulties

Questions 5 and 6 cover premigration difficulties. Determinants of mental health for refugees depend on both past trauma and postmigration stress (Silove and Ekblad 2002). Violence is a worldwide problem and takes multiple forms. State-sponsored military actions, civil wars, and ethnic cleansing have resulted in the deaths and wounding of thousands of people. Random, unpredictable paramilitary actions and religious conflict have added to the list of victims of violence. In addition, state-sponsored oppression and torture have affected millions of people. Some migrant patients have committed crimes prior to migration, the consequences of which may follow them (e.g., engaging in torture, terrorist activities, misrepresentation, drug smuggling).

The Immigrants and Refugees supplementary module can illuminate past traumatic experiences that have significant effects on individuals and families. The pervasive effects of hardship, persecution, and profound losses include not only trauma but also the disintegration of families and communities, the destruction of economic infrastructures, and the imposition of fear into daily life (Desjarlais et al. 1995; Summerfield 2000). Successive threats and human rights violations compound each other to challenge multiple adaptive systems at both individual and communal levels (Silove 1999).

Migration-Related Losses and Challenges

Questions 7–10 elicit information about migration-related losses and challenges. Common losses include separation from family and close friends and loss of a house, a job, or one's social network. Loss of a sense of control over the environment and social rules in a well-known culture may also occur. The following case of an Iranian woman who migrated to North America illustrates the challenges of separation, loss, and trauma experienced by many refugees and immigrants.

Case Vignette

"Am I bad woman? Doctor, do you think I am a bad woman?" Afsar asks her psychiatrist. She has been in Canada for 2 years as a refugee and has been dealing with severe depression. She was able to leave Iran when her husband was imprisoned for political reasons. From time to time, her parents are able to send her news about him. Over the past 2 years, every time she has heard about her husband, she has learned that his health continued to deteriorate. Recently, Afsar heard that he is in a hospital and is not expected to improve; her parents were told that there is no hope. Afsar was able to reach her husband at the hospital on his birthday (after more than a year of no contact), but he did not even recognize her on the phone. She has been trying to move forward with her own treatment and with her life in Canada. Afsar attends English classes, and her ability to communicate in English has improved considerably, so much so that an interpreter is no longer needed. However, every time she receives news about her husband, her depression worsens. Her reason to keep fighting is to be strong for her daughters. She has two daughters in Iran with whom she has daily contact through the Internet. Afsar wishes to be well one day because her daughters need her and she wants to be able to support them. She feels safe in Canada and happy she was able to escape, but at the same time she feels guilty for leaving her family behind.

Video 9 depicts the challenges of separation from family and functioning in a new social network after voluntary migration.

 Video Illustration 9: A small town, which is why I'm here (4:39)

In this video (highlighted in "Aspects of Cultural Identity Related to National, Ethnic, and Racial Background; Language; and Migration" also), a psychiatrist conducts an interview with a middle-aged Puerto Rican man who suffers from anxiety symptoms at work after his mother, who lives in Puerto Rico, has a stroke. The aim of the National, Ethnic, and Racial Background portion of the Cultural Identity supplementary module is to assess how a person's national, ethnic, and racial background affects his or her sense of self and his or her place in society and how these aspects of identity influence behavior. In this video, the clinician frames the purpose of the interview. This is an important part of any supplementary module, because it clarifies for the patient how the subsequent questions relate to the patient's reason for seeking help. In this case, the interviewer emphasizes that he wants to understand whether the patient's cultural identity influences his mental health problems and his expectations of care. The initial questions immediately reveal the reason for seeking help. The patient is experiencing substantial anxiety because his mother is in Puerto Rico in a town with limited access to the tertiary medical care she needs for her stroke. He feels pressure to return to the island to provide the care she needs, as seems to be expected of any good Puerto Rican son. In fact, if he does not go, his family might think less of him and perhaps even repudiate him to some extent. The conflict stems from the fact that his sense of himself is connected to being the kind of person who takes risks to become successful, including migrating to the United States for a better future. To complicate matters further, he fears that he could lose his job if he responds to what he and his community in Puerto Rico interpret as his filial duty. He appears puzzled by the reaction of his employers, who are unwilling to grant him leave from work to travel. He says, "At work they…kinda don't get this thing with family. I don't quite understand how it works over here, but it's almost like family isn't important, like you're supposed to go working anyway, you can't take any time off." His current predicament highlights the cultural differences between his new environment and key aspects of his identity, and this conflict appears to be heightening his anxiety.

Information on a patient's cultural identity can help clarify perspective on health, illness, and the mental health system. The way an individual represents himself to others, how he feels about his position in society, and how this relates to his mental health problems is useful information for the clinician. Starting from the information obtained in the video, the interviewer can proceed to elicit additional details. For example, the interviewer could obtain more information on the patient's role in his family. The clinician could ask if the patient is the eldest son, who is thought to have a special responsibility for his mother, or how his family reacted to his migration and to his drive to succeed, which may put extra pressure on him that could contribute to his symptoms. To help with the current situation at work, the clinician could inquire whether he has felt misunderstood there in other situations, whether there are other Puerto Rican coworkers, whether they have experienced the same kind of misunderstandings, and whether he is afraid to be discriminated against as a result of his ethnicity if he asks for unpaid leave.

Ongoing Relationship With Country of Origin

Some migrants keep strong connections with their country of origin, as examined in questions 11 and 12. Many are responsible for supporting family left behind. One or two parents may leave for better job opportunities to be able to send money back home to support their children, left in the care of family members. The Internet has facilitated contact and enables migrants to talk to and see family and friends, sometimes daily. Some migrants keep strong business connections with their country, or they may be working for a group or institution from their country of origin. These relationships may impede the acculturation process, reinforcing a strong connection with the homeland.

Resettlement and New Life

Challenges associated with resettlement are explored in module questions 13–15. The arrival in a new country can present difficult challenges, such as obtaining visas, citizenship, or refugee status. This complex process can be a huge obstacle for someone who has just arrived, is not yet fluent in the new language, and has no source of income.

Acculturating to a new country lasts throughout a lifetime. Age at migration can influence the extent to which a migrant acculturates to a new society. Other things being equal, younger age favors more thorough acculturation. Children's greater proficiency with the host country's language frequently leads to the reversal of traditional generational roles, as the children become the communication facilitators and culture brokers between the family and the majority society.

For migrants of an advanced age, acculturation may be minimal or superficial. After migration, elderly refugees may live with a diminished status both within families and in the society at large because of a lack of language proficiency, little or no formal education, and no relevant work. The willingness of the migrant to be assimilated and the willingness of the receiving culture to assimilate the migrant can also affect this process in deep and lasting ways.

Acculturation failure refers to the absence of reasonably functional acculturation, given the age of the migrant and the mutual assimilation processes of the migrating and receiving cultures (Westermeyer 1989b). Refugee children and adults may have suffered conditions—bullet, shrapnel, or blast wounds to the brain; malnutrition; infectious disease; torture; and other conditions—that impede acculturation by limiting the capacity to acquire new knowledge, skills, and attitudes (Ahearn and Athey 1991). Elderly refugees may lack the motivation or cognitive capacity to acquire a new language, as well as the innumerable skills and requisite knowledge to function in a new culture. Young and middle-aged migrants may have to alter life plans and change careers, while concurrently caring for their children and aging parents.

Successful acculturation requires affiliation with individuals and groups from the receiving culture. Through these relationships, migrants learn the new culture. This learning involves decisions regarding what new norms and skills to acquire and what to leave behind. Continued contact with expatriate friends and relatives, who have been undergoing the same process, serves critical functions in processing the changes, exploring moral and identity issues, and garnering support (Chance 1965; Leung and Boehnlein 2005).

Relationship With the Clinical Problem

Questions 16 and 17 explore the links between the migration experience, the current situation in the new country, and the clinical problem being assessed. Chronology of migration can affect the type of psychiatric condition that develops. Adjustment disorders usually occur within several months of relocation, but they can also occur years later if acculturation is delayed. Anxiety and mood disorders tend to appear within the first years of relocation, whereas substance use disorders typically appear several years or more after relocation (Krupinski 1967). Psychosis may occur at any time in relation to migration. Paranoid symptoms and disorders occur more often in migrant patients than in persons in their native-born community (Kendler 1982). Because paranoid symptoms, such as mistrust or projected hostility, can occur with most conditions, clinicians must beware of overdiagnosing paranoid disorders in migrants. Paranoid symptoms tend to abate gradually over the first decade following relocation (Westermeyer 1989a). However, paranoid disorders, like other psychoses, can appear at any time following relocation. Secondary relocations following migration may be salutary but also can complicate adjustment if resources are lost and adjustment challenges remain unchanged.

Future Expectations

Despite the difficulties involved in migration, migrants often view it as a new beginning and have hopes and plans for the future. Including question 18 at the end of the interview brings perspective to the situation—that as hard as migration may be, it can be seen as a transition to a better future. Successful resettlement can produce many personal and social gains. The individual matures and gains greater appreciation of the self and others. Enhanced competence may pervade many aspects of daily life.

Challenges in Assessment

Various challenges are involved in the assessment of immigrants and refugees. Clarifying the reasons and context for an initial assessment is usually helpful. Collaboration with interpreters is critical for both migrants and clinicians. For both partners in the clinical dyad, the addition of one person triples the interpersonal complexity: from patient-clinician to interpreter-patient, interpreter-clinician, and patient-clinician (Mirdal et al. 2012; Westermeyer 1990). Clinicians must appreciate the challenge of translating culturally embedded emotional and symbolic terms (e.g., anxiety, depression, morale) contrasted with terms describing universal physical or physiological experiences (e.g., tachycardia, diarrhea, nightmares). Inquiry into less-than-universal experiences (e.g., delusions, hallucinations, fugue, delirium) requires special phrasing for each language and dialect. Some cultures require that a family member be present or nearby, especially if the patient-clinician dyad differs by gender.

Cultural transference can intrude, for good or ill (Comas-Díaz and Jacobsen 1991). The patient may overvalue the clinician's culture, leading to unrealistic expectations, or the patient's culture may have an unsavory political history or class conflict with the clinician's presumed ethnic group, creating a barrier to trust. Clinicians may likewise manifest cultural countertransference, which can impede and/or augment the clinician's commitment to the migrant patient. Useful clinician attributes in assessing and treating migrants include curiosity, open-mindedness, flexibility, creativity, acceptance, and previous cross-cultural experience in adapting to another society. The questions in the Patient-Clinician Relationship supplementary module may help the clinician explore this important aspect of care.

Obstacles to assessing distress and psychiatric disorders across cultural groups include language barriers; variations in cognitive and emotional schemata, social traditions, and cultural beliefs; and continued change in these variables as acculturation occurs (Lu et al. 1995). Efficiently and comprehensively integrating social science and psychiatric perspectives is essential in interviewing refugees and immigrants so that assessment is accurate and treatment is effective. For example, understanding how a particular cultural group interprets the symptoms of an illness and its appropriate treatment can facilitate adherence with appropriate treatment after migration (Harwood 1981). A cross-cultural interview, while maintaining a systems perspective, also should not lose sight of the uniqueness of each individual or family who has migrated in search of safety, security, and a better life.

Conclusion

The CFI, including the Immigrants and Refugees supplementary module, provides access to clinically relevant information useful in the care of migrants. Assessment using these tools reassures patients by including salient queries critical to understanding migrants and their dilemmas. The CFI informs the clinician's assessment, setting a realistic foundation for treatment planning. It enables clinicians to make recommendations, undertake negotiations, promote acceptance and adherence, and achieve an optimal clinical outcome.

KEY CLINICAL POINTS

- Important factors that influence mental health among immigrants and refugees include premigration difficulties, exposure to violence and persecution, the historical time frame of migration, migration-related losses and challenges, continued ties to the country of origin, resettlement and life in the new country, and future expectations.
- A cross-cultural assessment, while maintaining a systems perspective, should not lose sight of the uniqueness of each individual and family.

Questions

1. What are the most common challenges that immigrants and refugees encounter after migration?

2. What is the relevance of premigration challenges for postmigration adjustment?

3. What are some frequent losses experienced by refugees and immigrants, regardless of country of origin?

4. What are some factors that influence successful or unsuccessful acculturation?

5. What are frequent obstacles for clinicians in being able to accurately and efficiently assess immigrant and refugee mental health status?

References

Ahearn FL, Athey JL (eds): Refugee Children: Theory, Research, and Services. Baltimore, MD, Johns Hopkins University Press, 1991

Berry JW, Kim V, Minde T, et al: Comparative studies of acculturative stress. Int Migr Rev 21:491–511, 1987

Chance NA: Acculturation, self-identification and personality adjustment. Am Anthropol 67:372–393, 1965

Comas-Díaz L, Jacobsen FM: Ethnocultural transference and countertransference in the therapeutic dyad. Am J Orthopsychiatry 61(3):392–402, 1991 1951646

De Jesús-Rentas G, Boehnlein J, Sparr L: Central American victims of gang violence as asylum seekers: the role of the forensic expert. J Am Acad Psychiatry Law 38(4):490–498, 2010 21156907

Desjarlais RL, Eisenberg L, Good B, et al: World Mental Health: Problems and Priorities in Low-Income Countries. New York, Oxford University Press, 1995

Finch BK, Vega WA: Acculturation stress, social support, and self-rated health among Latinos in California. J Immigr Health 5(3):109–117, 2003 14512765

Harwood A: Ethnicity and Medical Care. Cambridge, MA, Harvard University Press, 1981

Hollifield M, Warner TD, Jenkins J, et al: Assessing war trauma in refugees: properties of the Comprehensive Trauma Inventory-104. J Trauma Stress 19(4):527–540, 2006 16929508

Kendler KS: Demography of paranoid psychosis (delusional disorder): a review and comparison with schizophrenia and affective illness. Arch Gen Psychiatry 39(8):890–902, 1982 7103678

Krupinski J: Sociological aspects of mental ill-health in migrants. Soc Sci Med 1:267–281, 1967

Leung PK, Boehnlein JK: Vietnamese families, in Ethnicity and Family Therapy, 3rd Edition. Edited by McGoldrick M, Giordano J, Garcia-Preto N. New York, Guilford, 2005 pp 363–373

Lu F, Lim R, Mezzich J: Issues in the assessment and diagnosis of culturally diverse individuals, in American Psychiatric Press Review of Psychiatry, Vol 14. Edited by Oldham JM, Riba MB. Washington, DC, American Psychiatric Press, 1995 pp 477–510

Mirdal GM, Ryding E, Essendrop Sondej M: Traumatized refugees, their therapists, and their interpreters: three perspectives on psychological treatment. Psychol Psychother 85(4):436–455, 2012 23080532

Silove D: The psychosocial effects of torture, mass human rights violations, and refugee trauma: toward an integrated conceptual framework. J Nerv Ment Dis 187(4):200–207, 1999 10221552

Silove D, Ekblad S: How well do refugees adapt after resettlement in Western countries? Acta Psychiatr Scand 106(6):401–402, 2002 12392482

Summerfield D: War and mental health: a brief overview. BMJ 321(7255):232–235, 2000 10903662

Westermeyer J: Paranoid symptoms and disorders among 100 Hmong refugees: a longitudinal study. Acta Psychiatr Scand 80(1):47–59, 1989a 2763859

Westermeyer J: The Psychiatric Care of Migrants: A Clinical Guide. Washington, DC, American Psychiatric Press, 1989b

Westermeyer J: Working with an interpreter in psychiatric assessment and treatment. J Nerv Ment Dis 178(12):745–749, 1990 2246648

Suggested Readings

Birman D, Chan WY: Screening and Assessing Immigrant and Refugee Youth in School-Based Mental Health Programs. Washington, DC, Center for Health and Health Care in Schools, 2008. Available at: http://www.rwjf.org/content/dam/farm/reports/issue_briefs/2008/rwjf29520. Accessed February 16, 2015.

Centers for Disease Control and Prevention: Immigrant and Refugee Health, 2013. Available at: http://www.cdc.gov/immigrantrefugeehealth/. Accessed February 16, 2015.

U.S. Citizenship and Immigration Services: Refugees & Asylum, 2011. Available at: http://www.uscis.gov/humanitarian/refugees-asylum. Accessed February 16, 2015.

Supplementary Module 12: Caregivers

Ladson Hinton, M.D.

Rita Hargrave, M.D.

Iqbal Ahmed, M.D.

Caregivers often play a central role in the lives of persons with mental illness. Caregivers perform a diverse set of roles, including providing emotional support and helping with decision making, participating in clinic visits, and helping with patient adherence to mental health treatment. For clinicians to most effectively engage, mobilize, and support informal helpers (i.e., immediate family, extended family, friends), they must understand how culture shapes the meanings, values, and activities associated with the caregiving role. For example, a Vietnamese caregiver for a patient with dementia in the United States may draw on concepts from Buddhism and Catholicism (e.g., karma, God's will) to make sense of her relative's dementia, to experience the caregiving role as an act of sacrifice and compassion, and to cope with her own personal suffering (Hinton et al. 2008). Awareness of these cultural orientations to caregiving would help the clinician support the caregiver in a culturally congruent fashion and understand her resigned and accepting view of the illness and of treatment (often glossed over as "fatalism" by health professionals). The Caregivers supplementary module of the DSM-5 (American Psychiatric Association 2013) Cultural Formulation Interview (CFI) is a tool to assist clinicians in the cultural assessment of caregiving, with the ultimate goal of promoting accurate diagnosis and treatment that are both patient and family centered. In this subchapter, we describe the rationale for the Caregivers module, summarize its contents, and propose guidelines for its clinical use.

Rationale for the Supplementary Module

Mental illness is experienced, expressed, and responded to within an interpersonal context that often includes family members, extended family, and friends or neigh-

---

The views expressed in this publication are those of the authors and do not reflect the official policy or position of the Department of the Army, Department of Defense, or the U.S. government.

bors (i.e., informal social networks). In many situations, members of the patient's informal network will be sources of emotional, instrumental, and material support in dealing with psychiatric symptoms, treatment, and recovery. Assessing caregiver perspectives and roles in the lives of persons with mental illness and, when appropriate, engaging them in the treatment process can be very important.

Caregivers can, for example, extend and augment mental health treatment in powerful ways, such as by providing collateral information, helping with treatment adherence, and monitoring psychiatric symptoms and medication side effects (Lefley 1996). Because mental health problems can take a substantial emotional, social, and financial toll on caregivers, clinicians need to assess the caregiver levels of burden and to offer support so that they do not "burn out" or suffer adverse health and/or mental health outcomes. Family caregivers of persons with dementia, for example, are at increased risk for depression and psychological distress, adverse physical health outcomes, and even cognitive decline (Liu and Gallagher-Thompson 2009; Schulz and Beach 1999; Vitaliano et al. 2003). Although caregivers experience considerable stress, they also report positive feelings about caregiving, including a sense of family togetherness, reciprocity, and satisfaction about helping others (Zarit 2012). When clinicians assess caregiving dynamics and roles, they are in a better position to intervene when caregivers negatively impact patients' mental health treatment (e.g., by providing depression psychoeducation when family members and friends discourage treatment or view depression as a moral failing rather than an illness). Clinicians need to keep in mind that individual caregivers may sometimes be a "double-edged sword" in the sense that they are acting in ways that both promote and hinder mental health care (Hinton et al. 2014).

How members of a patient's social network interpret and respond to mental health problems reflects their own cultural conceptions of health and illness, social role expectations, styles and norms of verbal and nonverbal communication, and orientations to health and mental health care (Knight and Sayegh 2010). These reactions matter for the course of illness. For example, expressed emotion, including both critical comments and limited expressions of warmth, influences the likelihood of rehospitalization among patients with schizophrenia (Jenkins and Karno 1992; López et al. 2004). Knowing how best to support caregivers requires understanding the role of culture in shaping caregiving-related roles, values, and ethics (Hinton et al. 1999). Although these cultural orientations are often shared by the caregiver and patient, increasingly in pluralistic and multicultural settings there may also be important differences within informal social networks.

Caregiving systems are often complex in structure and dynamics. At any given point in time, for example, a person with mental illness may rely on more than one person for help and support in dealing with his or her mental health problem. For example, a young Latina with schizophrenia may be accompanied to mental health visits by her sister but rely on her elderly mother for day-to-day help at home with medication adherence and on her husband for assistance with decision making. Patterns of caregiving may change over time, resulting in changes in caregiving roles and levels of involvement. Awareness of the distribution of different aspects of caregiving—emotional, instrumental, and material—will help clinicians navigate these informal systems of support.

Overview of the Supplementary Module

The Caregivers supplementary module (provided in Appendix C in this handbook) allows clinicians to explore important psychosocial issues that affect caregivers, such as their willingness to assume and accept the role of care provider, their reactions to their perceived obligation or choice to provide care, and their preferences for how formal services should be organized and delivered (Family Care Alliance 2006.). In contrast to the CFI–Informant Version (Appendix B in this handbook), which focuses on a caregiver's views about the patient's problem, the questions in the Caregivers supplementary module permit more specific exploration of the type of support the caregiver provides and the associated meanings, motivations, challenges, and rewards associated with this support.

The Caregivers module emphasizes four domains of assessment. The initial section of the module (questions 1 and 2) allows the clinician to better understand the nature and history of the caregiving relationship, including its duration and the connection of the caregiver to the patient (e.g., immediate family, extended family or nonfamilial support, paid or unpaid caregiver). Questions 3–8 focus on caregiving activities and cultural perceptions of caregiving; the respondent is asked to describe the nature and extent of the assistance he or she provides to the care recipient and to identify the positive and challenging aspects of the caregiving relationship. This second section of the module also encourages the respondent to articulate how cultural traditions and practices may influence his or her approach to caregiving. The caregiver is asked to assess whether his or her current activities are consistent with or at odds with the role expectations of most caregivers in the community. The information in this section can highlight potential sources of care-related strain. The third section (questions 9–11) focuses on the social context of caregiving. The caregiver is encouraged to outline his or her current coping strategies for managing the care recipient and to describe the extent and adequacy of support and assistance that he or she receives from family members, friends, or neighbors. The module concludes with questions 12–14, which explore the caregiver's expectations of the mental health system and his or her caregiving preferences. The module may be used in its entirety, or the clinician may select specific questions to include in the assessment.

Guidelines for Clinical Use of the Module

The person-centered process of administering the CFI–Informant Version and the Caregivers supplementary module, as well as the collaborative dialogue between the care recipient, health practitioner, and caregiver, is intended to enhance the cultural validity of the assessment process, facilitate treatment planning, and promote the engagement and satisfaction of the patient, his or her caregiver, and the rest of the support network. The information obtained from the module and the CFI–Informant Version is complementary and should be integrated with other clinical material to form the basis of a collaborative plan that includes attention to caregiver issues and is comprehensive and culturally relevant.

Prior to administering the Caregivers module, clinicians must decide whether, when, and how to engage informal caregivers in the diagnostic and treatment process. To inform these decisions, clinicians should consider 1) the availability of care-givers in the patient's life, 2) the patient's preferences for involvement of an informal caregiver in clinical care, and 3) the real or potential adverse effects of informal care-giver involvement in clinical care. We briefly discuss each of these considerations.

First, the clinician must determine whether the patient is relying on a caregiver for help in managing his or her mental health problem. In some situations, it may be quite clear that the patient relies heavily on a family member or friend for assistance. A patient may, for example, ask that a family member or friend accompanying him or her to the clinic be included in the clinical interview. In other situations, the clinician may first become aware of the role of informal helpers through the core CFI. For ex-ample, a patient with schizophrenia may mention that he or she lives with family members who help with medications and who often accompany him or her to the clinic.

Second, the clinician should assess whether the patient prefers to have an informal helper involved in the clinical encounter. The clinician should initiate a discussion with the patient about the involvement of a caregiver both as a source of collateral in-formation on the patient's situation and in terms of the caregiver's own views and ex-periences as a provider of care. This consultation with the patient may help the clinician respect his or her desire for autonomy and privacy and explore the reasons why the patient may not want family to be involved. This discussion may illuminate, for example, sources of family friction or conflict. It is important to remember that family involvement is not all or nothing; it is possible for family to be involved only in certain aspects of the diagnosis or treatment process. With a flexible and open ap-proach, clinicians are more likely to successfully navigate these social relationships to benefit treatment while respecting the wishes of the patient.

Finally, the clinician needs to consider the possible adverse impact of family mem-bers or other informal helpers on the patient's mental health treatment. Family mem-bers can impede treatment in a variety of ways, including discouraging initial care seeking or adherence to treatment, criticizing the patient or expressing stigmatizing views of mental illness, and disrupting communication during clinic visits. In the most extreme cases, dysfunctional relationships with informal caregivers may actu-ally trigger or amplify mental health symptoms. During the process of diagnostic as-sessment, clinicians will want to evaluate the roles of family members, assess potential pitfalls of family involvement, and identify clinical interventions to address these issues in order to enhance care. For example, a psychoeducational intervention may help family members view mental illness in less stigmatizing ways and improve how they communicate with the patient. The recommendations of the Patient Out-comes Research Team study of schizophrenia suggest that persons with this disorder who have ongoing contact with their families, including relatives and significant oth-ers, should be offered a family intervention. This intervention has been found to sig-nificantly reduce rates of relapse and rehospitalization (Dixon et al. 2010).

The Caregivers supplementary module can be used in conjunction with other CFI components, particularly the CFI–Informant Version. These two instruments are quite complementary. Whereas the CFI–Informant Version assesses the informant's views on the patient's illness and other aspects of the presented problem—essentially gathering all of the core CFI information from the informant's perspective—the Caregivers module assesses the meaning and impact of caregiving itself. It is important, however, for clinicians to recognize that most, but not all, informants will also be caregivers.

The Caregivers module may be used during the diagnostic interview or later in the course of treatment. For example, the clinician may become aware that a caregiver is distressed and seek to better understand his or her experience and the impact of caregiving on his or her well-being. Other supplementary modules may also elicit information to complement the Caregivers module, including the Social Network and Psychosocial Stressors modules. The Social Network module helps the clinician gather information about the patient's broader social network, including caregivers. This might be useful, for example, if the clinician is trying to identify family members who are not engaged in caregiving but might be mobilized to assist with some aspect of treatment. The Psychosocial Stressors module may be used to examine negative aspects of caregiving relationships, such as interpersonal conflicts with the caregiver. Both of these modules are administered to the patient and may provide important contextual information to guide the assessment of caregiving issues.

Like the core CFI, the Caregivers module encourages clinicians to use follow-up or rephrased questions as needed to clarify the respondent's answers. This module was designed to be a practical and flexible guide to cultural assessment, an aid to the elucidation of the respondent's perspective on caregiving, and a tool to promote rapport building and collaboration between the caregiver and the clinician. The clinician may choose to use all or only part of the module, depending on what components of the instrument seem most relevant to clinical care. Also, the clinician may choose to administer the module during the same visit as the core CFI or at subsequent visits, depending on the clinical situation.

In situations with multiple family members or caregivers, pragmatic decisions must be made about whom to interview based on patient preferences as well as caregivers' knowledge of the patient and the extent to which they are involved in day-to-day caregiving activities. However, each caregiver may raise different important cultural issues affecting care. For example, caregivers from apparently similar cultural backgrounds may be acculturated to the larger culture to varying degrees in a racial/ethnic minority or immigrant family, especially if they are from different generations, as presented in the vignettes below.

Caregiver assessment can be beneficial to caregivers at any stage of treatment. The CFI Caregivers module, like other caregiver assessment tools, should be used in the early stages of treatment to engage the caregiver as an active participant in the treatment planning process and to identify unmet psychosocial and service needs (Family Care Alliance 2006.). Some authors conceptualize caregiver assessment as an ongoing process and recommend periodic reassessment of family helpers. Family caregivers are frequently engaged in the process for several years, and their views and experiences may be affected by changes in the care recipient's and a caregiver's health and level of functioning, as well as family economic resources. Regular collaborative dialogues between clinicians and caregivers, guided by instruments such as the CFI, may identify critical areas of the treatment plan that require modification, highlight unmet needs of the caregiver and his or her support network, and assist in the evaluation of the effectiveness of the existing treatment plan (Family Care Alliance 2006.). The following vignettes illustrate approaches that the clinician may find useful in working with caregivers.

Case Vignette 1

Beatrice is a 78-year-old African American woman suffering from Alzheimer's disease, hypertension, and diabetes mellitus who was admitted to the hospital for delirium and confusion after she sustained a fall at her home. Beatrice's husband had been her primary caregiver until his death 6 months earlier. Her son John flew into town after she telephoned and told him, in a moaning voice, that the nurses were abusing her, giving her the wrong medications, and trying to poison her. John was irritable and confrontational with nursing staff and demanded to speak with the hospital administrator to secure better care for his mother. Even though he lived in another state 1,000 miles away, as the youngest of four children, he had been raised to accept his role in the family as his mother's primary caregiver. He resisted asking his siblings to help by increasing their participation in their mother's care. Like his mother, John believed that his siblings were not capable or strong enough to be effective advocates for her; he alone felt he could be responsible for her care.

In this situation, the Caregivers supplementary module could help clarify the extent and availability of the caregiving network and the adequacy of the primary caregiver's coping strategies for managing the care recipient. Resulting recommendations might include psychoeducation of the caregiver on the needs of older adults with cognitive decline and joint development of a strategy to increase collaboration between the caregiver, his family, the patient, and the medical staff.

Case Vignette 2

An Asian Indian family that had immigrated to the United States decided to bring the husband's mother from India to help diagnose growing signs of cognitive impairment. The patient was depressed, claiming that her daughter-in-law—the main caregiver—was not sufficiently respectful and deferential toward her. The daughter-in-law, a college graduate, had been raised in a fairly westernized family in a large Indian city, whereas her husband, an engineer, had been raised in a traditional family in a small Indian town. The daughter-in-law shared the family view that she had a filial responsibility to care for her husband's mother, but she felt that the expectations from both her husband and her mother-in-law were unreasonable. This led her to feel resentful as well as guilty about these feelings; she felt that she should be more assertive about her own "psychological needs." The couple's two children had been raised in the United States and were in high school. Although they occasionally helped their mother in caregiving activities, they could not understand why a professional caregiver could not be brought in to help. The husband felt that his job consumed his time and that, in any case, it was really his wife's role to take care of his mother, as had been the case in the community in which he was raised. The clashing family views led to marital conflict. The couple had a handful of Indian friends but no friends from the larger community; they were ashamed to discuss their problems with their Indian friends and decided to seek help from a psychiatrist of Indian background because they felt he might understand the cultural issues involved.

In this situation, the core CFI, the CFI–Informant Version, and the Caregivers supplementary module could help the clinician appreciate and disentangle the cultural perspectives of the patient, the primary caregiver (the daughter-in-law), and the secondary caregivers (the son and grandchildren). A culturally appropriate intervention would need to be formulated to address the family conflict, which is driven at least in part by cultural expectations about caregiving, and the nature of interpersonal relationships, including intergenerational expectations.

Conclusion

Family involvement in mental health care is widely recognized as a critical element for strengthening mental health interventions and services (Sederer and Sharfstein 2014). The Caregivers supplementary module and the CFI–Informant Version can help clinicians better understand the cultural dimensions of caregiving and connect with the experience of informal caregivers, including immediate family, extended family, and nonfamily helpers. Armed with this knowledge, clinicians will be better positioned to mobilize these social relationships to advance care, mitigate any negative effects of these relationships, and support and strengthen the caregiving systems.

KEY CLINICAL POINTS

- Care of patients often occurs in a larger social context, including informal caregivers such as family members.

- Cultural factors impact the perception of the illness, the meaning and value of caregiving, the relationship between the patient and the caregiver, and the availability of social support, all of which can affect caregiver burden.

- By assisting in the evaluation of these cultural factors, the Cultural Formulation Interview can help enhance the quality of patient care and reduce caregiver burden, leading to the use of culturally informed approaches.

Questions

1. What four domains of assessment does the CFI Caregivers supplementary module emphasize?

2. Prior to administering the Caregivers supplementary module, what issues do clinicians need to consider to guide decisions about whether, when, and how to engage informal caregivers in the diagnostic and treatment process?

3. What other supplementary modules may also elicit information to complement the Caregivers module?

4. How does the Caregivers supplementary module differ from the CFI–Informant Version?

5. To best support caregivers requires understanding the role in culture in what aspects of caregiving?

References

American Psychiatric Association: Diagnostic and Statistical Manual of Mental Disorders, 5th Edition. Arlington, VA, American Psychiatric Association, 2013

Dixon LB, Dickerson F, Bellack AS, et al: The 2009 schizophrenia PORT psychosocial treatment recommendations and summary statements. Schizophr Bull 36(1):48–70, 2010 19955389

Family Care Alliance: Caregiver Assessment: Principles, Guidelines and Strategies for Change. Report From a National Consensus Development Conference, Vol 1. San Francisco, CA, Family Care Alliance, 2006. Available at: https://www.caregiver.org/national-consensus-report-caregiver-assessment-volumes-1-2. Accessed May 14, 2014.

Hinton L, Tran JN, Tran C, et al: Religious and spiritual dimensions of the Vietnamese dementia caregiving experience. Hallym Int J Aging HIJA 10(2):139–160, 2008 20930949

Hinton L, Apesoa-Varano EC, Unützer J, et al: A descriptive qualitative study of the roles of family members in older men's depression treatment from the perspectives of older men and primary care providers. Int J Geriatr Psychiatry August 11, 2014 [Epub ahead of print] 25131709

Hinton WL, Fox K, Levkoff S: Introduction: exploring the relationships among aging, ethnicity, and family dementia caregiving. Cult Med Psychiatry 23(4):403–413, 1999 10647942

Jenkins JH, Karno M: The meaning of expressed emotion: theoretical issues raised by cross-cultural research. Am J Psychiatry 149(1):9–21, 1992 1728192

Knight BG, Sayegh P: Cultural values and caregiving: the updated sociocultural stress and coping model. J Gerontol B Psychol Sci Soc Sci 65B(1):5–13, 2010 19934166

Lefley HP: Family Caregiving in Mental Illness. Thousand Oaks, CA, Sage Publications, 1996

Liu W, Gallagher-Thompson D: Impact of dementia caregiving: risks, strains, and growth, in Aging Families and Caregiving. Edited by Qualls SH, Zarit SH. Hoboken, NJ, Wiley, 2009, pp 85–112

López SR, Nelson Hipke K, Polo AJ, et al: Ethnicity, expressed emotion, attributions, and course of schizophrenia: family warmth matters. J Abnorm Psychol 113(3):428–439, 2004 15311988

Schulz R, Beach SR: Caregiving as a risk factor for mortality: the Caregiver Health Effects Study. JAMA 282(23):2215–2219, 1999 10605972

Sederer LI, Sharfstein SS: Fixing the troubled mental health system. JAMA 312(12):1195–1196, 2014 25122559

Vitaliano PP, Zhang J, Scanlan JM: Is caregiving hazardous to one's physical health? A meta-analysis. Psychol Bull 129(6):946–972, 2003 14599289

Zarit SH: Positive aspects of caregiving: more than looking on the bright side. Aging Ment Health 16(6):673–674, 2012 22746192

Suggested Readings

Ahmed I, Kramer E (eds): Ethnic Minority Elderly Curriculum. Arlington, VA, American Psychiatric Association, 2014. Available at: http://www.psychiatry.org/practice/professional-interests/diversity/diversity-resources. Accessed May 15, 2014.

Family Care Alliance: Caregiver Assessment: Principles, Guidelines and Strategies for Change. Report From a National Consensus Development Conference, Vols 1 and 2. San Francisco, CA, Family Care Alliance, 2006. Available at: https://www.caregiver.org/

national-consensus-report-caregiver-assessment-volumes-1-2. Accessed May 15, 2014.

Kleinman A: From illness as culture to caregiving as moral experience. N Engl J Med 368:1376–1377, 2013

National Alliance on Mental Illness: http://www.nami.org

Yeo G, Gallagher-Thompson D: Ethnicity and the Dementias, 2nd Edition. New York, Routledge, Taylor and Francis Group, 2006

CHAPTER 4

Clinical Implementation of the Cultural Formulation Interview

Planning and Assessment

Neil Krishan Aggarwal, M.D., M.B.A., M.A.

This chapter addresses implementation of the DSM-5 (American Psychiatric Association 2013) Cultural Formulation Interview (CFI) within clinical practice. *Implementation* has been defined as "the process of putting to use or integrating evidence-based interventions within a setting," and a formal *implementation strategy* has been defined as "the systematic processes, activities, and resources that are used to integrate interventions into usual settings" (Rabin and Brownson 2012, pp. 26–27). My colleagues and I have made the case elsewhere that the CFI is an intervention in development (Aggarwal et al. 2014) if we define *interventions* as purposive change strategies that target malleable risk factors to produce positive outcomes (Fraser and Galinsky 2010). In the case of the CFI, clinicians are encouraged to target the malleable risk factors of misdiagnosis, treatment disengagement, and patient dissatisfaction through change strategies of open-ended questions on patient cultural views for diagnosis and treatment planning (American Psychiatric Association 2013).

Clinicians, administrators, and patients may wonder why an entire chapter on CFI implementation is necessary. However, implementation often exposes the gap between researchers who develop interventions and the clinicians who use them. The words of an article by scientists from the National Institutes of Health (NIH)—the largest funder of biomedical research in the United States—remind readers that most funding is spent on developing interventions rather than studying their use: "[F]or each dollar spent in discovery, mere pennies are spent learning how interventions known to be effective can be better disseminated" (Glasgow et al. 2012, p. 1274). In fact, it takes 17 years to translate 14% of original research into interventions benefiting patient care (Balas and Boren 2000). At various points throughout this time period, granting priorities can change for research funding, publications may be rejected from peer-reviewed journals, study findings may not be synthesized in textbooks and practice guidelines, and interventions may not be disseminated even when they are found to produce positive outcomes (Green et al. 2009). Keeping in mind that the CFI represents a revision of the Outline for Cultural Formulation (OCF) that was originally published in DSM-IV (American Psychiatric Association 1994), one can appreciate the length of time needed to develop an intervention through iterative revisions and to achieve its eventual clinical implementation. In addition, overviews have discussed how clinical implementation is not simply a matter of "changing physician behavior." For example, clinic administrators have named general barriers to implementing interventions, such as the relevance of research interventions to real-world practices, scattered information about interventions, difficulties in assessing the quality of research evidence, training costs, provider resistance, and burdensome workloads (Proctor et al. 2007). Work from the DSM-5 field trial revealed that health providers report concerns about the unclear relevance of culture to treatment planning, training costs, and burdensome workloads as anticipated barriers to CFI use (Aggarwal et al. 2013b; American Psychiatric Association 2013). For this reason, my colleagues and I believe that a clear implementation strategy may help clinicians and administrators bridge the research-practice gap in introducing the CFI within clinical settings. The need to consider implementation issues from the beginning of developing an intervention around the CFI also falls in line with NIH funding priorities to consider real-world needs in all steps of research (Carroll and Rounsaville 2003; Nunes et al. 2010).

Aside from the research-practice gap, implementers of interventions also encounter structural barriers. The public health systems in many countries consist of a network of government health agencies with laws, regulations, and priorities that vary by administrative level (local, state, national), hindering implementation if there is not systematic coordination (Stamatakis et al. 2012). Clinical experience with the OCF has shown that implementation conforms to the exigencies of delivering care within service constraints. For example, although there is worldwide interest in the OCF (see Chapter 1, "Cultural Formulation Before DSM-5"), the lack of a coordinated implementation strategy has led to different service models for OCF use. These service models range from individual outpatient clinicians who ask patients direct questions through OCF-based interviews to an entire cultural consultation service with over 50 culture and linguistic brokers at McGill University in Montreal, Quebec, Canada. No data are available on whether the OCF has been used within private practice settings. This fractured approach to OCF implementation has prevented generalizations about clinician experience or standardization in the collection of research data (Lewis-Fernández et al. 2014).

This chapter, therefore, presents two possible CFI implementation strategies, one for clinicians and one for organizational teams, the two groups of stakeholders ultimately responsible for delivering culturally competent care to patients. Implementation research has grown over the past decade, with hundreds of researchers, thousands of peer-reviewed publications, and billions of research dollars awarded to such projects, many with competing theoretical backgrounds and implementation strategies (Colditz 2012). One systematic review identified 68 discrete strategies to plan, educate, finance, restructure, and evaluate the implementation of an intervention within general health care settings (Powell et al. 2012), although only 11 studies tested such strategies for mental health interventions (Powell et al. 2014). The tenet that connects this disparate work throughout implementation science is a focus on understanding what, why, and how interventions work in real-world clinical settings with populations that will ultimately be affected (Peters et al. 2013). Given the real-world emphasis in implementation work, the research climate has shifted from a previous model in which knowledge was seen to flow unidirectionally from researchers to clinicians and administrators in favor of a more equitable model of exchange in which all stakeholders contribute to and gain from collaboration (Proctor et al. 2009). Evidence-based practices originating from researchers must be combined with practice-based evidence originating from clinicians to promote valid research, policy, and practice (Chambers and Azrin 2013). Therefore, clinicians and administrators play crucial roles in the adoption of any CFI implementation strategy. In keeping with the multidisciplinary nature of implementation science, the goal in this chapter is not to favor one perspective over another but rather to provide two such CFI implementation strategies for clinicians, administrators, and researchers and the organizational teams they develop.

CFI Implementation Strategies for Individuals and Teams

Implementation strategies have been called the how-to component of changing health care practice when new interventions are introduced in clinical settings (Proctor et al. 2013). Proctor et al. (2013) have proposed minimum standards for implementation strategies containing sufficient detail that interventions can be adopted in practice, scientifically tested, and communicated clearly among clinicians, administrators, and researchers. This chapter uses these standards to envision a template for implementing the CFI in diverse clinical settings. Clinical settings in which the CFI is introduced may vary widely. Organizations have their own cultures and social structures, so administrators will need to assign personnel responsible for implementing the CFI successfully. However, certain characteristics are common across all settings: for example, it is the clinician who administers the CFI to the patient, not vice versa.

A crucial component in any implementation strategy is the extent to which the intervention has been delivered with fidelity, as intended by the developers of the intervention. If this fidelity is not evaluated, the impact of an intervention on health outcomes cannot be known: any effects on outcomes can result from the science of the intervention itself or from the strategy used to implement the intervention (Carroll et al. 2007). For this reason, monitoring and evaluating fidelity to an implementation strategy can point to both successful practices that should be retained and less successful practices eligible for quality improvement. The process of implementation can be divided into four phases: development, training, execution, and evaluation. Measuring fidelity through each phase can help to troubleshoot barriers as they arise and to identify unique threats to fidelity by phase. To assist measurement of CFI fidelity, the Cultural Formulation Interview–Fidelity Instrument (CFI-FI) is introduced, which has been tailored to the ultimate version of the core CFI included in DSM-5. The development and psychometric properties of the CFI-FI followed rigorous research standards, which are presented by Aggarwal et al. (2014). In this chapter, the focus is on measuring CFI fidelity throughout the implementation phases of training, execution, and evaluation. Fidelity should be measured effectively to assess desirable performance and efficiently to prevent resource strain (Schoenwald et al. 2011), and the CFI-FI accomplishes both tasks.

In line with Proctor et al.'s (2013) recommendations, CFI implementation strategies for individuals and teams along seven dimensions whose clarity would concretely operationalize implementation are discussed: 1) actors, 2) action, 3) action target, 4) temporality, 5) dose, 6) implementation outcomes affected, and 7) justification. Table 4–1 presents definitions for each of these seven dimensions. A side-by-side comparison demonstrates how an implementation strategy can differ for individual clinicians administering the CFI compared to a CFI implementation team with various stakeholders. Each dimension of these implementation strategies is explained below in greater detail.

Actor(s)

The actors involved in a CFI implementation strategy would differ for individual clinicians and implementation teams. Individual clinicians may wish to implement the CFI either without administrative support—as in private practice—or without organizational resources, such as time and funding, when they are not immediately obtainable. The actors involved in implementation strategies for individual clinicians would be the clinicians themselves. Implementation strategies for individual clinicians may provide direct performance feedback through the use of rating instruments such as the CFI-FI. At the same time, implementation strategies for individual clinicians may not consider organizational resources that can aid implementation through coordinated support from multiple actors.

Implementation strategies at the team level may involve actors from different backgrounds who wish to introduce the CFI throughout an organization. Different functions of a CFI implementation strategy may require individuals with different skill sets and professional backgrounds. For example, individual clinicians will be ultimately responsible for delivering the CFI to patients. At the same time, a CFI implementation team may be composed of various individuals, such as administrators who can oversee clinical use, outside consultants who may be involved in auditing, and payers who maximize financial resources to encourage implementation. Training needs could also

TABLE 4–1. Specification of sample Cultural Formulation Interview (CFI) implementation strategies

Dimension	Definition	Strategy: individual clinicians using the CFI	Strategy: CFI implementation team
Actor(s)	Stakeholder(s) who deliver(s) the implementation strategy	Individual clinicians who are trained to deliver the CFI to patients	A team of clinicians and administrators wishing to implement the CFI throughout an organization
Action	Steps, processes, and sequences of behavior outlined in the implementation strategy	Clinicians should be trained in the CFI and supervised to ensure that the CFI is delivered with fidelity.	CFI team should reflect on how the CFI is being implemented within the organization by sharing lessons learned, supporting learning and training programs, and proposing changes as necessary.
Target of action	Party thought to be affected by the implementation strategy	Individual clinicians using the CFI with patients; targets of action can be measured through the *clinician competence* and *intervention distinctness* subscales of the CFI-FI*	All clinicians trained in the CFI and organizational stakeholders such as administrators who ensure implementation
Temporality	Order or sequence of the implementation strategy	Clinicians should 1) be trained in the CFI, 2) be supervised for CFI fidelity with a test case soon after training, and 3) use the CFI in practice.	CFI implementation team would determine the exact order and schedule for the implementation.
Dose	Intensity of certain implementation components, such as the time spent in training and the frequency of audit or feedback	For training, dose is the amount of protected organizational time spent learning the CFI; for execution, dose is measured by the number of core CFI questions asked as rated by the CFI-FI*; for evaluation, dose is the amount of time that the organization provides feedback.	CFI implementation team would determine the time spent for each implementation step.
Implementation outcomes	Effects of deliberate and purposive actions to implement interventions in health care settings	CFI uptake, penetration among eligible patients, and fidelity of CFI implementation*	CFI uptake, penetration among eligible patients, fidelity to the CFI, long-term sustainability, and costs*
Justification	Justification or rationale for strategies used to implement an intervention	Asking patients about their cultural views on topics covered by the CFI may improve satisfaction with the provider and participation in treatment.	Cooperative learning theory may aid the entire team with implementation at the organizational level.

Note. CFI-FI=Cultural Formulation Interview–Fidelity Instrument.
*See subsection on this dimension in text.

vary depending on whether the organization hires employees to monitor needs internally or contracts training to outside parties. To optimize chances that clinicians will implement the CFI, administrators should assign implementation functions matched to knowledge, skills, and organizational responsibilities. The strengths of a team-based approach can be peer support and formal institutional policies around implementation, although more costs and personnel may be needed to implement the CFI at a team level than at the individual level. Individuals and organizations can determine which implementation strategies to use based on available resources to optimize successful CFI fidelity.

Action

Ideally, actions are itemized in detail before an implementation strategy is operational to increase the likelihood of successful implementation (Proctor et al. 2013). Training clinicians in the use of the CFI is an essential component for implementation strategies at both individual and team levels. Clinicians should be trained in the use of the CFI through a formal session that consists of four components: 1) reviewing the CFI's written guidelines in DSM-5, 2) observing a simulation of the CFI in use, 3) simulating the CFI through practice cases, and 4) asking questions for clarification. These four training modalities help guarantee that psychosocial and behavioral interventions are disseminated in a standard fashion with a training protocol that can be replicated in diverse organizations (Rounsaville et al. 2001). These modalities help to ensure that the CFI is delivered with fidelity through rigorous quality control.

Some have questioned whether all four modalities of training are actually necessary given the resources needed (e.g., opportunity costs of productivity), especially with the introduction of newer technologies that can scale up training (Beidas et al. 2011). Nonetheless, there is now consensus that passively watching presentations and video demonstrations—known as the "train and hope" approach (Henggeler et al. 2002)—may change clinician knowledge but do not necessarily change clinician behavior without behavioral simulations and small group discussions that provide feedback on active performance (Beidas et al. 2012; Dimeff et al. 2009; Miller et al. 2004). The gold standard array of passive and active learning modalities has been used in training clinicians for the DSM-5 CFI field trial. It is an open question whether a particular mix of training modalities improves clinician CFI fidelity, and organizations that implement the CFI may not have the resources to complete all four training modalities. In all instances, we recommend that the actors responsible for executing the CFI implementation strategy—whether individual clinicians or entire implementation teams—first identify training modalities that match their needs and resources.

After training has been completed, supervisors can assess clinicians on their fidelity to the CFI. Systematic reviews have shown that fidelity has been measured through the following five constructs (Dusenbury et al. 2003):

1. Clinician adherence to methods—the extent to which the implementation of intervention activities and methods corresponds with written instructions
2. Clinician competence—the extent to which a provider delivers intervention content in a way that is considered ideal by intervention developers

3. Participant responsiveness—the extent to which participants are engaged by and involved in the intervention
4. Intervention distinctness—core principles specified to ensure the uniqueness of an intervention so that it can be reliably differentiated from other interventions
5. Dosage—the amount of intervention received by participants

Researchers at the New York State Psychiatric Institute have tested how each of these five subscales could be used to measure CFI fidelity with New York City participants in the DSM-5 field trial. We found that raters who evaluated fidelity by listening to interviews independently (not with each other) reached the same score (*interrater reliability*) in over 60% of their ratings for the first four subscales: 1) clinician adherence to CFI question topic, 2) clinician competence throughout the overall interview, 3) participant (i.e., patient) responsiveness, and 4) intervention distinctness (Aggarwal et al. 2014). The value of 60% has traditionally been a benchmark of high interrater reliability that produces dependable ratings (Grove et al. 1981). (A full rater's manual is available via e-mail from the author.) Tables 4–2 and 4–3 present a revision of the CFI-FI keyed to the core CFI included in DSM-5; the field trial version differed slightly.

Modifications to interventions, training protocols, and fidelity measures should change based on ongoing intervention development; just as interventions change, so should fidelity measures because "one size cannot fit all" (Carroll and Nuro 2002). Consequently, the CFI-FI below has been updated to include topics that were added after completion of data collection in the DSM-5 field trial. Tables 4–2 and 4–3 make up the two parts of the revised CFI-FI. Table 4–2 rates fidelity by core CFI question, whereas Table 4–3 rates the quality of the clinician's delivery by examining general factors throughout the interview. My colleagues and I believe that both checklists should be used together for a holistic understanding of fidelity throughout the CFI session.

Different constructs of fidelity yield separate types of information, each of which is valuable in its own right. For example, it may be intuitive that clinician adherence to the CFI hews closely to the content and order of the CFI topics. In developing the CFI-FI, however, we found that patient responsiveness can affect clinician adherence because patients suffering from serious mental illness may not answer cultural questions relevantly because of cognitive burden (Aggarwal 2012); therefore, clinicians may eventually stop asking CFI questions if patients do not answer or if they provide answers that are not relevant (Aggarwal et al. 2014). In these situations, the CFI-FI allows clinicians and administrators to identify points throughout the CFI when adherence to individual questions waned based on patient responsiveness.

Similarly, the core CFI (see Appendix A of this handbook) has been designed with questions in a specific order and is intended to produce cultural information that influences the direction of the subsequent standard clinical assessment. The serial order of questions and the information covered in each cultural topic distinguish the core CFI from other types of intake interviews. The CFI-FI assumes that the CFI will be delivered in order and in its entirety. Future work can determine whether this approach is the best way to rate fidelity or whether there are better ways. For example, clinicians may find that interspersing sections of the standard clinical assessment with the

TABLE 4–2.   Cultural Formulation Interview–Fidelity Instrument subscales of clinician adherence and patient responsiveness

CFI-FI question based on core CFI topic	Clinician adherence: Did the clinician ask a core CFI question about...[a]	Patient responsiveness: Did the patient answer about...[b]
1. The patient's presented problem?		
2. The patient's description of the problem to members of the patient's social network?		
3. The severity of the problem? (The patient may not be experiencing any severity at all, and this should still be coded.)		
4. The causes of the problem from the patient's perspective?		
5. The causes of the problems from the perspective of the patient's social network?		
6. What makes the problem better?		
7. What makes the problem worse?		
8. The most important aspects of the patient's background or identity?		
9. How identity relates to the patient's presented problem?		
10. How identity relates to other concerns or difficulties?		
11. Self-coping?		
12. Past help seeking?		
13. Barriers to care?		
14. The patient's current treatment preferences?		
15. Current treatment preferences from the perspective of the patient's social network?		
16. Concerns about the clinician-patient relationship?		
Total		

Note.   CFI-FI=Cultural Formulation Interview–Fidelity Instrument.
[a]Ratings: 0=no; 1=yes.
[b]Ratings: 0=no; 1=response not relevant to core CFI topic; 2=response relevant to core CFI topic.

TABLE 4–3. **Cultural Formulation Interview–Fidelity Instrument subscales of clinician competence and intervention distinctiveness**

CFI-FI fidelity construct	Clinician score[a]
Clinician competence	
Empathy: Did the clinician paraphrase or name the patient's emotional state?	
Patient centeredness: Did the clinician maintain a nonjudgmental attitude (not arguing, confronting, or correcting the patient)?	
Clarification: Did the clinician ask follow-up questions to understand unclear patient responses?	
Illness narration: Did the clinician's interactions help the patient construct and explore a narrative account of illness, or did the clinician seem to rush through the core CFI?	
Total	
Intervention distinctness	
Drift: Did the clinician stick to the CFI questions and *not* ask about topics that typically belong to the standard clinical interview (history of present illness, current medications, detailed psychiatric or medical history, family history, social history, Mini-Mental Status Examination)?	
Order: Did the clinician ask about all topics in order as reflected in the core CFI clinician guidelines?	
Total	

Note. CFI-FI=Cultural Formulation Interview–Fidelity Instrument.
[a]Ratings: 0=no; 1=throughout less than half of the interview; 2=throughout more than half of the interview.

core CFI improves its implementation compared with asking all questions in strict, successive order.

Finally, the elements that measure clinician competence can be seen as the extent to which clinicians elicit complete and accurate responses to the CFI questions. Clinician competence is not rated by question because some patients answer questions to such a degree of completion that clinicians do not need to ask follow-up questions (Aggarwal et al. 2014). For example, patients may describe the problem from their point of view as well as from the perspectives of close associates such as family or friends, obviating the need for the clinician to ask this follow-up question. In addition, my colleagues and I realized that dose—measured as time length of the core CFI—was not a good measure of fidelity because some clinicians would not redirect patients who answered tangentially, thereby increasing the time needed to complete the core CFI and overall interview, whereas other clinicians could complete the core CFI and standard assessment within a typical 1-hour session (Aggarwal et al. 2014).

Because the constructs differ conceptually and by scoring method, spaces are provided on the CFI-FI for separate total scores rather than an overall score. Ratings are not tallied for the entire CFI-FI but for the individual constructs of clinician adherence, clinician competence, patient responsiveness, and intervention distinctness. We encourage raters to familiarize themselves with the CFI-FI before rating fidelity for more accurate ratings.

The CFI-FI assesses fidelity at the patient-clinician level. This fidelity measurement may suffice for implementation strategies tailored to individual clinicians. However, implementation strategies at the team level may require additional measures of fidelity. Proctor et al. (2013) specifically refer to audit and feedback measures to assess what has been completed and what remains to be done throughout all steps of the implementation process. Audit and feedback measures have been defined as summaries of clinical performance over a specified period of time, and they are particularly effective in situations where there is low baseline adherence to practice and when feedback can be delivered intensively (Jamtvedt et al. 2006). Audit and feedback measures influence clinical practice when information is presented close to the time of clinical decision making and when participants have agreed to receive such feedback rather than viewing it as an imposition (Mugford et al. 1991). My colleagues and I recommend that CFI implementation teams actively incorporate audit and feedback measures within implementation strategies to foster skill development and satisfaction among all organizational stakeholders.

Target of Action

Implementation strategies should specify the targets of an intervention to help focus the strategy and suggest how outcomes can be measured (Proctor et al. 2013). For this reason, the CFI implementation strategies presented in this section vary by emphases in their stated targets of action. An implementation strategy targeting individual clinicians using the CFI with individual patients could focus on training and fidelity. Training with the CFI is intended to increase practitioner knowledge and skill, whereas fidelity checklists evaluate competence in administering the CFI after training. The CFI-FI measures of clinician competence in Table 4–3 may fulfill this need.

In contrast, an implementation strategy at the team level may include several stakeholders. For instance, the organization may want information from patients and administrators as well as from clinicians. Information from patients may come in the form of satisfaction surveys and scales about clinicians' CFI use in practice. This type of information would communicate how the CFI was received among intended beneficiaries; this target of action differs from clinician training and fidelity. As another example, an implementation team may want to ask administrators about CFI use in an organizational context related to time needed for completion, potential scheduling concerns, billing procedures, and other practices that do not directly relate to the CFI as an intervention but are, nonetheless, instrumental to its implementation. Review of implementation and dissemination models has shown that implementation strategies typically target more than one stakeholder to provide comprehensive information (Tabak et al. 2012), and organizations implementing the CFI may find that information from multiple stakeholders clarifies decision making. For example, if clinicians deliver the CFI with fidelity but administrator feedback indicates difficulties with scheduling due to increased time spent per patient, then implementation teams can deliberate over how to use the CFI more efficiently.

Temporality

Temporality refers to the sequence of steps in an implementation strategy. An implementation strategy focused on clinicians might begin with CFI training, followed by supervision with one case through ratings of fidelity and then implementation with patients. This sequence of steps corresponds to general frameworks for introducing interventions to clinicians when fidelity is vital to prevent intervention drift (Carroll and Nuro 2002; Gearing et al. 2011; Rounsaville et al. 2001). Active feedback to clinicians through CFI-FI ratings may improve practice if provided soon after the first case. This temporality also may make intuitive sense: attempts to measure CFI fidelity may be met with resistance without a prior training session.

Similarly, a CFI implementation team may benefit from planning the sequence of steps necessary for an implementation strategy. Models of implementation can differ with respect to the number of exact steps needed to introduce and sustain an intervention in health care settings, but they all involve planning, executing, and evaluating (Proctor et al. 2013). A CFI implementation team can map out the sequence of steps with start and end dates to assess whether any step takes longer than anticipated and how members of the team can respond to implementation barriers.

Dose

A persistent question in research on intervention development and implementation science concerns the amount of the intervention delivered by clinicians and received by beneficiaries (Gearing et al. 2011; Rounsaville et al. 2001). Unlike medications, psychosocial interventions—including interviews such as the CFI and specialized forms of psychotherapy such as cognitive-behavioral therapy—do not come from a single manufacturer who can guarantee quality, so dose (or intensity) depends on the skills of the implementer (Carroll and Nuro 2002; Rounsaville et al. 2001). Researchers and practitioners involved with any intervention should measure dose so that others can learn about the minimal dose needed to achieve the strongest effect (Proctor et al. 2013).

A CFI implementation strategy can measure dose in two ways, depending on the level of implementation. For individual clinicians, dose can be measured by completing the CFI-FI checklist in Table 4–2, rating the clinician's adherence to asking each of the 16 questions in the core CFI. At the organization level, dose can be measured through the sequence of steps outlined in the "Temporality" section. Key variables include the time and intensity spent on training, the time and intensity of the phase when the CFI is implemented, and the time and frequency of audit and feedback measures (Proctor et al. 2013).

Implementation Outcomes

The multidisciplinary nature of implementation and dissemination science has led practitioners and researchers to propose multiple outcomes, often without clear definitions and means of measurement (Grimshaw et al. 2006). For this reason, implementation scientists have suggested a common taxonomy to measure *implementation outcomes*—defined as the effects of deliberate, purposive actions to implement new interventions—so that implementers can evaluate implementation success and intermediary processes (Proctor et al. 2011). This framework has informed analyses of CFI feasibility and acceptability among patients and clinicians in the DSM-5 field trial (Aggarwal et al. 2013a; Lewis-Fernández et al. 2014); Table 4–4 presents these outcomes based on the work of Proctor et al. (2011). The "Level of Analysis" column indicates at what levels this information can promote implementation strategies: consumer, clinician, and organization.

Implementation strategies need not target every single implementation outcome, but they should be explicit in which outcomes are selected, how they are measured, and at what phase of implementation they are measured (Proctor et al. 2013). This perspective can inform how CFI implementation teams select suitable outcomes for measurement. For example, in the planning phase of CFI implementation, interviews with clinicians and administrators may clarify outcomes of *acceptability* (whether people like the CFI) and *appropriateness* (whether the CFI is seen as relevant). In the execution phase, *fidelity* can be measured after training via CFI-FI ratings, *adoption* can indicate how many providers are using the CFI, and *feasibility* can suggest whether and which providers think that the CFI is practical or not within service constraints. In the evaluation phase, *penetration* may be measured by examining the numbers of providers who use the CFI or the numbers of patients with whom the CFI has been used after an initial trial period, whereas *sustainability* would focus on the integration and routinization of the CFI within everyday practice. At all implementation phases, administrators may want to assess *cost*.

Stakeholders may also differ in their perceptions of which implementation outcomes are pertinent (Proctor et al. 2011). For example, *cost* may be most important to service administrators, *feasibility* to providers, *acceptability* to patients, and *fidelity* to trainers and CFI developers. For this reason, the two sample CFI implementation strategies compared in Table 4–1 emphasize slightly different outcomes. Both implementation strategies would ideally address *CFI uptake, penetration among eligible patients,* and *fidelity of CFI implementation*. In addition, implementation strategies for CFI teams may also focus on *long-term sustainability* and *costs,* especially to address human resources issues that may not concern individual clinicians, such as ongoing staff training, staff attrition, and rehiring. Clarity about which implementation outcomes are being measured, at what implementation phase, and through which specific measurements may help CFI clinicians, administrators, and researchers to evolve a common language and comparative framework.

Justification

Proctor et al. (2013) recommend that clinicians, administrators, and researchers justify any intervention and associated implementation strategies so that potential needs, barriers, and facilitators related to implementation can be addressed to promote practice change. This rationale can be applied to the two implementation strategies focused on clinicians and organizations in Table 4–1. For example, research demonstrates that interventions by clinicians on patient cultural views increase patient participation throughout the interview, clinician-patient information exchange,

TABLE 4–4. Implementation outcomes for a Cultural Formulation Interview (CFI) implementation strategy

Implementation outcome	Definition	Level of analysis	Implementation stage	Methods for measurement
Acceptability	Perception among implementation stakeholders that the CFI is agreeable	Individual provider or individual consumer	All stages	Surveys, interviews, or administrative data
Adoption	Intention or initial decision to use the CFI in practice	Individual provider or organization	Early to middle	Surveys, interviews, or administrative data
Appropriateness	Perceived fit or relevance of the CFI for a given setting, provider, or consumer	Individual provider, individual consumer, or organization	Early (before actual adoption)	Surveys, interviews, or focus groups
Cost	Resources necessary to implement the CFI	Organization	All stages	Administrative data
Feasibility	Extent to which the CFI can be successfully used within practice constraints	Individual provider or organization	Early (during adoption)	Surveys, interviews, or administrative data
Fidelity	Degree to which the CFI was implemented as intended	Individual provider	Early to middle	Checklists (CFI-FI), observation, self-report
Penetration	Integration of the CFI within the service setting	Organization	Middle to late	Case audit, checklists
Sustainability	Extent to which the CFI is maintained or institutionalized in an ongoing, stable manner	Organization	Late	Case audit, interviews, checklists

Note. CFI-FI = Cultural Formulation Interview–Fidelity Instrument.
Source. Adapted from Proctor et al. 2011.

interpersonal rapport, and overall patient satisfaction (Newes-Adeyi et al. 2004; Paw-likowska et al. 2012; Roter et al. 2012; Tibaldi et al. 2011). In interviews with patients and clinicians participating in the DSM-5 field trials, the CFI was shown to improve patient satisfaction throughout the interview, obtain information necessary for diagnosis and treatment, elicit the patient's perspective, and help clinicians piece together information (Aggarwal et al. 2013a). My colleagues and I believe that these findings justify implementation of the CFI among clinicians. Similarly, organizational implementation strategies should be based on relevant theory, empirical evidence, and/or practical data (such as low costs or ease of implementation) (Proctor et al. 2013). Proctor et al. (2013) recommend cooperative learning theory as a justification for implementation strategies. Cooperative learning differs from competitive or individual learning in that stakeholders work together to accomplish common goals that are 1) explained through clear objectives, 2) discussed in small groups, and 3) emphasized through individual accountability (Johnson et al. 1998). We agree that this approach may help stakeholders advance CFI implementation. For example, groups of clinicians and administrators can separately discuss factors that enhance or detract from CFI implementation, sharing tips on what has worked and not worked to encourage positive information exchange and group interdependence. Groups meeting on a set schedule can serve as a mechanism for internal checks and balances in the form of an audit-and-feedback measure. CFI implementation strategies that are not based on a justification that convinces relevant stakeholders are likely to encounter resistance.

Conclusion

In this chapter, two sample CFI implementation strategies based on Proctor et al.'s (2013) guidelines to specify and report elements that are crucial to the implementation of any intervention have been recommended. My colleagues and I have selected this framework because it represents the first attempt to identify and standardize common elements of successful implementation strategies. Our purpose has not been to favor this framework over others but to evolve a common framework for clinicians, administrators, and researchers interested in the CFI. The use of CFI implementation strategies can help promote understanding of what steps and processes may be useful in implementing the CFI within particular contexts through detailed descriptions. Such understanding about which CFI implementation strategies work and why can inform clinical practice and future research questions on what needs adaptation to safeguard implementation success.

KEY CLINICAL POINTS

- Implementation science can help clinicians and administrators implement the Cultural Formulation Interview (CFI) within clinical practice.
- Implementation strategies can be customized for those responsible for implementing the CFI into their unique practice setting.

- Implementation strategies can predetermine what outcomes are most important to measure.
- The Cultural Formulation Interview–Fidelity Instrument can be used to measure how well and how completely the CFI was administered.

Questions

1. What is implementation science and how can it help with implementing the CFI in practice settings?

2. What are implementation strategies and how can they be used to implement the CFI?

3. What are the seven dimensions common to all implementation strategies?

4. How do implementation strategies for the CFI differ for individual clinicians and implementation teams?

4. What are the subscales of the Cultural Formulation Interview–Fidelity Instrument?

References

Aggarwal NK: The psychiatric cultural formulation: translating medical anthropology into clinical practice. J Psychiatr Pract 18(2):73–85, 2012 22418398

Aggarwal NK, DeSilva R, Nicasio AV, et al: Does the Cultural Formulation Interview for the fifth revision of the Diagnostic and Statistical Manual of Mental Disorders (DSM-5) affect medical communication? A qualitative exploratory study from the New York site. Ethn Health Nov 2013a [Epub ahead of print]

Aggarwal NK, Nicasio AV, DeSilva R, et al: Barriers to implementing the DSM-5 Cultural Formulation Interview: a qualitative study. Cult Med Psychiatry 37(3):505–533, 2013b 23836098

Aggarwal NK, Glass A, Tirado A, et al: The development of the DSM-5 Cultural Formulation Interview-Fidelity Instrument (CFI-FI): a pilot study. J Health Care Poor Underserved 25(3):1397–1417, 2014 25130248

American Psychiatric Association: Diagnostic and Statistical Manual of Mental Disorders, 4th Edition. Washington, DC, American Psychiatric Publishing, 1994

American Psychiatric Association: Diagnostic and Statistical Manual of Mental Disorders, 5th Edition. Arlington, VA, American Psychiatric Publishing, 2013

Balas EA, Boren SA: Managing clinical knowledge for health care improvement, in Yearbook of Medical Informatics 2000. Edited by van Bemmel JH. Stuttgart, Germany, Schattauer, 2000, pp 65–70

Beidas RS, Koerner K, Weingardt KR, et al: Training research: practical recommendations for maximum impact. Adm Policy Ment Health 38(4):223–237, 2011 21380792

Beidas RS, Edmunds JM, Marcus SC, et al: Training and consultation to promote implementation of an empirically supported treatment: a randomized trial. Psychiatr Serv 63(7):660–665, 2012 22549401

Carroll C, Patterson M, Wood S, et al: A conceptual framework for implementation fidelity. Implement Sci 2:40–49, 2007 18053122

Carroll KM, Nuro KF: One size cannot fit all: a stage model for psychotherapy manual development. Clinical Psychology: Science and Practice 9:396–406, 2002

Carroll KM, Rounsaville BJ: Bridging the gap: a hybrid model to link efficacy and effectiveness research in substance abuse treatment. Psychiatr Serv 54(3):333–339, 2003 12610240

Chambers DA, Azrin ST: Research and services partnerships: partnership: a fundamental component of dissemination and implementation research. Psychiatr Serv 64(6):509–511, 2013 23728600

Colditz GA: The promise and challenges of dissemination and implementation research, in Dissemination and Implementation Research in Health: Translating Science to Practice. Edited by Brownson RC, Colditz GA, Proctor EK. Oxford, UK, Oxford University Press, 2012, pp 3–22

Dimeff LA, Koerner K, Woodcock EA, et al: Which training method works best? A randomized controlled trial comparing three methods of training clinicians in dialectical behavior therapy skills. Behav Res Ther 47(11):921–930, 2009 19695562

Dusenbury L, Brannigan R, Falco M, et al: A review of research on fidelity of implementation: implications for drug abuse prevention in school settings. Health Educ Res 18(2):237–256, 2003 12729182

Fraser MW, Galinsky MJ: Steps in intervention research. Designing and developing social programs. Res Soc Work Pract 20:459–466, 2010

Gearing RE, El-Bassel N, Ghesquiere A, et al: Major ingredients of fidelity: a review and scientific guide to improving quality of intervention research implementation. Clin Psychol Rev 31(1):79–88, 2011 21130938

Glasgow RE, Vinson C, Chambers D, et al: National Institutes of Health approaches to dissemination and implementation science: current and future directions. Am J Public Health 102(7):1274–1281, 2012 22594758

Green LW, Ottoson JM, García C, et al: Diffusion theory and knowledge dissemination, utilization, and integration in public health. Annu Rev Public Health 30:151–174, 2009 19705558

Grimshaw J, Eccles M, Thomas R, et al: Toward evidence-based quality improvement. Evidence (and its limitations) of the effectiveness of guideline dissemination and implementation strategies 1966–1998. J Gen Intern Med 21 (suppl 2):S14–S20, 2006 16637955

Grove WM, Andreasen NC, McDonald-Scott P, et al: Reliability studies of psychiatric diagnosis: theory and practice. Arch Gen Psychiatry 38(4):408–413, 1981 7212971

Henggeler SW, Schoenwald SK, Liao JG, et al: Transporting efficacious treatments to field settings: the link between supervisory practices and therapist fidelity in MST programs. J Clin Child Adolesc Psychol 31(2):155–167, 2002 12056100

Jamtvedt G, Young JM, Kristoffersen DT, et al: Audit and feedback: effects on professional practice and health care outcomes. Cochrane Database Syst Rev 2(2):CD000259, 2006 16625533

Johnson DW, Johnson RT, Smith KA: Cooperative learning returns to college: what evidence is there that it works? Change 30:27–35, 1998

Lewis-Fernández R, Aggarwal NK, Bäärnhielm S, et al: Culture and psychiatric evaluation: operationalizing cultural formulation for DSM-5. Psychiatry 77(2):130–154, 2014 24865197

Miller WR, Yahne CE, Moyers TB, et al: A randomized trial of methods to help clinicians learn motivational interviewing. J Consult Clin Psychol 72(6):1050–1062, 2004 15612851

Mugford M, Banfield P, O'Hanlon M: Effects of feedback of information on clinical practice: a review. BMJ 303(6799):398–402, 1991 1912809

Newes-Adeyi G, Helitzer DL, Roter D, et al: Improving client-provider communication: evaluation of a training program for Women, Infants and Children (WIC) professionals in New York State. Patient Educ Couns 55(2):210–217, 2004 15530756

Nunes EV, Ball S, Booth R, et al: Multisite effectiveness trials of treatments for substance abuse and co-occurring problems: have we chosen the best designs? J Subst Abuse Treat 38 (suppl 1):S97–S112, 2010 20307801

Pawlikowska T, Zhang W, Griffiths F, et al: Verbal and non-verbal behavior of doctors and patients in primary care consultations——how this relates to patient enablement. Patient Educ Couns 86(1):70–76, 2012 21621365

Peters DH, Adam T, Alonge O, et al: Implementation research: what it is and how to do it. BMJ 347:f6753, 2013 24259324

Powell BJ, McMillen JC, Proctor EK, et al: A compilation of strategies for implementing clinical innovations in health and mental health. Med Care Res Rev 69(2):123–157, 2012 22203646

Powell BJ, Proctor EK, Glass JE: A systematic review of strategies for implementing empirically supported mental health interventions. Res Soc Work Pract 24(2):192–212, 2014 24791131

Proctor EK, Knudsen KJ, Fedoravicius N, et al: Implementation of evidence-based practice in community behavioral health: agency director perspectives. Adm Policy Ment Health 34(5):479–488, 2007 17636378

Proctor EK, Landsverk J, Aarons G, et al: Implementation research in mental health services: an emerging science with conceptual, methodological, and training challenges. Adm Policy Ment Health 36(1):24–34, 2009 19104929

Proctor E, Silmere H, Raghavan R, et al: Outcomes for implementation research: conceptual distinctions, measurement challenges, and research agenda. Adm Policy Ment Health 38(2):65–76, 2011 20957426

Proctor EK, Powell BJ, McMillen JC: Implementation strategies: recommendations for specifying and reporting. Implement Sci 8:139–150, 2013 24289295

Rabin BA, Brownson RC: Developing the terminology for dissemination and implementation research, in Dissemination and Implementation Research in Health: Translating Science to Practice. Edited by Brownson RC, Colditz GA, Proctor E. Oxford, UK, Oxford University Press, 2012, pp 23–51

Roter DL, Wexler R, Naragon P, et al: The impact of patient and physician computer mediated communication skill training on reported communication and patient satisfaction. Patient Educ Couns 88(3):406–413, 2012 22789149

Rounsaville BJ, Carroll KM, Onken LS: A stage model of behavioral therapies research: getting started and moving on from Stage I. Clinical Psychology: Science and Practice 8:133–142, 2001

Schoenwald SK, Garland AF, Chapman JE, et al: Toward the effective and efficient measurement of implementation fidelity. Adm Policy Ment Health 38(1):32–43, 2011 20957425

Stamatakis KA, Vinson CA, Kerner JF: Dissemination and implementation research in community and public health settings, in Dissemination and Implementation Research in Health: Translating Science to Practice. Edited by Brownson RC, Colditz GA, Proctor EK. Oxford, UK, Oxford University Press, 2012, pp 359–383

Tabak RG, Khoong EC, Chambers DA, et al: Bridging research and practice: models for dissemination and implementation research. Am J Prev Med 43(3):337–350, 2012 22898128

Tibaldi G, Salvador-Carulla L, García-Gutierrez JC: From treatment adherence to advanced shared decision making: new professional strategies and attitudes in mental health care. Curr Clin Pharmacol 6(2):91–99, 2011 21592062

Suggested Readings

McGill University: CCS Cultural Formulation. Montreal, Canada, McGill University, 2014. Available at: http://www.mcgill.ca/iccc/resources/cf. Accessed September 15, 2014. McGill University hosts this Web site on how the CFI's precursor, the OCF, has been implemented in different service settings around the world.

National Information Center on Health Services Research and Health Care Technology (National Institutes of Health): Health Services Research Information Central. Bethesda, MD, National Institutes of Health, 2014. Available at: http://www.nlm.nih.gov/hsrinfo/implementation_science.html. Accessed September 15, 2014. The National Institutes of Health hosts this Web site, which acts as a clearinghouse for different tools, instruments, meetings, and conferences on implementation.

New York State Office of Mental Health, Center of Excellence for Cultural Competence: Cultural Formulation Interview Project, 2013. Available at: http://nyculturalcompetence.org/research-initiatives/initiative-diagnosis-engagement/cultural-formulation-interview-project/. Accessed September 15, 2014. This site hosts publications, videos, and training modules on the CFI.

Use of the Cultural Formulation Interview in Different Clinical Settings

Renato D. Alarcón, M.D., M.P.H.

Johann Vega-Dienstmaier, M.D.

Lizardo Cruzado, M.D.

Two basic and complementary premises set the stage for the content of this subchapter: 1) culture has a pervasive presence in every level, aspect, and setting of a clinical activity, and 2) the clinician needs to ascertain the impact of culture on the patient's suffering and the evaluation process (Alarcón 2009; Kirmayer et al. 2003). The Cultural Formulation Interview (CFI) is a semistructured instrument that can help clinicians elicit and document the cultural aspects of any patient's diagnosis and treatment plan arrived at through a comprehensive evaluation. As discussed throughout this volume, the purpose of the CFI is to expand on the clinical information obtained through standard diagnostic assessments of the patient's explanatory, coping, and help-seeking efforts and to elicit more information about the social context that can reveal both pathogenic and potentially therapeutic factors (Alarcón et al. 2009) (see subchapters "Supplementary Module 1: Explanatory Model" and "Supplementary Module 7: Coping and Help Seeking").

The diagnostic process does not take place in a vacuum. The clinical setting in which the evaluation occurs can play a decisive role in the way patients and their relatives tell their story. Aspects of the setting that influence the clinical encounter include its physical environmental characteristics; the type and roles of professional and ancillary staff present; the dynamic interactions between professionals, patients, and their entourage; and institutional norms and procedures. Furthermore, the pathways to care affect the setting. Many patients come to hospitals or clinics after a complex process of self-negotiations and interactions with people they trust, whereas others are brought against their will because of the overwhelming nature of their clinical symptoms and as a result of decisions made by persons they have never met.

The differences in pathways to care and among the settings where the clinical encounter takes place may require variations in the use of the CFI. To illustrate this variation, we focus in this subchapter on emergency departments (EDs), consultation-liaison services (i.e., inpatient medical and surgical units in general hospitals), outpatient clinics, as well as urban and rural community health centers. We describe each setting in terms of its environmental and patient- and staff-related features; clinical vignettes illustrate key issues. We also discuss technical aspects of the application of the CFI and its potential use in the context of collaborative or integrated care approaches to the provision of health and mental health services.

Emergency Departments

Clinical work in EDs is characterized by time urgency, especially the pressure to conduct a relatively thorough evaluation of the patient in a short period of time (Jarvis 2014). Cases seen in ED settings usually reflect disparities between patients' clinical needs related to complex symptomatology and the coping resources available in their immediate surroundings (including family and social support and financial options) (Allen et al. 2002; Hart and Alarcón 2006). These characteristics can make the ED environment, on occasion, seem chaotic. ED work has been described as the highest expression of multidisciplinary activity in the field of medicine, because of the presence of patients from all walks of life who have multiple, complex, and sometimes dramatic pathologies (Lettich 2004). In recent decades, because of increased demands for medical services in general and mental health problems in particular, EDs have become the entry point for patients with all kinds of conditions regardless of severity, thus making the atmosphere even more fluid and unpredictable. The circumstances of each patient's arrival and the presence of family members bring important cultural dimensions to assessment and care in this setting (Chanmugam et al. 2013).

The most frequently seen psychiatric presentations in EDs are psychotic crises or psychomotor agitation episodes of different origins, suicidal behaviors, and complications from drug or alcohol intoxication. From the sociodemographic perspective, an ED becomes a sort of "final common pathway," a setting in which patients of all social classes, educational levels, and ethnic origins converge for care of similar clinical conditions. This feature makes the setting eminently multicultural. Migration phenomena of all kinds contribute to this diversity, particularly in urban general hospitals.

Video 18 depicts a portion of the core CFI interview in the ED setting.

 Video Illustration 18: I've been feeling really frustrated (4:20)

> This video illustrates the use of the core CFI in the ED through an interview with a young man of Guatemalan descent who is being evaluated for suicidal ideation after the death of his baby daughter. The interview shows how the core CFI functions well in a situation of acute symptomatology. Despite his intense frustration and anger, the patient answers every question. He elaborates on being "out of control" and how he feels that nobody understands. He describes his ambivalence toward his main source of support, his wife, "The only person who understands me right now is my wife, and I don't know why she brought me here, I don't know why she pushed me to get here." He is able to communicate his sense of urgency, but he also evidences a perhaps unacknowledged willingness to seek help by talking about his family disagreements and the distressing nature of his suicidal ideation, shame, and emotional confusion. The core CFI questions also elicit more information that could help the ED cli-

nicians calibrate the level of severity of the situation and arrive at a treatment recommendation. The ED is probably the setting where patients' causal attributions emerge more loaded with feeling and also more spontaneously. In this case, the patient feels "God is trying to test me…to see if I am strong enough to deal with what happened right now, with losing my baby. To be honest, I don't feel strong…. I feel at times really upset, and I feel like I don't have the control to move on, and to push forward." The dissonance between his sense of a loving God and of himself as a strong man and his current feeling of abandonment, of existential emptiness, likely contributes to his suicidal ideation. His family is supportive, particularly his wife, but most of his relatives are far away in Guatemala, and in any case, he is not sure they "would understand." The core CFI offers an opportunity for the patient to describe his situation in his own terms, and what emerges in this case is a rich account of the patient's suffering, his distressing interpretations of his condition, and his lack of support. It also gives the patient a chance to express himself more fully, unburdening himself of his internal turmoil. The patient himself seems to acknowledge his need for help; despite his angry responses, he never asks to be discharged from the ED.

Tools such as the core CFI are extremely relevant to ED work because of the cultural impact on the psychiatrist's primary tasks of diagnosis and disposition, which involve assessing complex situations that may generate psychological and somatic symptoms as well as variable behavioral responses (Chincilla Moreno 2012; Triplett and DePaulo 2013). The core CFI is a flexible instrument, adaptable to the vicissitudes of the ED setting. The following two clinical examples illustrate its potential utility.

Case Vignette 1

Carlos, age 18, was brought by a paternal aunt to the ED of the local hospital in a mid-size Andean city in Peru. He felt "ashamed and humiliated" after his father strongly admonished him in front of his friends. He then experienced acute nausea and headaches and felt "physically ill." Examinations by an internist and several specialists and a variety of laboratory tests were negative. He received symptomatic medications but experienced no relief. The patient demanded intravenous fluids; when the doctors refused, he lost consciousness for a short period. The ED psychiatrist was then called in.

The patient appeared shy, fearful, and anxious but provided coherent information. He reported similar problems in the past, did not verbalize suicidal or homicidal ideas, and did not have psychotic symptoms. When asked about the cause of his problems, Carlos recognized the triggering impact of the "shame" he experienced after his father's reproaches and reaffirmed his belief that intravenous fluids would alleviate this. The psychiatrist then talked with the patient's aunt, a registered nurse who suggested that the "diagnosis" of her nephew was possibly *chucaque*, a cultural concept of distress described in some Andean countries. Encouraged by the psychiatrist's attention, she explained that this term was accepted in her cultural milieu of origin but that she was afraid to endorse this explanation, much less to suggest it, because as a nurse she knew that "doctors don't believe in *chucaque*." The psychiatrist's empathetic interaction with the patient afterward actually "validated" the patient's understanding of the problem and supported a culturally acceptable management that resulted in a significant improvement of Carlos's clinical condition.

Case Vignette 2

Carmen, a 45-year-old widow who has lived her entire life in a remote region of a Latin American country plagued by massive political violence, arrived at the ED of a city hospital after a long and arduous journey. She came in accompanied by several members of her family, who provided a recent history of social isolation, refusal to leave the house, neglect of her usual activities, anxiety, and distrustfulness. She only spoke her native language, Quechua, and as the ED clinician spoke only Spanish, the interview had to take place with the assistance of a nurse interpreter, a circumstance that made the patient even more reticent. To the question of whether Carmen had been seen "talking to herself," the relatives responded affirmatively, but the impression of the interviewing clinician was that because of their timidity, they seemed ready to answer "yes" to every question and were unwilling to contradict the doctors. Another relative, a young man who had migrated earlier to the urban coastal region of the country, reported that Carmen had been a teacher in the local school, but in recent years had been doing her work at home; she was afraid to leave it because she had been repeatedly threatened during the period of terrorist violence. Further questioning allowed the clinical team to rule out schizophrenia and focus on a possible posttraumatic stress disorder. They were also able to identify some cultural factors that had contributed to the delay in seeking professional help. These included mutual distrust and suspiciousness of neighbors who identified themselves as supporters of the people who had threatened Carmen and her own conception of her problem as *susto* (fright illness), an emotional condition subsequent to the experience of intense emotions.

The use of several sections of the core CFI would likely have helped in the task of evaluating the cultural aspects of the clinical and diagnostic realities of these two patients. In Carlos's case, for instance, eliciting the patient's cultural definition of the problem and the cultural perception of the cause and employing the use of specific local, colloquial terms (i.e., *chucaque*) might have facilitated a faster rapport. The patient had not sought help in the past, and exploring the absence of previous help seeking could have broadened the understanding of a complicated cultural background, which also strongly influenced his father's attitude and behaviors. The aunt's cautious approach changed after the psychiatrist entered into the family's cultural world by asking clinical questions in concrete cultural terms, as the CFI suggests. In Carmen's case, social and political realities had pushed the patient into a state of isolation, doubt, rumination, and overwhelming fear. The family's support was heartfelt but, because of the same fears and doubts, expressed itself through a help-seeking process of limited scope and resulted in longer delays in treatment for Carmen than for patients who follow more conventional pathways.

These two patients and their relatives conducted their relationships with the providers in an ambiguous manner, particularly initially. In this connection, the core CFI could also have helped to clarify crucial issues of cultural identity that influenced the clinician-patient interactions. Carlos was an adolescent subordinated to an authoritarian parental style but was able to respond to an empathetic approach that used his own cultural-syndromic language. Carmen was a member of a population attached to their original language, customs, traditions, habits, and beliefs and was distant and distrustful of city-based providers, all the more so because of her traumatic experiences. Fortuna et al. (2009) explain the advantages of a culturally informed model that can help assess factors "that affect the experience and interpretation of illness as understood by the patient, the family and the social network" (p. 434). In Peru, epidemiological investigations conducted by the country's National Institute of Mental Health have found a high prevalence of cultural concepts of distress such as *susto* and *chucaque* (Bernal-García 2010a, 2010b), supporting the inclusion of these well-established entities in the process of differential diagnosis in order to enhance diagnostic accuracy. The core CFI can play a decisive role in such epidemiological investigations.

The participation of interpreters is an important aspect of intercultural clinical work in emergency psychiatric settings. The cultural information provided by the interpreter in Carmen's case may have unintentionally obscured the meaning of some behaviors, including the coping activities aimed at helping her overcome her *susto*-like experience, which were not highlighted in the original translation. In ED settings in particular, interpreters' accuracy in conveying certain cultural phenomena, such as the nuances of an experience that might be construed as a delusion (particularly of the religious type), is crucial, because the clinician's conclusion in this regard may frame how he or she calibrates the severity of certain behavioral manifestations, understands the patient's coping mechanisms, and directs (or redirects) management interventions.

In addition to a well-conducted interview based on the core CFI in the ED setting, the supplementary modules can serve as useful clinical tools. For example, Carmen could have benefited from an adapted version of the Immigrants and Refugees supplementary module. The choice to deepen the inquiry in some sections of the core CFI will depend on the clinician's appropriate use of all the CFI components and correct understanding of the patient's cultural context.

Consultation-Liaison Psychiatry

By providing specialized services in the context of medical and surgical units in general hospitals, consultation-liaison (CL) psychiatry represents a historically progressive move toward comprehensive care (Kimball 1979). Cultural psychiatric consultation in medical settings, the newest addition to the CL approach, constitutes both a challenge and an opportunity to explore many aspects of the illness experience (Dominicé Dao and Kirmayer 2014).

The overall environment of general hospital CL settings is profoundly different from that of psychiatric units, not only for the nature of the clinical problems under treatment but also because of the presence of team staff members whose immediate attention is focused on medical conditions. The psychiatric consultant is called to see patients with overt physical problems, some of which are severe and exhausting; referral to a mental health specialist can be experienced as an additional stressor that makes these patients feel misunderstood, even humiliated. "I didn't come to see a shrink!" is a very common greeting from patients, who thereby raise a crucial barrier to their engagement with the psychiatrist; the situation may be further complicated by the presence of relatives who are equally or more insistent on a strictly medical approach. This concern, related to the dualism of biomedicine (Miresco and Kirmayer 2006), has a lot to do with cultural preconceptions about causality, course, and outcome of the disease. It also raises feelings of demoralization defined by subjective incompetence, denial, breakdown of the patient's "assumptive world," and subsequent distress (De Figueiredo and Gostoli 2013; Frank and Frank 1991). Although the presence of family poses challenges, the problem may be more complicated if, contrarily, no relatives are involved and the patient's feelings of abandonment, neglect, loneliness, and bitterness challenge the rapport-building efforts of the CL psychiatrist.

Furthermore, the psychiatrist often has limited time for the consultation and must focus on the clinical symptomatology to assess the case and recommend interventions for the problems identified by the referring physician. Given the complexity of CL cases, the psychiatrist should not come with preconceived diagnostic notions of "reactive depression," "illness anxiety disorder," or "psychiatric disorder due to a medical condition." Psychiatric problems commonly seen in CL settings include mood, cognitive, and adjustment disorders, but in many cases, they involve what have been called "ambiguous requests for consultation" (Arbabi et al. 2012). In not a few cases, the reasons for a referral stem from problems in the relationship between the patient and the clinical team or the institution. The use of the CFI can help to uncover such systemic issues, including discrepancies between the patient's understanding of the problem and the assumptions of the treatment team.

In addition to clarifying the specific issues described in the consultation request, the task of the CL psychiatrist requires examining cultural factors, both immediate and distant, that are affecting the clinical encounter. The importance of these factors is suggested by Collins et al.'s (1992) findings about differences in rates of and reasons for referral, overall prevalence of psychiatric disorders, and specific diagnoses among patients from different U.S. ethnic groups. These differences include lower rates of referral for Latinos than for whites, African Americans, and Asians; more frequent diagnoses of depression and suicide for Latinos; more notations of "grossly abnormal mental status" for blacks; and more diagnoses of adjustment disorder for Latinos, "primary thought disorder" and delirium among African Americans, and dementia for white patients (Collins et al. 1992). It must be kept in mind, however, that these variations may not reflect genuine cultural differences among the patient groups but rather biases in assessment and diagnostic practices.

Finally, broader health-related factors, such as the patient's age, may be decisive considerations in CL settings. Approaches such as Liaison Old Age Psychiatry (LOAP) have been shown to effectively reduce the overutilization of health resources through early identification of delirium, depression, and dementia (Nogueira et al. 2013). A similar reduction in overutilization may be observed as a result of CL services provided to children and adolescents. Kitts et al. (2013) report high satisfaction with the service of consultants, the effectiveness of their communication, the pertinence of their recommendations, and, above all, the helpfulness of interventions provided to both parents and youth. The issues of comprehensiveness of care and prevention are crucial for this type of service.

Although any of the core CFI sections and any of the supplementary modules may be particularly relevant in specific cases, the following components of the core CFI appear to be especially important in CL settings:

Cultural Perceptions of Cause, Context, and Support: The psychiatric component of the patient's illness may be seen by the patient and members of his or her social network mostly as a reaction to the stressor of the illness—that is, an unwanted complication—rather than a health problem in its own right. The evaluator should discreetly attempt to go beyond these arguments to identify deeper concerns, including fears, uncertainties, and related demoralization. This process highlights the value of exploring illness explanations, meanings of physical/somatic symptoms, and their interaction with emotional states.

Cultural Factors Affecting Self-Coping and Past Help Seeking: Understanding patients' coping or stress management styles is important for identifying individual vulnerabilities and sources of resilience that can be mobilized. Similarities with and differences from previous illness experiences should be explored in an effort to reinforce successful strategies that can be used again. Previous experiences in health care settings provide clues to a patient's perceptions of and response to the current hospitalization, as well as his or her understanding of the circumstances and meaning of the consultant's visit to the medical or surgical inpatient unit.

Cultural Factors Affecting Current Help Seeking: Relationships with the consultant as well as members of the referring clinical team are relevant. At times, the referral reveals a certain degree of "imposition" by the professional staff who requested the consultation. Acknowledging this and identifying the nature of the patient's relationship with the staff members of the referring unit may provide reassurance about the objectives and focus of the consultation and contribute to improving clinical care.

CL psychiatry services are expanding globally. Reports from different continents and countries (Aghanwa 2002; Botega 1992; Maharajh et al. 2008; Ularntinon 2012; Wand et al. 2009) indicate that this modality has become an essential component of everyday hospital work. Comparative studies of CL practice across different regions (Huyse et al. 2000; Kishi et al. 2007) confirm this trend. The cultural ingredients of CL psychiatry entail many dimensions of identity and context beyond categories of race and ethnicity. In particular, awareness of religious factors can enhance CL interventions (Waldfogel and Wolpe 1993). The disparities in quality of care observed in several studies (Delphin-Rittmon et al. 2012) reaffirm the need for comprehensive assessments with tools such as the CFI.

Outpatient Settings

Most of the issues examined in this section are based on work with the core CFI at the National Hospital Cayetano Heredia (HNCH) in Lima, Peru, one of the sites of the DSM-5 international field trials (American Psychiatric Association 2013; Lewis-Fernández et al. 2014). The main clinical conditions affecting those regularly attending the HNCH psychiatric outpatient department were depressive and anxiety disorders, schizophrenia, family or marital dysfunction, and the consequences of sexual abuse (Barrón-Del Solar et al. 2012). The CFI field trial included 36 patients with major depression, anxiety disorders (mainly panic disorder), substance use disorders (particularly alcohol and cocaine), or eating disorders; two patients with somatoform disorders; and one patient with gender identity disorder.

A psychiatric ambulatory care facility inserted in a general urban hospital must address the diversity of its patients in terms of help-seeking patterns, referral modalities, clinical presentations, and cultural features, including geographical origin, language, religion, migration status, and socioeconomic condition (Kinzie and Leung 2004). This was the case with the field trial sample, except for socioeconomic status, which was more uniform. Most patients had 8–10 years of education, came from lower-middle-class or working-class backgrounds, and were generally underemployed. Although most of the patients were self-referred or referred by other mental health professionals, a substantial minority came to the outpatient department following the advice of nonpsychiatric health professionals who perceived the primarily emotional or psychiatric nature of their complaints. The outpatient department tends to be a somewhat less hectic place than the ED; the staff typically has more time to evaluate the patients, although a variety of logistical demands make the availability of time an unpredictable feature of the setting.

The information gathered through the use of the core CFI in an outpatient department covers most or all areas of the interview. Patients in this setting tend to assert particular beliefs about what are the causes of their health problems, who must conduct the treatment, and how it must be done; all of these views affect patients' eventual adherence to the therapeutic regimen. A study conducted in Lima before the DSM-5 field trial, using clinical vignettes of typical cases of major depression, panic disorder, and schizophrenia, identified some beliefs that could interfere with the appropriate management of these conditions in an outpatient setting (Castro-Cuba Torres et al. 2013). For instance, study participants presented with vignettes of individuals with panic disorder often assumed that the case descriptions were of people with a physical illness that had not yet been diagnosed, so they expected little or nothing of value from a psychiatrist's intervention. Similarly, the belief that depression is caused by "weakness of character" combined with "everyday life problems" led study participants to make management suggestions such as leaving home; having fun; taking vitamins, magnesium, or nutritional supplements; or, as a "last resort," seeing a psychologist (but not a psychiatrist). The reasoning was very similar even in cases of schizophrenia; the illness was usually attributed to stressful experiences, and treatment was expected to be delivered by a psychologist first and a psychiatrist only later.

The Lima field trial delineated areas of the core CFI that were particularly relevant in the outpatient setting (Lewis-Fernández et al. 2014). The main results pointed out that the core CFI had these positive outcomes:

- Strengthening of the provider-patient relationship. Patients felt listened to and better understood and felt that the doctor's interest was more genuine and greater than expected. This, in turn, led to more openness on the patient's part.
- Detection of and facilitation of a prompt discussion of potential sources of distrust and prejudice, such as the fact that the patient was from a different ethnic group than the psychiatrist. It also allowed discreet inquiries about topics as varied as religious beliefs, bewitchment, psychosomatic symptoms, and personality styles.
- Encouragement of open expression of patients' views about their disorders and treatment and of awareness and acceptance of factors such as family, social, and financial resources that could impact access to care, treatment adherence, and clinical course.

- Elicitation of information to help guide the modality of psychotherapy recommended (individual, couple, or family oriented).

Our experience with the core CFI in the psychiatric outpatient setting showed that it could be extremely valuable in exploring connections between the cultural aspects of the patient's illness experience and medically unexplained physical symptoms (Fiestas-Teque and Vega-Dienstmaier 2012; García-Campayo et al. 2008). This connection is clearly important in certain cultures, such as those in Latin America or Africa (Bagayoyo et al. 2013; Gureje et al. 1997), where clinical somatization and related features are often interpreted following traditional beliefs about health and disease. Moreover, it is equally relevant to understand the illness experience in any patient struggling to make sense of persistent symptoms (Kirmayer and Sartorius 2009).

Urban and Rural Community Health Centers

In addition to traditional health centers, the practice of community psychiatry encompasses settings such as halfway houses, ambulatory home services, rehabilitation centers, and other venues. These services emphasize coverage of a geographical area or territory, continuity of care, multidisciplinary health care teams, and active community participation. In fact, they have been recognized as the antecedents of current efforts to develop integrated or collaborative care (Diez-Canseco et al. 2014). In these contexts, cultural aspects of the individual and his or her social surroundings may transcend other considerations, and the cultural competence of the psychiatrist and other providers becomes a sine qua non of clinical practice.

Cultural competence—the knowledge, familiarity, and understanding of the way of life of communities or minority populations and the skills needed to deal with all kinds of patients—is a compelling requirement in settings that are more closely situated "inside the community" (Kirmayer 2012). Instruments such as the CFI can facilitate work in such settings, both by identifying important contextual aspects of the patient's experience and by engaging other community members, for example, through the use of the CFI–Informant Version with people in the patient's entourage or, when appropriate, members of the larger community. When the focus is on patients' lives in the community context, issues such as cultural identity and explanatory models, as well as help-seeking patterns, levels of functioning, and family or social support, may become paramount in the evaluation process.

Certain aspects of urban and rural community settings can add to the complexity of the cultural assessment. A wide range of behaviors are seen in the community that ordinarily may not reach clinical attention. For instance, phenomena usually described as "hallucinations" may be more prevalent and regarded as normal by different ethnic and cultural groups, particularly those strongly influenced by religious beliefs. Similarly, paranoid ideation may be seen more frequently among groups victimized by systematic persecution and discrimination. If contextual factors are neglected in the evaluation of community populations, the result may be erroneous diagnoses and deleterious treatments, an example of an undue pathologization of everyday behaviors (Alarcón et al. 1999).

In community settings, an important assessment step may involve gathering data, through the CFI, from relatives, community leaders, and other important people in the patient's everyday life. This is illustrated by the following vignette.

Case Vignette 3

A traveling clinical team working in a rural village in Peru's mountains was asked to visit a family home to assess the grandmother, who was showing depressive symptoms and possibly mild cognitive deterioration. Judging from the modest appearance of the home, the style of dress of two accompanying adolescent grandchildren, and the family's ethnoracial complexion, the team assumed that the family was culturally "traditional" and started to explore common cultural beliefs in the community (including bewitchment, or *brujería*) to use the information later in the psychoeducation process. During the second home visit, however, the team discovered that several family members who worked outside the village had been visiting frequently and had become the most consistent source of support for the grandmother. Most importantly, the family had adopted urban, Western-based views about her mood problems. Identifying the explanatory models used by those involved in the patient's care was essential to devising an appropriate treatment plan.

This vignette illustrates the dilemmas of stereotyping and of assuming cultural homogeneity even in remote communities. It is evident that had the CFI been available to the team, direct questioning of the patient and key family members about help-seeking patterns, explanatory models, and specific contacts with family support resources could have situated the mood symptoms and the cognitive manifestations in a more accurate context. The CFI postulates the exploration of local meanings of symptoms and behaviors and of the role of family members; this is especially valuable in rural communities not easily reachable by conventional health care services (Kirmayer et al. 2014). Such perspective also points to the potential value of using the CFI and other resources in combination with new communication technologies in telemedicine and telepsychiatry (Cotton et al. 2014).

Technical Aspects of CFI Applicability in Different Settings

Consideration of the role of culture in psychiatric conditions faces two potential problems that are critically opposed to each other: overvaluation and undervaluation. *Overvaluation* attempts to explain every symptom or clinical manifestation as a product of culture, whereas *undervaluation* excludes culture as an important source of contributing factors in the production and interpretation of unusual behaviors and psychopathology (Committee on Cultural Psychiatry 2002). Determining when and how to incorporate and validate cultural data as pathogenic and pathoplastic factors in clinical phenomena is a challenge that the use of the CFI can help clinicians successfully address.

The CFI can be used by nonpsychiatrist health professionals trained to perform multifaceted roles. This is the case, for example, with advanced practice psychiatric nurses (or clinical nursing specialists), who, as documented by Fung et al. (2014), can perform relevant cultural assessment functions as part of psychosocial interventions and the development of partnerships with non–mental health service providers. In a study by Dawber (2013), nurses and midwives who engaged in a process-focused CL psychiatric training group reported a positive impact on clinical practice, self-awareness, and resilience.

A potential misuse of cultural information during patient evaluation is *stereotyping*—the tendency to view all people belonging to a group as similar in their cultural beliefs and practices. In every community or population, there are wide individual variations due to biological, psychological, and environmental factors. Rather than reproducing stereotypes, the CFI can help clarify this variation. Although some patients may perceive certain CFI topics or questions as intrusive, most welcome the clinician's interest in their perspectives and the details of their lifeworld. However, patient concerns about intrusiveness should not be dismissed but rather should be met with discrete and opportune formulation of the CFI questions and clear explanations as to their potential relevance to the patient's care.

One challenge to the applicability of the CFI in many clinical settings is the length of time it requires to complete. Each setting has its particular dynamics (in which cultural factors also play an important role), but one shared aspect is that the time allotted for a cultural evaluation in CL, emergency, or outpatient departments may not be longer than 15 or 20 minutes. Depending on the complexity of the case, the core CFI itself may require from 20 to 60 minutes. A practical response to these time constraints could be to administer the CFI only in cases in which useful and relevant findings could be expected or to use only a few CFI questions or components (Caballero-Martínez 2009). The use of the CFI may be especially indicated when there are culturally based provider-patient relationship issues; a history of poor adherence; definite ethnic, socioeconomic, or religious discrepancies between patient's and provider's illness representations or treatment expectations; specific indications for psychotherapy; or significant problems in differential diagnosis.

In several of the settings discussed in this subchapter, a significant problem (not exclusive to psychiatry) is the distrust by patients and families of government and other official agencies. The nature of psychiatric symptoms and conditions, particularly their culturally based features, may intensify these feelings of distrust and lead to rejection of services when patients feel their traditional perspectives about health and disease, religion, and communal life are threatened or neglected. The CFI can help clarify these concerns and address them by opening up a collaborative discussion of diagnostic and treatment expectations.

Conclusion

Table 4–5 summarizes some distinguishing characteristics of the different clinical settings reviewed in this subchapter. The table outlines some of the environmental aspects of each setting, the diagnoses of patients more commonly seen in them, and the core CFI sections that may need greater emphasis in the evaluation process to arrive at a more cogent diagnosis and treatment plan. Further research is needed to examine the adaptation of various CFI components to different settings and to refine the instrument so that it can more fully realize its promise.

TABLE 4–5. Characteristics of different clinical settings relevant to the use of the core Cultural Formulation Interview (CFI)

Setting	Environmental characteristics	Main diagnoses	Main core CFI sections
Emergency departments	Quick-paced, "chaotic" multidisciplinary interactions Overt socioeconomic diversity	Psychomotor agitation Psychotic episodes Suicidal behaviors Psychiatric complications of medical conditions Drug or alcohol intoxications Cultural concepts of distress	Cause, context, and support Past and current help-seeking patterns
Consultation-liaison services	Nonpsychiatric units Less common psychiatric occurrences Well-delineated consultation rules	Psychiatric complications of medical or surgical conditions Psychiatric comorbidities Depressive and anxiety disorders	Cause, context, and support Past and current help-seeking patterns Clinician-patient relationship
Outpatient clinics	Regularly scheduled referrals and time assignments Independent assessments Mild to moderate severity levels	Mood disorders Anxiety disorders Personality disorders First-episode psychoses	Cultural identity Cultural definition of the problem Cause, context, and support Past and current help-seeking patterns
Urban and rural community health centers	Minority or immigrant patients Cultural diversity Socioeconomic homogeneity Moderate sense of urgency	Depressive and anxiety disorders Somatoform disorders Family or interpersonal conflicts	Cultural definition of the problem Cause, context, and support Self-coping activities Clinician-patient relationship

KEY CLINICAL POINTS

- Clinicians' awareness of the influence of culture on every patient, type of clinical encounter, and service setting is a basic ingredient of a comprehensive diagnostic evaluation.

- The clinical setting of a psychiatric evaluation can play a culturally decisive role if factors such as physical environment, types and assignments of professional and ancillary staff, and institutional norms and procedures are taken into account as a background of dynamic interactions between clinicians and patients and their families.

- The core Cultural Formulation Interview (CFI) is relevant for work in emergency departments because it can help assess complex situations, as well as clarify the cause and context of the clinical condition, past help seeking, current treatment expectations, and sources of support.
- Patients seen in outpatient settings and in urban and rural community health centers may benefit from use of the CFI to explore cultural identity and cultural definition of the clinical problem, including sociodemographic characteristics, illness severity levels, and perceived sense of urgency.

Questions

1. What factors must be taken into account when applying the CFI in different clinical settings?

2. What are two of the main consequences of misusing cultural information in different clinical settings?

3. What kinds of cultural elements can affect the presentation and management of psychiatric conditions in emergency department, consultation-liaison, outpatient, and urban and rural community health settings?

4. What are the main psychiatric diagnoses with significant cultural implications that can be seen in the different clinical settings mentioned above?

5. What are some of the challenges that need to be overcome in order to implement the CFI in each type of clinical setting?

References

Aghanwa H: Consultation-liaison psychiatry in Fiji. Pac Health Dialog 9(1):21–28, 2002 12737413

Alarcón RD: Culture, cultural factors and psychiatric diagnosis: review and projections. World Psychiatry 8(3):131–139, 2009 19812742

Alarcón RD, Westermeyer J, Foulks EF, et al: Clinical relevance of contemporary cultural psychiatry. J Nerv Ment Dis 187(8):465–471, 1999 10463063

Alarcón RD, Becker AE, Lewis-Fernández R, et al: Issues for DSM-V: the role of culture in psychiatric diagnosis. J Nerv Ment Dis 197(8):559–660, 2009 19684490

Allen MA, Forster P, Zealberg J, et al, American Psychiatric Association Task Force on Psychiatric Emergency Services. Report and Recommendations Regarding Psychiatric Emergency and Crisis Services: A Review and Model Program Descriptions. Arlington, VA, American Psychiatric Association, 2002. Available at: http://www.psychiatry.org/File%20Library/Learn/Archives/tfr2002_EmergencyCrisis.pdf. Accessed March 16, 2014.

American Psychiatric Association: Diagnostic and Statistical Manual of Mental Disorders, 5th Edition. Arlington, VA, American Psychiatric Association, 2013

Arbabi M, Laghayeepoor R, Golestan B, et al: Diagnoses, requests and timing of 503 psychiatric consultations in two general hospitals. Acta Med Iran 50(1):53–60, 2012 22267380

Bagayoyo IP, Interian A, Escobar JI: Transcultural aspects of somatic symptoms in the context of depressive disorders, in Cultural Psychiatry. Edited by Alarcón RD. Basel, Karger, 2013, pp 64–74

Barrón-Del Solar L, Romero-Sandoval K, Saldaña-Vásquez N, et al: Perfil clínico y epidemiológico del paciente que acude al Consultorio Externo de Psiquiatría del Hospital Nacional Cayetano Heredia, durante el periodo de Octubre a Diciembre de 2011. Rev Neuropsiquiatr 75:7–18, 2012

Bernal-García E: Estudio epidemiológico y síndromes folklóricos en cinco ciudades de la selva peruana: prevalencia de vida, asociación con tres síndromes psiquiátricos. Anales de Salud Mental 26:49–57, 2010a

Bernal-García E: Síndromes folklóricos en cuatro ciudades de la sierra del Perú: prevalencia de vida, asociación con tres síndromes psiquiátricos y sistemas de atención. Anales de Salud Mental 26:39–48, 2010b

Botega NJ: Consultation-liaison psychiatry in Brazil. Psychiatric residency training. Gen Hosp Psychiatry 14(3):186–191, 1992 1601294

Caballero-Martínez L: DSM-IV-TR cultural formulation of psychiatric cases: two proposals for clinicians. Transcult Psychiatry 46(3):506–523, 2009 19837784

Castro-Cuba Torres P, Segura-Carrillo R, Tordoya-Lizárraga G, et al: Conocimientos y estigmas sobre salud mental en familiares de pacientes que acuden a consultorio externo del Hospital Nacional Cayetano Heredia. Acta Médica Peruana 30:63–69, 2013

Chanmugam A, Triplett P, Kelen G (eds): Emergency Psychiatry. New York, Cambridge University Press, 2013

Chinchilla Moreno A (ed): Práctica Psiquiátrica en Atención Primaria. Madrid, Nature Publishing Group Iberoamérica, 2012.

Collins D, Dimsdale JE, Wilkins D: Consultation/liaison psychiatry utilization patterns in different cultural groups. Psychosom Med 54(2):240–245, 1992 1565759

Committee on Cultural Psychiatry, Group for the Advancement of Psychiatry: Cultural Assessment in Clinical Psychiatry. Washington DC, American Psychiatric Publishing, 2002

Cotton ME, Nadeau L, Kirmayer LJ: Consultation to remote and indigenous communities, in Cultural Consultation: Encountering the Other in Mental Health Care. Edited by Kirmayer LJ, Guzder J, Rousseau C. New York, Springer, 2014, pp 223–244

Dawber C: Reflective practice groups for nurses: a consultation liaison psychiatry nursing initiative: part 2—the evaluation. Int J Ment Health Nurs 22(3):241–248, 2013 23020828

De Figueiredo JM, Gostoli S: Culture and demoralization in psychotherapy, in Cultural Psychiatry. Edited by Alarcón RD. Basel, Karger, 2013, pp 75–87

Delphin-Rittmon M, Andres-Hyman R, Flanagan EH, et al: Racial-ethnic differences in referral source, diagnosis, and length of stay in inpatient substance abuse treatment. Psychiatr Serv 63(6):612–615, 2012 22422017

Diez-Canseco F, Ipince A, Toyama M, et al: Integration of mental health and chronic noncommunicable diseases in Peru: challenges and opportunities for primary care settings [in Spanish]. Rev Peru Med Exp Salud Publica 31(1):131–136, 2014 24718538

Dominicé Dao MD, Kirmayer LJ: Cultural consultation in medical settings, in Cultural Consultation: Encountering the Other in Mental Health Care. Edited by Kirmayer LJ, Guzder J, Rousseau C. New York, Springer, 2014, pp 313–331

Fiestas-Teque L, Vega-Dienstmaier JM: Síntomas físicos en pacientes con trastornos de ansiedad y depresión que acuden a la Consulta Externa de Psiquiatría del Hospital Nacional Cayetano Heredia. Rev Neuropsiquiatr 75:47–57, 2012

Fortuna LR, Porche MV, Alegría M: A qualitative study of clinicians' use of the cultural formulation model in assessing posttraumatic stress disorder. Transcult Psychiatry 46(3):429–450, 2009 19837780

Frank JD, Frank JB: Persuasion and Healing: A Comparative Study of Psychotherapy, 3rd Edition. Baltimore, MD, Johns Hopkins University Press, 1991

Fung YL, Chan Z, Chien WT: Role performance of psychiatric nurses in advanced practice: a systematic review of the literature. J Psychiatr Ment Health Nurs 21(8):698–714, 2014 DOI: 10.1111/jpm 24299195

García-Campayo J, Ayuso-Mateos JL, Caballero L, et al: Relationship of somatic symptoms with depression severity, quality of life, and health resources utilization in patients with major depressive disorder seeking primary health care in Spain. Prim Care Companion J Clin Psychiatry 10(5):355–362, 2008 19158973

Gureje O, Simon GE, Ustun TB, et al: Somatization in cross-cultural perspective: a World Health Organization study in primary care. Am J Psychiatry 154(7):989–995, 1997 9210751

Hart D, Alarcón RD: Cultural issues in the emergency room setting. Psychiatr Times 5:23–26, 2006

Huyse FJ, Herzog T, Lobo A, et al: European consultation-liaison services and their user populations: the European Consultation-Liaison Workgroup Collaborative Study. Psychosomatics 41(4):330–338, 2000 10906355

Jarvis GE: Cultural consultation in general hospital psychiatry, in Cultural Consultation: Encountering the Other in Mental Health Care. Edited by Kirmayer LJ, Guzder J, Rousseau C. New York, Springer, 2014, pp 293–313

Kimball CP: Liaison psychiatry as a systems approach to behavior. Psychother Psychosom 32(1–4):134–147, 1979 398997

Kinzie JD, Leung PK: Culture and outpatient psychiatry, in Cultural Competence in Clinical Psychiatry. Edited by Tseng WS, Streltzer J. Washington, DC, American Psychiatric Publishing, 2004, pp 37–52

Kirmayer LJ: Rethinking cultural competence. Transcult Psychiatry 49(2):149–164, 2012 22508634

Kirmayer LJ, Sartorius N: Cultural models and somatic syndromes, in Somatic Presentations of Mental Disorders: Refining the Research Agenda for DSM-V. Edited by Dimsdale JE, Patel V, Xin Y, et al. Washington, DC, American Psychiatric Publishing, 2009, pp 23–46

Kirmayer LJ, Groleau D, Guzder J, et al: Cultural consultation: A model of mental health services for multicultural societies, Can J Psychiatry 48(3):145–153, 2003 12728738

Kirmayer LJ, Rousseau C, Jarvis GE, et al: The cultural context of clinical assessment, in Psychiatry, 4th Edition. Edited by Tasman A, Maj M, First MB, et al. New York, John Wiley and Sons, 2014, pp 54–66

Kishi Y, Meller WH, Kato M, et al: A comparison of psychiatric consultation liaison services between hospitals in the United States and Japan. Psychosomatics 48(6):517–522, 2007 18071099

Kitts RL, Gallagher K, Ibeziako P, et al: Parent and young adult satisfaction with psychiatry consultation services in a children's hospital. Psychosomatics 54(6):575–584, 2013 23453126

Lettich L: Culture and the psychiatric emergency service, in Cultural Competence in Clinical Psychiatry. Edited by Tseng WS, Streltzer J. Washington, DC, American Psychiatric Publishing, 2004, pp 53–66

Lewis-Fernández R, Aggarwal NK, Bäärnhielm S, et al: Culture and psychiatric evaluation: operationalizing cultural formulation for DSM-5. Psychiatry 77(2):130–154, 2014 24865197

Maharajh HD, Abdool P, Mohammed-Emamdee R: The theory and practice of consultation-liaison (CL) psychiatry in Trinidad and Tobago with reference to suicidal behavior. ScientificWorldJournal 8:920–928, 2008 18836659

Miresco MJ, Kirmayer LJ: The persistence of mind-brain dualism in psychiatric reasoning about clinical scenarios. Am J Psychiatry 163(5):913–918, 2006 16648335

Nogueira V, Lagarto L, Cerejeira J, et al: Improving quality of care: focus on liaison old age psychiatry. Ment Health Fam Med 10(3):153–158, 2013 24427182

Triplett P, DePaulo JR: Assessment and general approach, in Emergency Psychiatry. Edited by Chanmugam A, Triplett P, Kelen G. New York, Cambridge University Press, 2013, pp 1–24

Ularntinon S: Child psychiatric consultation to pediatric inpatient services in Thailand. Pediatr Int 54(4):566–568, 2012 22591509

Waldfogel S, Wolpe PR: Using awareness of religious factors to enhance interventions in consultation-liaison psychiatry. Hosp Community Psychiatry 44(5):473–477, 1993 8509080

Wand AP, Corr MJ, Eades SJ: Liaison psychiatry with Aboriginal and Torres Strait Islander peoples. Aust NZ J Psychiatry 43(6):509–517, 2009 19440882

Suggested Readings

Alarcón RD (ed): Cultural Psychiatry (Advances in Psychosomatic Medicine, Vol 33). Basel, Switzerland, Karger, 2013

Chanmugam A, Triplett P, Kelen G (eds): Emergency Psychiatry. New York, Cambridge University Press, 2013

Kirmayer LJ, Guzder J, Rousseau C (eds): Cultural Consultation: Encountering the Other in Mental Health Care. New York, Springer, 2014

Tseng WS, Streltzer J (eds): Cultural Competence in Cultural Psychiatry. Washington, DC, American Psychiatric Publishing, 2004

Administrative Perspectives on the Implementation and Use of the Cultural Formulation Interview

Kavoos Ghane Bassiri, M.S., LMFT, LPCC, CGP

Angela Tang Soriano, M.S.S.W., LCSW

In this subchapter, we discuss administrative perspectives on the implementation and use of the DSM-5 (American Psychiatric Association 2013) Cultural Formulation Interview (CFI). It may seem unusual to include a section on administrative perspectives when presenting a new assessment tool such as the CFI. However, there are always administrative issues and changes that need to be considered in attempts to successfully implement a new procedure or protocol in any organizational setting, from smaller practices to midsize agencies and large institutions. Lack of attention to administrative issues and operational needs at every organizational level may result in poor uptake, fidelity, integration, and outcomes. In the sections that follow, we address 1) organizational purpose and need, 2) use and benefits, 3) implementation strategies, and 4) implementation challenges and potential solutions.

Organizational Purpose and Need

Cultural competence in health care provision is increasingly a necessity rather than an option or choice in practice. Cultural competence operates at all levels of health care delivery, from that of patient-provider interaction to the levels of health care organizations, service systems, and society. The focus in this subchapter is on the role of the CFI in promoting the concrete application of organizational cultural competence.

In thinking about organizational cultural competence, it is useful to review some fundamental concepts, such as *culture, cultural competence, cultural humility, culturally competent system of care,* and *organizational cultural competence,* which are defined in Table 4–6. Cultural competence is relevant to all institutions, not only those in which the patient population is composed of immigrants or those who speak a different language; moreover, to be effective, principles of cultural competence must be integrated systemwide (Aggarwal et al. 2013). To support organizational and practitioner integration, the U.S. Department of Health and Human Services developed the National Standards for Cul-

TABLE 4–6.   Fundamental concepts for cultural competency

Concept	Definition
Culture	"Systems of knowledge, concepts, rules, and practices that are learned and transmitted across generations…includes language, religion and spirituality, family structures, life-cycle stages, ceremonial rituals, and customs, as well as moral and legal systems" (American Psychiatric Association 2013, p. 749)
Cultural competence	"A set of congruent behaviors, attitudes, and policies that come together in a system, agency, or among professionals and enables…[it]…to work effectively in cross-cultural situations" (Cross et al. 1989, p. 13)
Cultural humility	Commitment to self-evaluation and self-critique and development of self-awareness and a respectful attitude toward diverse points of view (abstracted from Tervalon and Murray-García 1998, p. 117)
Culturally competent system of care	A system that "acknowledges and incorporates—at all levels—the importance of culture, the assessment of cross-cultural relations, vigilance towards the dynamics that result from cultural differences, the expansion of cultural knowledge, and the adaptation of services to meet culturally unique needs" (Cross et al. 1989, p. iv)
Organizational cultural competence	A systemic perspective of cultural competence that is operationalized at the meso (institutional and programmatic) level (abstracted from Fung et al. 2012, p. 167)

turally and Linguistically Appropriate Services in Health and Health Care (U.S. Department of Health and Human Services, Office of Minority Health 2010, revised 2013). Implementation of the CFI can help address several of these 15 standards.

To achieve cultural competence, an institution needs to make diversity a core value and engage in regular self-assessment, while enhancing staff cultural knowledge and maintaining a culturally humble stance. Cultural competence practices must be integrated in the culture of the work setting and the institution itself. This integration involves an ongoing process of learning, reflection, and repeated self-assessment, framed from the starting point of cultural humility—the recognition of the limits of one's own cultural understanding. To aid in culturally competent psychiatric assessment, the DSM-5 Cross-Cultural Issues Subgroup developed an updated Outline for Cultural Formulation (OCF) and the CFI, a specific set of assessment questions that can be used to apply the OCF in routine practice. Richmond Area Multi-Services (RAMS), an organization located in San Francisco, California, served as one of the field trial sites. Throughout this subchapter, we draw examples from the experience of RAMS in administering the core CFI to illustrate how the process of implementing the CFI can promote organizational cultural competence.

Founded in 1974, RAMS is a not-for-profit mental health agency with a mission to advocate for and provide community-based, culturally competent, and consumer-guided comprehensive services to meet the behavioral health, social, residential, vocational, and educational needs of the diverse San Francisco community, with a special focus on Asian and Pacific Islander Americans and Russian speakers, who represent a substantial proportion of the local population. Many of the agency's patients are recent immigrants and refugees in need of bilingual, bicultural mental health services. RAMS approaches cultural competency as a highly collaborative and ongoing process by which the principles are consistently applied and integrated into the development and implementation of policies and procedures (e.g., satisfaction surveys, client council, personnel recruitment and performance evaluation, training and supervision). Annually, RAMS serves about 18,000 adults, children, youth, and families, most of whom have extremely limited resources and receive public health benefits. The agency offers a wide array of mental health and social services in 30 languages at over 90 locations (including outpatient programs, schools, and child care sites). For the CFI study, RAMS engaged Cantonese-speaking Chinese American clients and clinicians, translating the core CFI questions into Chinese.

Use and Benefits

Psychiatric practice in cross-cultural settings faces several challenges, including practitioner-patient differences in ethnicity and culture that affect the therapeutic relationship. This, in turn, may lead to increased risk for bias and stereotyping, impeding the clinician's understanding of the patient and hindering a meaningful and effective clinical relationship (Scarpinati Rosso and Bäärnhielm 2012). In institutions striving to be culturally competent, administrators and supervisors seek ways to promote cultural competence and humility by engaging the institution's workforce in the process and by utilizing approaches and tools tailored for this purpose. Administrators in particular may be responsible for devising effective implementation processes and procedures to promote cultural competence. Implementation of the DSM-IV (American Psychiatric Association 1994) OCF was hampered because it relied heavily on the preexisting cultural knowledge, skills, and intuitions of the individual practitioner and/or group leadership (department/unit management). With the development of the DSM-5 CFI, an organization's or practitioner's ability to integrate culturally competent assessment has been significantly enhanced because the CFI offers 1) standardization of a qualitative method of assessment, 2) scalability and accessibility, and 3) a focus on information that can contribute to clinically relevant results and outcomes.

Standardization

The CFI operationalizes the OCF for clinicians by offering a structured format with a specific process and practical approach by which a patient assessment and/or interview can proceed, using field-tested wording and sequencing of questions. In many practice settings, clinicians are presented with an assessment form that is composed primarily of symptom checklists and/or rating scales. Clinicians may then use a wide variety of approaches to solicit the requisite information from patients. The CFI enables an organization and practitioner to standardize this qualitative aspect of patient interviewing, in a culturally competent manner, using a sequence of questions that foster a respectful, engaging, and thoughtful process to explore relevant issues.

Practitioners must assess cultural nuances with each patient because these nuances vary from person to person and affect how a patient thinks about mental health, wellness, and illness (Warren 2013). This assessment process can be difficult to carry out, however. In a qualitative study by Kai et al. (2007) on how health professionals experience and perceive their work, findings highlighted considerable uncertainty and disempowerment among practitioners in responding to the needs of patients of different ethnicities from their own; the study suggests interventions to empower professionals, which include shifting away from a cultural expertise model toward greater emphasis on each patient as an individual by soliciting patients' own viewpoints and experience. The CFI is not tailored to specific cultures but instead provides a generic format for cultural evaluation and therefore may help an organization support its practitioners in working with individuals and families from diverse and emerging communities and varying cultural experiences, potentially resulting in improved clinician satisfaction and morale. The standardization of assessment will likely increase diagnostic accuracy, treatment planning, and care coordination, leading to shorter treatments and savings for the organization (e.g., the health care plan may accommodate more patients) and the patient (e.g., lower out-of-pocket expenses).

Scalability and Accessibility

The CFI process is scalable in its training methodologies and accessible by organizations and practitioners. In addition to being included in DSM-5, the CFI components are provided in the appendixes in this handbook and are available free of charge from the American Psychiatric Association Web site (http://www.psychiatry.org/practice/dsm/dsm5/online-assessment-measures). The CFI can be implemented by organizations of any size and/or by specific units or departments. It may also be used by a wide range of practitioners (e.g., psychiatrists, psychiatric nurses, social workers, therapists, case managers, cultural brokers) with a range of clinical experiences (e.g., graduate students or seasoned clinicians; practitioners working with less familiar patient populations). The CFI does not require extensive training and knowledge to be used as an assessment tool. In RAMS's experience of training in the core CFI, many practitioners indicated that the questions were straightforward and familiar and could easily be integrated into their current practice. Practitioners were also open to using the core CFI because RAMS's organizational culture embodies and integrates, at all levels, cultural competence principles and practices. For example, RAMS conducts an organizational assessment of its integration of culturally and linguistically appropriate services and uses it to develop agency and programmatic objectives. Discussions about how to work with culturally diverse populations regularly take place both during formal sessions (e.g., weekly didactic trainings) and informally among practitioners. Our experience with the DSM-5 field trial is that the core CFI's comprehensive approach to engaging the patient and the sequencing of the questions prompt the patient to offer the information needed by the clinician to complete a typical diagnostic assessment. The design of the CFI supports RAMS's ability to easily integrate the CFI into many of its programs and departments, including its outpatient clinic, school-based services, welfare-to-work counseling program, and residential facility.

The CFI can be used for cultural competence training with residents in several medical fields (e.g., psychiatry, internal medicine, family medicine) as well as with interns and other trainees in various mental health disciplines. At RAMS, cultural competence training is conducted regularly throughout the year. For example, with graduate-level interns the training includes an overview of cultural competence concepts, an introduction to the OCF, and instruction on the CFI and how to incorporate it into the assessment process. We find the CFI to be a practical way of developing the clinical skills of trainees new to the health care field by teaching them to apply the theories and conceptual frameworks they learned in school. Being easy to teach facilitates its uptake by personnel from many disciplines. The CFI offers a common framework for the treatment team to foster communication between providers. As Dinh et al. (2012) reported on the use of the OCF, the parent framework for the CFI, "Case conceptualization starts out as multidisciplinary but becomes interdisciplinary, through the recognition, utilization and integration of the expertise and perspectives of the various professions represented in the group" (p. 13).

Information Relevant for Clinical Outcomes

The core CFI can be used at the beginning of the clinical encounter, as well as at any stage of treatment, because its application leads to a better understanding than standard clinical interviews of how the patient is embedded in a particular sociocultural context, which, in turn, may enhance the patient-practitioner relationship (Rohlof et al. 2009). The CFI seems to elicit the patient's own narrative of the situation to a greater extent than do symptom checklists. The CFI helps the clinician explore the patients' identity and understand how culture shapes everyday practices such as diet, living arrangements, emotional expressions, and decision-making processes (Aggarwal et al. 2013). Comprehensive, patient-centered assessment such as the CFI is expected to enhance practitioner-patient rapport and communication, diagnostic accuracy, treatment planning, treatment adherence, treatment outcome, and patient satisfaction.

Implementation Strategies

When introducing new tools and/or practices, administrators can consider the implementation strategy in terms of three main phases: 1) planning, including identification of goals and potential challenges (e.g., need for training to enhance culturally competent care and identification of potential obstacles) and selection of desired course of action (e.g., specific systemic changes and interventions, and methods of implementation); 2) implementation, including communication, allocation of roles, and mobilization of resources; and 3) evaluation, comprising review of effectiveness, benefits, and modification of the integration process as needed (Table 4–7).

Planning

To apply these strategic phases to the integration of the CFI in a health care system or organization, the administrator can first consider the organization's history, current cultural competence, and past ways of handling comparable changes in practice or procedures. Questions such as these may be useful: Has the organization recently undergone many procedural changes? What concerns have practitioners expressed about former or existing assessment tools? What is the awareness and level of com-

TABLE 4–7. **Cultural Formulation Interview (CFI) implementation checklist**

Task	Stage(s)
Assess organizational culture and readiness	Planning
Engage and identify implementation team and resources	Planning
Achieve buy-in	Planning
Develop implementation plan (e.g., training, time line, policy, workflow adjustments)	Planning
Integrate into workflow	Implementation
Provide training	Implementation
Roll out (possibly initially as a pilot)	Implementation
Communicate bidirectionally (e.g., reporting, feedback, disseminating data)	Implementation, evaluation
Make adjustments to implementation plan, as needed	Implementation, evaluation
Monitor and review for quality assurance	Evaluation
Provide ongoing support and additional training for sustained CFI use	Evaluation

mitment toward cultural competence initiatives shown by the organization, the funder(s), and the policymakers? What experience have the practitioners had with the application of the OCF? By anticipating challenges or obstacles, the administrator can more thoughtfully develop an appropriate and effective implementation plan.

A key component of planning and implementation is communication. It is important to approach this component horizontally by engaging the staff in ongoing discussions and collaboration rather than vertically by having administrators dictate use of the new protocol. Also, administrators must be aware of their own attitudes and level of enthusiasm about the implementation of the CFI so they can respond appropriately to feedback. Practitioners must be able to ask questions and have an open dialogue. Administrators and middle managers—including department/program directors, managers, and supervisors—must ensure that there is time to discuss the usefulness of the CFI, what did or did not work during its initial application and what challenges emerged in using the CFI to gather patient information. As a result, practitioners will be more receptive to hearing the administrator's presentation of the benefits and "added value" of CFI. The administrator's open and flexible stance can positively influence the effective implementation, fidelity, and sustained use of the CFI.

Along with these efforts to establish communication with practitioners and other providers, the administrator should also initially engage middle managers in developing the implementation plan. In RAMS's experience, there was an initial discussion with supervisors who provided feedback on the core CFI, focusing on how the tool would be beneficial, how patients might respond, and what would be the potential challenges to its use. The dialogue led to the development of an implementation plan, taking into account the identified issues, such as the timing of training and rollout, and potential end-user reactions. Practitioner engagement can also be channeled through the formation of a committee of key organization members who volunteer to take part in the implementation process and whose work would be affected by implementation of the CFI (e.g., middle management and end users such as psychiatrists and social workers). These individuals can function as intervention "champions" or people to go to when questions arise. Middle managers can support the messaging of the organizational goals to direct service practitioners and can provide the day-to-day support needed at the front line by listening to concerns and addressing any implementation dilemmas as they come up. It is crucial that middle managers be motivated to use the CFI and be supported by administrators who solicit their feedback throughout each stage of planning, implementation, and evaluation. To support this collaborative effort, the administrator can present the core implementation goals while granting the committee some flexibility in their application. Specific committee recommendations could focus on time line, scheduling, enrollment, and implementation deadlines as well as on scaling the rollout (e.g., which program[s] should implement it first). An implementation plan should include clear goals (e.g., process and outcome objectives) along with identified individuals and groups that are responsible for different aspects of the process.

It is also important for administration to support the integration of the CFI into existing clinical workflow and documentation procedures. For instance, how do the day-to-day logistics need to change to accommodate the use of the CFI? How should the CFI be integrated into existing documentation systems? Addressing these issues early on might include streamlining the revision of existing forms to include the domains covered by the CFI, with careful review to prevent duplication of information. For example, a so-called road map can be developed that illustrates how each core CFI question may lead to answering particular sections of a required form. Then a work group can be convened to combine the existing forms and the core CFI into a single document. At the same time, there should be consideration of how the core CFI and other CFI components can be incorporated into the management information systems and other data collection processes.

As part of the planning phase, administrators must also consider staff training needs and develop a training plan. It may be beneficial to facilitate the CFI training process by integrating it into existing training and/or staff meeting schedules (e.g., by holding the CFI training during a regular seminar). Because the CFI is used to improve the quality and cultural competence of the assessment process, it is more beneficial when used as part of a larger cultural competence and humility standards framework than when used in isolation. It is important that organizations develop policies and procedures to integrate cultural competence into everyday practice. For example, at RAMS, cultural competence principles are integrated as part of the orientation and training curriculum and performance evaluation process.

Implementation

CFI trainings may include role-playing and review opportunities. The usefulness of the CFI can be illustrated through case conferences, which can show how the information gathered can be used for case formulation, which, in turn, can lead to more accurate diagnosis, identification of the patient's strengths and need for community resources, appropriate intervention strategies, and comprehensive treatment planning. For example, existing case conferences can include the CFI within the presentation outline and discussion. For middle managers, there can be specific training on how to integrate the CFI as an educational and training tool and how to support continued utilization for practitioners. CFI training can offer additional incentives such as continuing education credits and/or educational training accommodations.

In larger organizations, it may be helpful initially to pilot test the CFI integration with a smaller group of practitioners before integrating it across the entire department, program, or system. Administrators can ask practitioners to volunteer for this pilot testing; having staff involved in this way may reduce some of the implementation challenges. Ideally, middle management and/or administrators can be included in the pilot test. Following this initiative, the administrator can obtain feedback from all middle managers and practitioners regarding the benefits and challenges that emerged so as to make further suggestions for integration. With each instance of feedback and/or suggestion, there needs to be consistent accountability for addressing any concerns or questions. For example, feedback sessions may include meeting notes with action items that indicate individuals responsible for follow-up; at the next meeting, updates in relation to each action item can be discussed. The administrators, middle managers, and/or practitioners involved can in turn share their experience with the CFI and its clinical utility, which may further motivate other practitioners to integrate it into practice.

Evaluation

To evaluate the usefulness of the CFI, administrators can develop feedback mechanisms such as in-person meetings (with individuals or large or small groups), consultations with the implementation committee, focused discussions with middle managers, and/or written evaluation protocols for practitioners and/or patients to complete. For example, anonymous patient satisfaction surveys can focus on changes in practitioner engagement. Key performance indicators may include, among others, increased rates of patient engagement following intake/assessment (e.g., higher attendance rates, fewer premature terminations), improved treatment adherence, improved patient satisfaction, improved practitioner skills in serving diverse communities (e.g., avoiding misdiagnosis), enhanced or adjusted service array, and improved organizational cultural competence.

It is also very helpful to share data with practitioners about the benefits and challenges of using a new tool. Administrators often develop and implement policies and then move on to other projects without obtaining staff feedback or even informing staff of the impact of the new procedures. It is crucial to have follow-up meetings to solicit feedback from the end users. Feedback should focus on whether the information gathered via the CFI assisted in diagnosis, engagement, care planning, and referral.

Implementation Challenges and Potential Solutions

When integrating new tools or practices, administrators must remain flexible so as to cope with unanticipated challenges, while simultaneously anticipating potential obstacles and developing solutions to overcome them. Adjustments to clinical procedures may be needed at all organizational levels (frontline staff to leadership) for a variety of reasons, including in response to serving an emerging cultural community. Although the administrative considerations are similar in most settings, they also vary depending on organization size, culture, and environment (e.g., funding stream, political climate). Implementation requires paying attention to challenges that emerge at least at these three levels: 1) overarching policy, funding, and reporting requirements; 2) organizational routines, procedures, and practices within the health care system and institutions; and 3) practitioner skills, roles, and activities.

Overarching Policy, Funding, and Reporting Requirements

Although there are compelling reasons for developing cultural competence in health care provision, the health care field is continually beset by increasing demands for heightened scrutiny, compliance with regulations, rigorous reporting and documentation, and patient satisfaction. There are federal, state, and local government policies that support enhancement and integration of cultural competence. However, funding tends to be limited for such efforts, particularly for administrative functions. For example, health insurance plans and public benefits programs such as Medicaid tend to reimburse for practitioner-patient direct service time but not for expanded organizational planning and clinician training. As a result, organizations may reallocate and/or seek additional resources. Although the CFI constitutes an investment of resources (e.g., staff time for training), we at RAMS expect an overall return on investment through the maximization of effective outcomes. In fact, most of the resources are needed in the initial implementation stages; once the CFI is fully integrated into the organization's routine, substantially fewer resources may be needed because the foundation of the procedures and structure has been established. Policies and funder requirements may also include specific assessment tools that must be used and/or mandates relating to the length of time allocated for sessions. However, the core CFI questions cover many of the same topics evaluated in a routine clinical assessment, albeit from a cultural perspective, making it possible to comply with requirements for existing instruments while still incorporating the CFI. If more information is needed, the 16-item core CFI can easily be supplemented with additional questions, including those from the supplementary modules also developed during the DSM-5 process (see Chapter 3, "Supplementary Modules," and Appendix C in this handbook).

Organizational Routines, Procedures, and Practices

The organization must consider how implementing the CFI will impact the clinical workflow and billing practices as well as how to streamline documentation of the information obtained. It also needs to consider how using the CFI might impact the assessment sessions (e.g., whether the intake appointment duration should increase or decrease, whether the initial patient chart packet needs to be updated). In our experience with implementing the core CFI at RAMS, some staff members noted that the core CFI includes assessment areas they might not otherwise have investigated during the interview (e.g., regarding the clinician-patient relationship). As such, the patient health record forms—whether paper based or electronic—must be reviewed to ensure that there are sections where the practitioner can note responses to the CFI questions (e.g., regarding suggested kinds of help). Because the core CFI can easily be integrated as part of the general intake assessment or treatment planning, billing for the CFI is streamlined (e.g., when an intake assessment incorporates the CFI, the total time can be considered assessment billing). The organization should also assess its capacity to adjust its management information systems accordingly.

The organization must also consider organizational policy issues regarding the administration of the CFI: Is CFI usage required by organizational leadership? Do providers need to adhere strictly to administering the entire set of core CFI questions? If assessments are collaboratively conducted by a multidisciplinary team, which specific practitioner would administer the CFI? In addition, the organization needs to consider training-related questions such as these: Who will coordinate the logistics of the training (e.g., initial rollout, ongoing training)? Who will conduct the training? How will competence in CFI be assessed? Moreover, if there are multiple trainers across different departments or sectors, other issues arise: How could cross-communication take place (e.g., shared training experience, consolidated feedback)?

The organization may also need to consider its protocol related to translations. Although CFI translations are forthcoming (e.g., through foreign-language translations of the full DSM-5), administering the CFI with non-English-speaking patients may present complications. Field trials were conducted in several countries, supporting the core CFI's translatability, ease of use, and applicability across diverse cultures (see Chapter 2, "The Core and Informant Cultural Formulation Interviews in DSM-5," and subchapters "Use of the Cultural Formulation Interview in Different Clinical Settings" and "Application of the Cultural Formulation Interview in International Settings" in the current chapter). At the same time, translation may introduce variations in how the questions are interpreted. For example, RAMS translated the core CFI to written Chinese, but there was ongoing discussion regarding word choice and phrasing, which are dependent on factors such as which Chinese language is used (e.g., Cantonese or Mandarin) and emigration area (e.g., mainland China or Hong Kong) of the patient. Agency administrators needed to remain flexible about how to use the translations, so that clinicians and interpreters can use a translation as a guide rather than adhering strictly to it. Documenting translation difficulties should be part of quality assurance.

Practitioner Skills, Roles, and Activities

As an organization implements the CFI, some clinician ambivalence (e.g., lack of motivation or buy-in) and/or "comfort in routine" may present in various ways. In RAMS's experience, some practitioners indicated that incorporating the core CFI added time to the existing assessment process. They also noted, however, that the core CFI offered a more comprehensive patient-centered interview. Some clinicians may view the introduction of the CFI as suggesting that the organization does not endorse the clinicians' typical approach and instead views it as ineffective or not culturally competent. This concern presents an opportunity for administrators to engage the clinicians, being careful not to reject their current way of assessing patients. Use of the CFI may be suggested, not required, while the administrator takes the opportunity to learn what the clinicians' current assessment approach is and how it is different from or compatible with the CFI.

Clinicians may also express difficulty accommodating to certain patient preferences and/or addressing resource needs. This can be responded to through supervision, case conferences, and ongoing training, as well as by developing collaborative partnerships in the community. Furthermore, in RAMS's experience, the utilization of case management and peer support services has been very helpful in dealing with some resource limitation issues. Of course, better engagement with patients may initially lead to greater demands for services, and it is important for the system of care to be prepared to respond appropriately.

Conclusion

Clinically sound and culturally competent service delivery, high standards of care, patient satisfaction, and clinical and administrative efficiency are important goals in any health care system and organization. Although implementation of the CFI may require initial resources, the benefits we are starting to see from its use at RAMS are important (Table 4–8). The CFI not only can improve our work with patients in meaningful ways but also can enhance the quality and outcomes of the health care services we deliver.

TABLE 4–8. **Lessons learned from implementing the Cultural Formulation Interview (CFI) at Richmond Area Multi-Services**

Lesson	Specifics
Organizations must integrate cultural competence practices in order to meet the needs of a continually diversifying population.	The DSM-5 CFI can contribute to culturally competent practice by providing a structured yet flexible assessment framework. The CFI fosters a person-centered dialogue about a patient's mental health concerns experienced in a specific cultural context, which is expected to lead to more accurate diagnosis and collaborative treatment planning.
The CFI offers many potential benefits at the organizational level.	Benefits include standardization of a qualitative method of assessment, scalability in its training methodologies, accessibility by organizations and practitioners, and potentially effective results and outcomes.
Implementation strategies should initially develop an implementation plan.	A small group of middle managers and practitioners can develop an initial plan that includes CFI pilot testing; ongoing training for practitioners and middle managers; case conferences; and integration with clinical workflow, documentation, and management information systems.
The implementation process should be flexible and open to feedback from all stakeholders.	This open process should help in developing feedback mechanisms and evaluative measures and in sharing results with practition-ers in order to support effective integration and fidelity of the CFI.
Implementation challenges will arise that can be addressed through a planning process that includes multiple stakeholders.	Implementation challenges typically involve policy and funding requirements, organizational routines and procedures, and practitioner skills and roles.

KEY CLINICAL POINTS

- The DSM-5 Cultural Formulation Interview (CFI) is expected to enhance an organization's or clinician's ability to integrate culturally competent assessment because the CFI offers 1) standardization of a qualitative method of assessment, 2) scalability and accessibility, and 3) a focus on information that can contribute to clinically relevant results and outcomes.
- When introducing new tools and/or practices, administrators can consider the implementation strategy in terms of three main phases: 1) planning, 2) implementation, and 3) evaluation.
- Key components of the implementation strategy are communication and remaining flexible to cope with both anticipated and unanticipated challenges.

Questions

1. What are the main phases and key components of an implementation strategy?

2. What communication approaches can help integrate the CFI into a health care system or organization?

3. How could the DSM-5 CFI enhance an organization's or clinician's ability to integrate culturally competent assessment into routine practice?

4. What issues are to be considered when integrating the CFI into a health care system or organization?

5. What key performance indicators may be used to evaluate the usefulness of the CFI?

References

Aggarwal NK, Nicasio AV, DeSilva R, et al: Barriers to implementing the DSM-5 Cultural Formulation Interview: a qualitative study. Cult Med Psychiatry 37(3):505–533, 2013 23836098

American Psychiatric Association: Diagnostic and Statistical Manual of Mental Disorders, 4th Edition. Washington, DC, American Psychiatric Association, 1994

American Psychiatric Association: Diagnostic and Statistical Manual of Mental Disorders, 5th Edition. Arlington, VA, American Psychiatric Association, 2013

Cross T, Bazron B, Dennis K, et al: Towards a Culturally Competent System of Care, Vol 1. Washington, DC, Georgetown University Child Development Center, CASSP Technical Assistance Center, 1989

Dinh NM, Groleau D, Kirmayer LJ, et al: Influence of the DSM-IV Outline for Cultural Formulation on multidisciplinary case conferences in mental health. Anthropol Med 19(3):261–276, 2012 22309357

Fung K, Lo HT, Srivastava R, et al: Organizational cultural competence consultation to a mental health institution. Transcult Psychiatry 49(2):165–184, 2012 22508635

Kai J, Beavan J, Faull C, et al: Professional uncertainty and disempowerment responding to ethnic diversity in health care: a qualitative study. PLoS Med 4(11):e323, 2007 18001148

Rohlof H, Knipscheer JW, Kleber RJ: Use of the cultural formulation with refugees. Transcult Psychiatry 46(3):487–505, 2009 19837783

Scarpinati Rosso M, Bäärnhielm S: Use of the Cultural Formulation in Stockholm: a qualitative study of mental illness experience among migrants. Transcult Psychiatry 49(2):283–301, 2012 22508638

Tervalon M, Murray-García J: Cultural humility versus cultural competence: a critical distinction in defining physician training outcomes in multicultural education. J Health Care Poor Underserved 9(2):117–125, 1998 10073197

U.S. Department of Health and Human Services, Office of Minority Health: National Standards for Culturally and Linguistically Appropriate Services in Health and Health Care. Rockville, MD, U.S. Department of Health and Human Services, 2010. Available at: https://www.thinkculturalhealth.hhs.gov/Content/clas.asp. Accessed March 1, 2014.

Warren BJ: How culture is assessed in the DSM-5. J Psychosoc Nurs Ment Health Serv 51(4):40–45, 2013 23451737

Suggested Readings

Burke WW: Organization Change: Theory and Practice, 4th Edition (Foundations for Organizational Science). Thousand Oaks, CA, Sage, 2013

U.S. Department of Health and Human Services, Office of Minority Health: Think Cultural Health: Advancing Health Equity at Every Point of Contact. Rockville, MD, U.S. Department of Health and Human Services, 2013. Available at: http://www.thinkculturalhealth.hhs.gov/. Accessed August 25, 2014.

U.S. Department of Health and Human Services, Office of Minority Health: The Center for Linguistic and Cultural Competency in Health Care. Rockville, MD, U.S. Department of Health and Human Services, 2014. Available at: http://www.minorityhealth.hhs.gov/omh/browse.aspx?lvl=2&lvlid=34. Accessed August 25, 2014.

Application of the Cultural Formulation Interview in International Settings

Sofie Bäärnhielm, M.D., Ph.D.

David M. Ndetei, M.B.Ch.B., D.P.M., MRCPsych, FRCPsych, M.D., D.Sc.

Hans Rohlof, M.D.

K. Musa Misiani, B.Sc. Hons

Victoria M. Mutiso, M.Sc., Ph.D.

Abednego M. Musau, M.B.Ch.B.

Rhodah Mwangi, B.A.

Smita Neelkanth Deshpande, M.D., D.P.M.

Mental health care faces the global challenge of integrating awareness of culture and context into psychiatric diagnosis and treatment planning. In this subchapter, we discuss whether the Outline for Cultural Formulation (OCF) and the Cultural Formulation Interview (CFI) are useful tools for addressing cultural diversity in clinical diagnostic practice outside the United States and Canada. Our discussion is based on experience in India, Kenya, the Netherlands, and Sweden and other Nordic countries. These settings were chosen because they are culturally, socially, and geographically different from each other and all have experience using the OCF and the CFI.

The international usefulness of the CFI can easily be questioned. The OCF and the CFI are included in a diagnostic system presenting a psychiatric nosology developed in the United States. The idea that Diagnostic and Statistical Manual (DSM) nosology has universal validity, when the research supporting it has been based mainly in North America and Western Europe, has been criticized (Gone and Kirmayer 2010). In most nations, psychiatric diagnostic practice and documentation have been developed according to the International Classification of Diseases (ICD), the official international diagnostic system (World Health Organization 1992). The desk reference edition (American Psychiatric Association 2013a) of DSM-5 (American Psychiatric Association 2013b) diagnostic criteria has been translated into several languages, but DSM-5, which includes the OCF and the CFI, is available in fewer languages. Therefore, access to the OCF and the CFI, as well as to the introductory texts about culture included in DSM-5 and the text about cultural variation in relation to diagnostic criteria, is restricted.

Despite these limitations, clinical experience suggests that the OCF, the core and informant versions of the CFI, and the CFI supplementary modules can be usefully and relevantly applied in international settings. These tools offer a valuable person-centered approach for taking culture and context into account in an individualized and nonstereotyping way. In this subchapter, we discuss our experience with the OCF and the CFI in several countries, potential modifications of the CFI for use in international settings, and the role that psychiatric practice in other countries may play in continuing to refine the CFI.

Experiences With the CFI in India

India is the second most populous country on earth, with 1.25 billion inhabitants and enormous cultural diversity (Datanet India 2014). Health care depends on both free government health care facilities available to all and private out-of-pocket expenditures for those who are able to access private health care services. India was the first low- and middle-income country to implement a national mental health program to decentralize and deprofessionalize mental health care (Directorate General of Health Services 1982). However, India continues to have a dearth of trained mental health professionals, including psychiatrists (only about 4,000 are in the whole country, mostly in urban areas), clinical psychologists, psychiatric social workers, and psychiatric nurses (less than 2,000). Indian students use standard Western textbooks during their medical training, although the students themselves may be deeply rooted in an Indian ethos. Several leading Indian psychiatrists have described Indian cultural concepts of distress, such as *dhat* syndrome and possession states (Gautam and Jain 2010; Malhotra and Wig 1975). Although Indian educators do emphasize the role of cultural and social issues in diagnosis and management, most students find it easier to follow the textbook. ICD-10 is the official diagnostic system adopted by the Indian government, but textbooks refer to DSM, so students are also familiar with the DSM system and use it frequently.

Two Indian clinical sites, in New Delhi and Pune, were part of the DSM-5 field trial of the core CFI. Our experience at the New Delhi site is described in this subchapter. The clinical setting was the Post-Graduate Institute of Medical Education and Research (PGIMER), at the Dr. Ram Manohar Lohia Hospital, one of the oldest free tertiary-care teaching institutions run by the government. The department of psychiatry is housed in a general hospital psychiatry unit serving metropolitan New Delhi as well as nearby North Indian states. The unit treats 200–250 outpatients per day and had more than 10,000 new patients in 2012 and 2013. Faculty members participate in the teaching and academic activities of Guru Gobind Singh Indraprastha University in Delhi, with which PGIMER is affiliated. The department has a strong tradition of research in major mental disorders and associated social and psychological issues (Post-Graduate Institute of Medical Education and Research, Dr. Ram Manohar Lohia Hospital 2014), which led to its inclusion in the CFI field trial.

Patients presenting to the New Delhi site hail from several North Indian states and have widely varying cultures and languages. People from the hills, tribes, and urban and rural areas in and around Delhi, as well as people from South Indian states, present every day. Although Hinduism is the dominant religion and Hindi the dominant language, other religions are practiced and languages spoken by at least half the patients admitted. Belief in Indian systems of medicine, such as Ayurveda, Unani, homeopathy, faith healing, and home remedies, runs high. The view is prevalent that modern medical treatment is synonymous with medications, and patients tend to be skeptical of modern nonmedical interventions. Stigmatization of mental illness is frequent. Although expression of mental symptoms in physical terms is common among rural or less psychologically sophisticated populations, the urban or more educated people verbalize their mental distress in psychological terms. The educational background of the mental health personnel who administered the core CFI is rooted in Western traditions, textbooks, and scientific paradigms.

Experiences From the CFI Field Trial

The design of the field trial is described in Chapter 2, "The Core and Informant Cultural Formulation Interviews in DSM-5." Thirteen clinicians at the New Delhi site, including psychiatrists, clinical psychologists, and psychiatric social workers, were trained through two didactic lectures and two interactive workshops. Several clinicians also participated in the CFI translation process. Only new outpatient admissions registering for the first time were enrolled in the study. Their diagnoses were not known beforehand and included psychoses, drug abuse, childhood problems, and "minor" psychiatric disorders, such as anxiety, mild depression, and relationship issues. Both patients and clinicians provided quantitative and qualitative feedback on the core CFI–enhanced diagnostic interview, and investigators also gathered the impressions of several colleagues who participated in the trial.

Participants

The consent process and CFI process were novel for participants, many of whom had come from remote areas. All 68 participants in the field trial appreciated the clinician's efforts to obtain more information through the CFI, which emphasized that their cultural background was important for their ailments. All said that the questions were helpful and that the doctor gave a lot of time and "asked everything." The vast majority of patients used the word *good* to describe the experience, and they were impressed with the clinician's behavior. However, some found it difficult to comprehend questions on their "cultural background" because it was something they had never considered or been asked about. Some felt that they should have been asked about their economic situation, relations with their spouse, or childhood experiences. The time and opportunity for free communication during the CFI was most valued. Most patients reported that a great burden had been taken off their minds, because "everything had been asked." They felt that the clinician showed caring involvement or relatedness (or *apnapan,* which is Hindi for intimacy, affinity, kinship) by eliciting cultural details. Those who were advised to seek psychotherapy and nonmedication treatments such as yoga were even more appreciative. They felt that the doctor had gotten to the root of their problem by not merely focusing on medications and that they would get well. Because of the detailed interview process, they could be frank so that the doctor understood them better and this would help their recovery. However, the majority said that they had come to the hospital because of their illness and expected medication.

Because this was their first visit to the clinic, patients had difficulty articulating what help they wanted. Almost all felt that a clinician's cultural background mattered little because the clinicians were professionals and were "supposed to know" about the correct treatment. Notably, they felt that the information from the CFI would significantly improve mental health care not only for themselves but for patients in general.

Clinicians

Participating clinicians felt that the CFI was most useful for developing rapport, clarifying the patient's psychosocial background, and obtaining information on issues affecting illness expression. They said that it significantly improved communication, "bonding," and the clinician-patient relationship and that it was helpful in comprehensively eliciting all symptoms, thus aiding in diagnosis, treatment planning, and adherence. Even issues of daily living could be better investigated. Some said that the CFI yielded information about the patient's economic status. The CFI was described as not being helpful in cases of drug abuse or withdrawal syndromes, as well as with uncooperative or disorganized patients.

Most clinicians felt that the initial questions on the nature of the patient's concerns were most informative and immediately established rapport and that the questions on clinician background and "how can we help" also helped improve communication. However, some thought that the original question on the patient-clinician relationship included in the field trial version of the core CFI inquired unnecessarily about clinician background and made participants uncomfortable. This question was later revised for the DSM-5 version.

Summary of Indian Experience

The importance of culture in psychiatric evaluation and the potential usefulness of the core CFI were recognized by both clinicians and patients participating in the field trial. The overall response was positive. The core CFI seemed to facilitate the inclusion of patients' language of symptom expression in the diagnostic process and the involvement of patients as active partners in treatment planning by attending to their cultural concerns. When clinicians took the time to patiently ask about cultural and personal issues, important facts emerged. Overall, professional participants were most sensitive to how cultural background shapes illness expression and treatment adherence. Department members became more aware of local symptom expression, and senior members' teaching of the importance of cultural factors in management grew more emphatic. The result of the field trial was greater emphasis on the Indian experience and expertise in teaching. However, the time needed for the core CFI is likely to constrain its general use. Perhaps, as some clinicians suggested, only the most relevant questions can be woven into the general psychiatric history–taking process. To be useful for regular clinical use in Indian contexts, the core CFI will need to be shortened significantly.

Experiences With the CFI in Kenya

Kenya, with a population of 43 million people, is one of the poorest countries in the world, ranked 144th out of 177 countries in the human development index. Nairobi, the country's capital, is home to one of the largest slum areas in Africa: Kibera, a vast shanty city with 170,000 to 1 million inhabitants (Central Intelligence Agency 2013). Provision of health services in Kenya is predominantly government funded. It is broadly structured into six levels: national referral hospitals (level 6), provincial general hospitals (level 5), district hospitals (level 4), health centers (level 3), dispensaries (level 2), and volunteer community health workers (level 1) (Republic of Kenya Ministry of Health 2005). Mental health care remains extremely limited in terms of infrastructure, staffing, and finances. Specialist care is largely delivered by psychiatric nurses in outpatient clinics at the district level and in inpatient units and outpatient clinics at the provincial level. Psychiatrists, on the other hand, provide specialized care in the national referral hospitals at Mathari National Teaching and Referral Hospital, Kenyatta National Hospital/University of Nairobi, and recently the Moi Teaching and Referral Hospital. The total number of mental health hospital beds for the entire Kenyan population was 1,114 in 2009, a bed-to-population ratio of approximately 1:200,000 (In2MentalHealth 2013).

Kenya has a training program for psychiatrists at the University of Nairobi; at least six new psychiatrists graduate per year. There are currently about 80 Kenyan psychiatrists; however, most are sequestered in urban centers, with about a quarter (21 of 80) working in education. Another quarter live and work outside the country. Effectively, this means that outside of Nairobi, the psychiatrist-to-population ratio is 1:3,000,000– 5,000,000. Compounding this extreme dearth of psychiatrists is the fact that of the 500 trained psychiatric nurses, only 250 are currently deployed in psychiatry. Seventy are deployed to Mathari National Teaching and Referral Hospital, leaving 180 nurses to work in the districts and provinces. The result is that there is less than one psychiatric nurse per district. Many of the rest have retired, died, left the country, or gone to work for nongovernmental organizations. The future is as gloomy as the present because the number of new applicants for mental health nurse training is declining.

Local Need for Cultural Awareness

The indigenous Kenyan population consists of approximately 42 tribes or ethnic groups. Despite their cultural diversity, the various groups' cultural perceptions about the causes of mental illness are quite similar. The vast majority believe that mental illnesses are caused by supernatural powers such as evil spirits. Many think that those who develop mental disorders do so to atone for sins committed against ancestors or as a result of being bewitched (Kiima et al. 2004). Kenyans who have adopted Christianity and Islam have abandoned some of these traditional cultural beliefs. However, some sects within the Christian faith, especially among Protestants, believe in faith healing. These sects attract some psychiatric patients, especially those whose mental illnesses are colored by religious experiences. Usually, Muslim patients are taken to their sheikhs; these faith healers often use the cultural attitudes toward mental illness prevalent in their communities to offer spiritual intervention through prayer (Kiima et al. 2004).

The culture-sensitive nature of psychiatric phenomenology has been explored by several authors. In a hospital-based study of psychiatrically ill African immigrants in a London hospital, Ndetei (1988) noted that paranoia, religious phenomenology, and hallucinations (in particular, auditory hallucinations and first-rank symptoms of schizophrenia) do not necessarily have the same clinical significance in various cultural groups. Many Africans when ill seek not only treatment but an explanation for their affliction and guidance toward spiritual well-being (Offiong 1999). They may engage in Western treatment to cure the illness but then enlist the aid of a traditional healer to seek an explanation for the cause of the illness. For many, health is not merely the absence of disease; it signifies peace with the ancestors and spirits (Lambo 1962). In Kenya, this practice cuts across all cultural groups regardless of educational status or position in society (Odhalo 1962; Otsyula 1973). The health-related actions, beliefs, traditions, and ways of thinking of Kenyans and other Africans can be seen to follow local explanatory models and notions of illness causality. This is evident in the tendency to attribute misfortune or disease to the actions of witches or evil people and to react with paranoid ideation to certain threatening situations (Ndetei 1988). These examples inform the need for culture-tailored diagnostic tools such as the CFI.

Experiences From the CFI Field Trial

At the Kenyan site of the field trial, the core CFI was administered to 30 patients in an outpatient psychiatric clinic in Nairobi. All of the patients were adult indigenous Kenyans who had been referred for psychiatric management. Patients' CFI interviews were recorded and analyzed qualitatively. Two main findings emerged: 1) the core CFI helped improve clinicians' understanding of the patients' conditions, and 2) patients reported feeling that they had expressed themselves better. These findings were noted especially for patients being evaluated for psychotic illnesses. The following case vignette illustrates this point.

Case Vignette

Simon, a 37-year-old man from a large coastal city, presented with a 2-month history of constant low mood, anhedonia, and "unusual" behavior that included singing loudly and shouting at night. After reassuring him that the goal was to understand his specific problem, experience, and ideas and that there were no wrong or right answers, the interviewer asked what problems or concerns brought him to the clinic. Simon replied that he was fine until he lost his job. He then began to display behavior that he insisted was not abnormal but that his relatives perceived to be "unusual," and they referred him to a traditional healer. When asked what he thought was the cause of his problem, Simon said that he felt he was being tormented by evil spirits. On further probing, he attributed his predicament to family conflicts involving property and to the fact that he came from a minority ethnic community in coastal Kenya. He said that his relatives and siblings had contributed to his condition because they sent the evil spirits to him. He also said that what helped him cope with his condition was praying to God and watching music videos.

Use of the core CFI enabled further probing of Simon's cultural belief system, resulting in a diagnosis of depression and not paranoid schizophrenia. It is important to appreciate that in many communities in Kenya, any apparent bad luck that befalls someone (e.g., the loss of a job) will tend to be attributed to perceived enemies' use of black magic and evil spirits. The apparent persecutory delusions reported by this patient might have been mistaken for symptoms of psychosis if they were not understood within the patient's sociocultural context. The core CFI was useful in obtaining information about the context and the meaning of the patient's symptoms and concerns, which, combined with the interviewer's background knowledge of the societal norms, helped clarify the diagnosis.

Summary of Kenyan Experience

In Kenya, implementation of the core CFI started among clinicians working in research. Because Kenya is officially an English-speaking country, the original English version of the core CFI could be used by clinicians. However, a majority of Kenyans do not use English as their first language or as the primary language of communication. We translated the core CFI to Kiswahili, the national language. The diversity of languages in a multilingual society such as Kenya, however, poses considerable difficulty in implementing this tool, because Kiswahili is still a second language to many Kenyans. Nevertheless, the core CFI has gained considerable traction, especially because Kenya was among the countries that participated in the CFI field trial.

Because of its inclusion in DSM-5, the CFI has been integrated into the curriculum at Kenya's only psychiatric training institution, the University of Nairobi. The DSM-IV (American Psychiatric Association 1994) OCF had been used extensively in training in this institution, which eased the introduction of the CFI as an integral part of training. This process is gaining momentum because the CFI is now a compulsory part of training for graduate students specializing in psychiatry. With additional funding to develop appropriate teaching materials, the use of the CFI could penetrate into daily clinical practice through its adoption in continuing medical education to train practitioners in mental health care in outpatient clinics and in primary care or even psychiatric units in any of the other national psychiatric hospitals.

Experiences With the CFI in the Netherlands

The Netherlands is a country of 17 million people, of whom about 1 million are Muslim. Since the 1960s, the ethnic diversity of the Dutch population has grown enormously. The number of people from a foreign background, first and second generation, is currently about 20% of the population and is expected to grow to 30% by 2060 (Stoeldraijer and Garssen 2011). In the west of the country, where 7 million people live close together in the so-called City of Holland, foreign-born individuals are becoming the majority of the inhabitants.

These demographic shifts have important repercussions for mental health care. The proportion of immigrants in the mental health care system, which before 1990 was lower than the percentage of immigrants in the general population, has gradually increased to an equal percentage, although some groups are seen mainly in emergency departments or forensic settings (Dieperink et al. 2007). Recognition of the need for more cultural awareness has increased in response to studies showing that poor communication with patients from a different cultural background leads to less effective treatment, premature treatment discontinuation, and poor adherence (Blom et al. 2010; Fassaert et al. 2010). Large mental health institutions, mainly in the west of the country, have started to show interest in more culturally competent care for migrants.

Mental health care in the Netherlands is well developed, with universally available outpatient services, inpatient services, and other services such as day clinics, foster homes for chronic psychiatric patients, and day activity centers. DSM is used as the standard diagnostic system. In 2008, the financial structure of mental health care was completely changed, with payment transferred from government-funded health insurance to private health insurance companies. The purpose of the switch was to reduce costs and improve efficiency through competition. This has resulted in a more diverse system, in which different regional care providers compete with local care providers. For the individual patient, this change has resulted in more freedom of choice. However, the general costs of mental health care have increased substantially, and the government is trying to raise some barriers to mental health care use. A routine outcome monitoring system requires caregivers to monitor changes in symptoms and functioning and to provide outcome data to the health insurance companies.

Experiences With the CFI Field Trial

Three centers in the Netherlands took part in the DSM-5 CFI field trial: a specialized clinic for refugees, a typical mental health institution, and a psychotrauma clinic. Clinicians were generally satisfied with the feasibility and acceptability of the version of the core CFI used in the field trial. They were more satisfied with its impact on improving contact with the patient than with its usefulness for diagnosis and treatment planning. Patients viewed the core CFI more positively than did clinicians, particularly in terms of its potential clinical utility, but were somewhat less satisfied with the length of the interview and its clarity. Some questions were considered unclear or too similar to other questions. Discussions by the international research group led to changes in the final version of the core CFI for DSM-5. In addition, some of the most experienced clinicians found the structure of the core CFI overly constraining. To address this concern, the final version of the core CFI notes that the questions should be regarded as examples that need not be followed verbatim as long as the content of each question is examined.

It is worth noting that the core CFI was useful for working with native Dutch patients as well as migrants. For example, when asked about belonging to a certain group, one Dutch person responded, "My group is the group of veterans. I only feel at ease in the company of other veterans. I have noticed that you have a veterans program in your clinic. I only accept other veterans in my company, and I hope that all the therapists will have a veteran background too." A woman who appeared to be of Dutch origin remarked, "I've lived in the Netherlands for 50 years, but I still feel myself East Indian." She came from the former colony of the Dutch East Indies, now Indonesia. People born there, who are often of mixed ethnic background, are not considered immigrants in the Netherlands but, nevertheless, have their own culture with strong family bonds, distinctive food, and Asian ways of handling difficult emotions by maintaining equanimity; Dutch clinicians not from their background sometimes find it difficult to diagnose the presence of depressed mood because of their usual smiling demeanor.

Summary of Dutch Experience

Researchers and clinicians in the Netherlands were pioneers in the implementation of the DSM-IV OCF, prior to the development of the CFI. In the late 1990s, a group of Dutch clinicians began to use the DSM-IV OCF and prepared a book in Dutch with chapters on theory and case vignettes (Borra et al. 2002). The concluding chapter noted that the OCF needed further operationalization. To that end, a cultural interview based on the DSM-IV OCF was developed and used in the clinic to get a better understanding of refugees, who are sometimes culturally very distant from their caregivers (Rohlof et al. 2002). The interview was well tolerated by patients and yielded excellent information about their cultural backgrounds but generally took about 90 minutes to complete (Rohlof and Ghane 2003); hence, there were attempts to reduce the number of questions. An abbreviated cultural interview was developed, which required about half the time to administer. Patients showed better acceptance of the shorter version, and the information gathered was comparable to that obtained with the longer interview (Groen and Laban 2011). Further refinements and applications of this work were carried out, both in psychiatry and general health care and in clinical practice and education, resulting in a book in Dutch describing the various cultural interviews and their applications, including in forensic and child psychiatry settings (van Dijk et al. 2012). In the Netherlands, the original cultural interview (the Rohlof version) and the abbreviated cultural interview (the Groen version) based on the DSM-IV OCF have been widely used in the training of psychiatric residents (in the national training module), clinical psychologists, social psychiatric nurses, nurse-practitioners, and general practitioners (Bruggeman and Busser 2012). Implementation of these cultural interviews in education has been a success, but their routine use in clinical practice has proven more difficult. The Dutch experience with disseminating and implementing the local cultural interviews serves as a useful precedent for the CFI; many of the same barriers as well as principal uses and settings of initial uptake apply to implementation of the CFI.

Experiences From Sweden and Other Nordic Countries

Sweden and other Nordic countries (Denmark, Norway, and Finland) were relatively culturally homogeneous until World War II, when immigration of laborers and refugees started to increase the cultural diversity of Nordic countries. At present, 15% of the Swedish population of 9.6 million is foreign born, and first- and second-generation immigrants make up 20.1% of the population; 53% of the immigrants are from non-European countries (Statistics Sweden 2013). Migration has also transformed other Nordic countries, although the percentages of foreign-born immigrants in these other countries are lower than in Sweden: 8.1% of the Danish population of 5.6 million (Danmarks Statistik 2013), 10.8% of the Norwegian population of 4.9 million (Vasileyva 2011), and 4.3% of the Finnish population of 5.4 million (Vasileyva 2011).

Sweden and other Nordic countries have tax-funded health care systems that provide equal rights to care for migrants who have been granted a residency permit. For asylum seekers, undocumented migrants, and uninsured European Union citizens, there are restrictions governing access to care. In Sweden, as in other European Union countries, health care disparities between native-born inhabitants and migrants increase the vulnerability of migrants to poor mental health (Rechel et al. 2013). Despite equal rights to care, barriers to mental health treatment for migrants include poor fluency in Nordic languages, stigmatization, limited knowledge of the health care system, and a lack of cultural sensitivity in the mental health care system.

ICD-10 is the official national diagnostic system of the Nordic countries. In clinical care, however, DSM is sometimes used in parallel with ICD. Moreover, DSM is often used in research, education, and training and has a substantial impact on professional and public discussions on mental health and mental health care. Attention to cultural variations in ICD-10 is limited. Regional versions of ICD-10 from China, Japan, Cuba, and Latin America represent attempts to adapt the nosology to local cultural and social realities (Mezzich et al. 2001). The ICD model, with regional geographical adaptations, is not helpful in addressing cultural awareness regarding psychiatric care in the Nordic countries. This limitation has promoted interest in DSM-IV and DSM-5, which address culture in the core definition of mental disorder, culture-related issues in relation to diagnostic criteria, the OCF, and (in DSM-5) the CFI as a practical diagnostic tool for taking culture into account.

Local Need for Cultural Awareness

Few clinical service models in Sweden address cultural aspects of mental illness and treatment. This situation persists despite the fact that some efforts have been made to address cultural aspects of care with interpreters, in clinics for traumatized refugees, and in various development projects. However, the concerns about culture have not been enough to cope with the diversity of needs. The clinical challenge in addressing culture and context in psychiatric diagnosis has directed attention to the OCF, first in DSM-IV and now in DSM-5. The clinical contexts of other Nordic countries share various similarities with the Swedish situation.

Experiences With the DSM-IV OCF

There were no Swedish sites in the CFI field trial; however, Swedish clinicians and researchers have been at the forefront of developing a standardized interview for the OCF. A Swedish interview guide for how to use the DSM-IV OCF was prepared to facilitate its clinical use (Bäärnhielm et al. 2007). This guide, which is quite similar to the core CFI and the supplementary modules in DSM-5, was evaluated in a multiple-case study with immigrant and refugee patients, most of whom came from the Middle East, at an outpatient clinic for nonpsychotic disorders (Scarpinati Rosso and Bäärnhielm 2012). Patients' narratives were transcribed and analyzed. Results showed that all the narratives were solidly grounded in their everyday lives, highlighting the importance of contextualizing symptoms to aid clinical understanding. The narrative format of the OCF facilitated interviewers' use of open-ended questions to probe the contextual details of patients' experience (Bäärnhielm and Scarpinati Rosso 2009). In this study, an interview operationalizing the OCF was conducted after the ordinary clinical psychiatric diagnostic evaluation. Its use led to a revision of psychiatric disorder diagnostic groupings for 13 of the 23 patients (56%) (Bäärnhielm et al. 2014). Most of the changes involved identifying missed cases of anxiety disorders and posttraumatic stress disorder, but some of the changes resulted from revisions of specific anxiety diagnoses and from reassessing a misdiagnosis of posttraumatic stress disorder. In a different study, cultural analysis based on the DSM-IV OCF was carried out with 20 women at a substance abuse outpatient clinic in Sweden (DeMarinis et al. 2009). The cultural assessment revealed that these patients constructed their identity around alcohol use, developing elaborate drinking rituals and behaviors related to consumption, with implications for service delivery and intervention.

Summary of Nordic Experience

In Sweden, clinical implementation of the DSM-IV OCF started with clinicians working in marginalized, multicultural communities. As diversity increased nationwide, interest in cultural formulation expanded to include a broader segment of the mental health care system. A key factor in this wider interest was the inclusion of the core CFI in DSM-5, which will be translated into Swedish and made available to all free of charge by the local publisher. Recent psychiatric textbooks in Swedish include information about the CFI. To support clinical use of the Cultural Formulation approach in the greater Stockholm area, terms to document social and cultural information are included in the shared information technology system for medical records (www.transkulturelltcentrum.se/vara-kunskapsomraden/transkulturell-psykiatri/journalforing-i-takecare/).

In Stockholm, information about the OCF and CFI is also included in guidelines for care and on official psychiatric Web sites. Experiences implementing the CFI in Sweden indicate the importance of combining clinical application with training and consultative support. The ethnographic approach of the CFI, which involves eliciting contextual information through open-ended questions, can be somewhat unfamiliar for clinicians, because much current diagnostic interviewing has become narrowly symptom focused. Interpreting a patient's narrative involves a process of translating from the patient's system of meaning to a medical framework. To use the CFI in a flexible way, creating a natural narrative flow, it is important that clinicians understand the purpose of the questions. This facilitates the reformulation of questions to ensure that they are comprehensible to the patient, as well as probing for clarification and elaboration.

There is also interest in the CFI in the other Nordic countries. The Swedish interview guide was translated into Norwegian and Finnish, and a Danish guide was also developed (Østerskov 2011). Clinical implementation of the CFI in the Nordic countries will require its translation into local languages. Although initially only the diagnostic criteria of DSM-5 and not the whole text were published in Nordic languages, the CFI and some other assessment measures will be translated into Swedish.

The Transcultural Center of the Stockholm County Council initiated training in the DSM-IV OCF in 2003. Currently, in Sweden, standard training in the use of DSM-5 and in transcultural psychiatry is starting to incorporate the CFI. In Norway, the National Norwegian Center for Minority Health Research has organized several training events on the DSM-IV OCF, and the CFI is included in transcultural training activities during psychiatric residency. In Copenhagen, training for mental health professionals has begun on the use of the Danish interview guide.

Conclusion

Our experience in four distinct cultural settings suggests that the OCF and CFI substantially improve awareness of culture and context internationally in an individualized nonstereotyping way in psychiatric diagnostic practice. The CFI represents a fundamental paradigm shift in psychiatric nosology, highlighting social and cultural influences on psychiatric phenomenology. By integrating a medical anthropological framework, the CFI provides a richer background for diagnosis. It is important to emphasize, however, that the use of the CFI requires a flexible approach that is tailored to each patient's peculiarities rather than a verbatim reading of the questions to the patient. The use of the CFI does not in any way replace the traditional tools and skills useful for understanding each patient.

For implementation of the CFI in non-English-speaking countries, translations into local languages are necessary, including the development of local training materials. To support clinical implementation, there is a need for research on the contribution of the CFI to diagnostic validity and to improving care in different cultural settings. More information on how patients understand the various domains and questions of the CFI can facilitate its use and may contribute to additional clinical impact. On the basis of our experiences, the application of the CFI requires training followed by practical support in how to use it. Consultative support in clinical cases can be valuable. International experiences can contribute to refining the DSM-5 CFI for diverse populations in different settings. Furthermore, these experiences may also enhance knowledge about how culture and context influence mental distress and coping strategies.

KEY CLINICAL POINTS

- The person-centered, nonstereotyping approach of the Cultural Formulation Interview (CFI) makes it a useful tool for routine clinical practice outside North America and helps establish trust and rapport between patient and clinician.
- Clinical implementation of the CFI requires local training and ongoing support.
- Clinicians need to understand the meaning and purpose of the CFI questions in order to adapt them to the local context and individual encounters.
- Clinical use of the CFI in non-English-speaking settings requires its translation into local languages and potential simplification of some terms.
- Clinical application of the CFI may require health system resource supports and changes in procedures, such as incorporation into clinical guidelines and medical record documentation formats.
- International experience can contribute to refining the CFI for diverse populations in different settings.

Questions

1. How should use of the CFI in routine clinical practice be promoted in international settings?

2. What are the pros, cons, and anticipated challenges involved in using the CFI globally?

3. On the basis of experience with the tool in diverse settings, what procedures, refinements, and adaptations may be needed to use the CFI internationally?

4. What can international experience contribute to the development of the field of cultural assessment and cultural psychiatry more generally?

5. How can international use of the CFI contribute to awareness of local symptom expressions?

References

American Psychiatric Association: Diagnostic and Statistical Manual of Mental Disorders, 4th Edition. Washington, DC, American Psychiatric Association, 1994

American Psychiatric Association: Desk Reference to the Diagnostic Criteria From DSM-5. Arlington, VA, American Psychiatric Association, 2013a

American Psychiatric Association: Diagnostic and Statistical Manual of Mental Disorders, 5th Edition. Arlington, VA, American Psychiatric Association, 2013b

Bäärnhielm S, Scarpinati Rosso M: The Cultural Formulation: a model to combine nosology and patients' life context in psychiatric diagnostic practice. Transcult Psychiatry 46(3):406–428, 2009 19837779

Bäärnhielm S, Scarpinati Rosso M, Pattyi L: Kultur, Kontext och Psykiatrisk Diagnostik. Manual för Intervju Enligt Kulturformuleringen i DSM-IV [Culture, Context and Psychiatric Diagnosis. Interview Manual for the Outline for Cultural Formulation in DSM-IV]. Stockholm, Sweden, Transkulturellt Centrum, Stockholms läns landsting, 2007

Bäärnhielm S, Åberg Wistedt A, Rosso MS: Revising psychiatric diagnostic categorization of immigrant patients after using the Cultural Formulation in DSM-IV. Transcult Psychiatry Dec 9, 2014 25492265 [Epub ahead of print]

Blom MBJ, Hoek HW, Spinhoven P, et al: Treatment of depression in patients from ethnic minority groups in the Netherlands. Transcult Psychiatry 47(3):473–490, 2010 20688800

Borra R, van Dijk R, Rohlof H (eds): Cultuur, Classificatie en Diagnose: Cultuursensitief Werken met de DSM-IV [Culture, Classification and Diagnosis: Culture-Sensitive Work With DSM-IV]. Houten, The Netherlands, Bohn Stafleu Van Loghum, 2002

Bruggeman L, Busser G: Cultureel interviewen en de huisartsopleiding: scenes uit een huwelijk [Cultural interviewing and the training of general practitioners: scenes of a marriage], in Het Culturele Interview [The Cultural Interview]. Edited by van Dijk R, Beijers H, Groen S. Utrecht, The Netherlands, Pharos, 2012, pp 148–160

Central Intelligence Agency: Kenya: country profile, in The World Factbook. 2013. Available at: https://www.cia.gov/library/publications/the-world-factbook/geos/ke.html. Accessed March 10, 2014.

Danmarks Statistik: Invandrare i Danmark 2013 [Immigrants in Denmark 2013], 2013. Available at: http://www.dst.dk/da/Statistik/Publikationer/VisPub.aspx?cid=17961. Accessed August 6, 2014.

Datanet India: Indiastat.com (Web site). Available at: http://www.indiastat.com/default.aspx. Accessed August 4, 2014.

DeMarinis V, Scheffel-Birath C, Hansagi H: Cultural analysis as a perspective for gender-informed alcohol treatment research in a Swedish context. Alcohol Alcohol 44(6):615–619, 2009 19047017

Dieperink C, van Dijk R, de Vries S: Vijftien jaar GGZ gebruik door allochtonen: groei en diversiteit [Fifteen years' care use by migrants: growth and diversity]. Maandblad Geestelijke Volksgezondheid 62:710–721, 2007

Directorate General of Health Services: National Mental Health Programme (NMHP) for India. New Delhi, Ministry of Health Government of India, 1982. Available at: http://mohfw.nic.in/WriteReadData/l892s/9903463892NMHP%20detail.pdf. Accessed August 8, 2014.

Fassaert T, Peen J, van Straten A, et al: Ethnic differences and similarities in outpatient treatment for depression in the Netherlands. Psychiatr Serv 61(7):690–697, 2010 20592004

Gautam S, Jain N: Indian culture and psychiatry. Indian J Psychiatry 52 (suppl 1):S309–S313, 2010

Gone JP, Kirmayer LJ: On the wisdom of considering culture and context in psychopathology, in Contemporary Directions in Psychopathology: Scientific Foundations of the DSM-V and ICD-11. Edited by Millon T, Krueger RF, Simonsen E. New York, Guilford, 2010, pp 72–96

Groen S, Laban K: Beter Begrepen, Sneller Bereikt [Better Understood, Quicker Reached]. Beilen, The Netherlands, De Evenaar, 2011

In2MentalHealth: Eight encounters with mental health care Kenya. In2MentalHealth, 2013. Available at: http://in2mentalhealth.com/2013/02/14/eight-encounters-with-mental-health-care-kenya/. Accessed March 11, 2014.

Kiima DM, Njenga FG, Okonji MM, et al: Kenya mental health country profile. Int Rev Psychiatry 16(1–2):48–53, 2004 15276937

Lambo TA: African traditional beliefs, concepts of health and medical practice. Lecture presented at Philosophical Society, University College, Ibadan, Nigeria, October 1962

Malhotra HK, Wig NN: Dhat syndrome: a culture-bound sex neurosis of the Orient. Arch Sex Behav 4(5):519–528, 1975 1191004

Mezzich JE, Berganza CE, Ruipérez MA: Culture in DSM-IV, ICD-10, and evolving diagnostic systems. Psychiatr Clin North Am 24(3):407–419, 2001 11593853

Ndetei DM: Psychiatric phenomenology across countries: constitutional, cultural, or environmental? Acta Psychiatr Scand Suppl 344:33–44, 1988 3227985

Odhalo J: A report on the Luo culture and health. East Afr Med J 39:694–701, 1962 13939472

Offiong DA: Traditional healers in the Nigerian health care delivery system and the debate over integrating traditional and scientific medicine. Anthropol Q 72:118–130, 1999

Østerskov M: Kulturel Spørgeguide [Cultural Interview Guide]. Copenhagen, Videnscenter for Transkulturel Psykiatri, 2011

Otsyula W: Native and western healing: the dilemma of East African psychiatry. J Nerv Ment Dis 156(5):297–299, 1973 4704221

Post-Graduate Institute of Medical Education and Research, Dr. Ram Manohar Lohia Hospital: Indo-U.S. Programme for Genetics and Psychoses. New Delhi, India, 2014. Available at: rmlh.nic.in. Accessed June 15, 2014.

Rechel B, Mladovsky P, Ingleby D, et al: Migration and health in an increasingly diverse Europe. Lancet 381(9873):1235–1245, 2013 23541058

Republic of Kenya Ministry of Health: Reversing the Trends: The Second National Health Sector Strategic Plan of Kenya—NHSSP II: 2005–2010. Nairobi, Kenya, Ministry of Health, Health Sector Reform Secretariat, 2005. Available at: http://www.nacc.or.ke/attachments/article/102/NHSSP%20II-2010.pdf. Accessed March 10, 2014.

Rohlof H, Ghane S: Het culturele interview [The cultural interview], in Cultuursensitief Werken met de DSM-IV [Culture-Sensitive Working With DSM-IV]. Edited by van Dijk R, Sönmez N. Rotterdam, The Netherlands, Mikado, 2003, pp 49–52

Rohlof H, Loevy N, Stassen L, et al: Het culturele interview [The cultural interview], in Cultuur, Classificatie en Diagnose: Cultuursensitief Werken met DSM-IV [Culture, Classification and Diagnosis: Culture-Sensitive Work With DSM-IV]. Edited by Borra R, van Dijk R, Rohlof H. Houten, The Netherlands, Bohn Stafleu Van Loghum, 2002, pp 251–261

Scarpinati Rosso M, Bäärnhielm S: Use of Cultural Formulation in Stockholm: a qualitative study on mental illness experiences among migrants. Transcult Psychiatry, 49(2), 283–301 2012 22508638

Statistics Sweden: Statistical Yearbook of Sweden, 2014. Örebro, Sweden, SCB, 2013

Stoeldraijer L, Garssen J: Prognose van de bevolking naar herkomst 2010–2060 [Population prognosis viewed at origin 2010–2060], in Bevolkingstrends [Trends in Population], Jaargang 59, 2e Kwartaal. The Hague, The Netherlands, Centraal Bureau voor de Statistiek, 2011, pp 24–31

van Dijk R, Beijers H, Groen S (eds): Het Culturele Interview [The Cultural Interview]. Utrecht, The Netherlands, Pharos, 2012

Vasileyva K: 6.5% of the EU population are foreigners and 9.4% are born abroad. Eurostat: Statistics in Focus. Issue 34/2011, 2011. http://ec.europa.eu/eurostat/documents/3433488/5579176/KS-SF-11-034-EN.PDF/63cebff3-f7ac-4ca6-ab33-4e8792c5f30c. Accessed August 7, 2014.

World Health Organization: Mental and behavioural disorders, in International Statistical Classification of Diseases and Related Health Problems, 10th Revision. Geneva, World Health Organization, 1992 pp 311–387

Suggested Readings

Chavan BS, Gupta N, Arun P, et al (eds): Community Mental Health in India. New Delhi, India, Jaypee Brothers, 2012

Okpaku SO (ed): Clinical Methods in Transcultural Psychiatry. Washington, DC, American Psychiatric Press, 1998

Yilmaz AT, Weiss MG, Riecher-Rössler A: Cultural Psychiatry: Euro-International Perspectives. Basel, Switzerland, Karger, 2001

Danish

Kompetencecenter for Transkulturel Psykiatri (Web site): Available at: http://www.ctp-net.dk. Accessed February 18, 2015.

Dutch

Borra R, van Dijk R, Rohlof H (eds): Cultuur, Classificatie en Diagnose [Culture, Classification and Diagnosis]. Houten, The Netherlands, Bohn Stafleu Van Loghum, 2002

van Dijk R, Beijers H, Groen S (eds): Het Culturele Interview [The Cultural Interview]. Utrecht, The Netherlands, Pharos, 2012

Finnish

Paksalahti A, Huttunen MO (eds): Kulttuurit ja Lääketiede [Culture and Medicine]. Helsinki, Finland, Duodecim, 2010

Norwegian

Javó C: Kulturens Betydning for Oppdragelse og Atferdsproblemer [The Impact of Culture on Upbringing and Behavioral Problems]. Oslo, Norway, Universitetsforlaget, 2010

National Center for Minority Health, Oslo, Norway (Web site): Available at: http://www.nakmi.no. Accessed February 13, 2015.

Swedish

Bäärnhielm S: Transkulturell Psykiatri [Transcultural Psychiatry]. Stockholm, Sweden, Natur och Kultur, 2014

Transkulturellt Centrum, Stockholm County Council, Stockholm, Sweden (Web site): Available at: http://www.transkulturelltcentrum.se. Accessed February 13, 2015.

CHAPTER 5

Cultural Competence in Psychiatric Education Using the Cultural Formulation Interview

Russell F. Lim, M.D., M.Ed.

Esperanza Díaz, M.D.

Hendry Ton, M.D., M.S.

The DSM-5 (American Psychiatric Association 2013a) Cultural Formulation Interview (CFI) offers medical educators an important opportunity to incorporate culturally appropriate assessment techniques into existing curricula and teaching approaches. In this chapter, we review current regulations and published guidelines on the teaching of culturally appropriate assessment in medical student education, resident education, and continuing medical education (CME) and suggest how the CFI can be incorporated into these efforts.

Regulations and Guidelines on Teaching Cultural Assessment

Education in cultural competence is mandated in medical school and adult psychiatric residency programs, as well as in some U.S. states for practicing psychiatrists. Training physicians in cultural competence must start at the level of medical student education, when basic medical knowledge, skills, and attitudes are developed and solidified. The Association for American Medical Colleges and the Liaison Committee on Medical Education, which provide oversight to medical schools in Canada and the United States, require cultural competence training as part of the accreditation process. According to ED-21 and ED-22 of the Standards for Accreditation of Medical Education Programs Leading to the M.D. Degree (Liaison Committee on Medical Education 2013), medical students must know that the patient's ethnic background can influence diagnostic assessment and treatment planning, and they must also develop the ability to self-assess their levels of bias and stereotyping that may lead to health and mental health disparities. Training medical students in the use of the CFI can help address both of these objectives (e.g., via core CFI questions 4 and 5 and 15, respectively).

For psychiatric resident education, the Accreditation Council of Graduate Medical Education (ACGME) incorporates cultural competence principles in its Guidelines for Six Core Competencies and the Psychiatry Milestone Project (Accreditation Council of Graduate Medical Education and American Board of Psychiatry and Neurology 2013; Ling et al. 2013). Residents must see a sufficient variety of patients to be trained in how to assess different ethnic minority groups. Specifically, new milestones in the professionalism section guide educators in rating residents' ability to understand how patient diversity affects patient care, in developing a care plan that bridges patient and physician health beliefs, and in discussing their own cultural background and beliefs and how these affect their patient interactions. For example, the professionalism 1 domain in these milestones focuses on "compassion, integrity, respect for others, sensitivity to diverse patient populations" (Accreditation Council of Graduate Medical Education and American Board of Psychiatry and Neurology 2013). Although the ACGME does not specifically use the term *cultural competence* in the milestones, its principles have been included in the reviews of accreditation criteria.

CME training in cultural competence is required to renew physicians' licenses in six states: California, Connecticut, New Jersey, New York, Ohio, and Washington (National Consortium for Multicultural Education for Health Professionals 2009). Each state's requirement is different. For example, California Assembly Bill 1195 requires all CME programs to address cultural competence, and New Jersey's CME requirements specifically mandate cultural competence education in all medical schools in the state and a one-time, 6-hour certification in cultural competence for all physicians licensed in New Jersey. The CFI can help physicians meet these training requirements, especially via items focusing on cultural illness beliefs (cultural conceptualizations of distress) and the impact of culture on the doctor-patient relationship (Lewis-Fernández et al. 2014).

Medical Student Education

Integration

Efforts to implement cultural competence in medical student education typically use an "additive" approach in which cultural concepts, themes, and perspectives are added to the general curriculum without significant integration or ongoing reinforcement, commonly done by assigning an article or module as an adjunct to the core curriculum. The results are cultural competence curricula that are fragmented, uncoordinated, and at times redundant. Unfortunately, this method of curriculum development marginalizes the role of cultural competence and limits the opportunity for ongoing curricular development and application to clinical practice (Betancourt 2003; Reitmanova 2011).

Recognizing the risk of stereotyping and cultural oversimplification that comes from focusing only on content descriptions of racial and ethnic differences (Kai et al. 1999), many educators now base their training efforts on multiculturalism, integrating sexual orientation, migration histories, spirituality, unconscious bias, social determinants of health, and other cultural concepts into a coherent framework. The CFI offers an excellent approach for designing and implementing a medical student curriculum based on multiculturalism. First, the CFI definition of *culture* stresses how cultural views emerge from patients' engagement with a great diversity of social groups in their background, not only as a result of their race and ethnicity. Second, the CFI emphasizes how certain aspects of the person's background come to the fore as primary elements of the patient's identity vary at different times and in different contexts (e.g., at home, at school). Finally, the CFI can help medical students apply these complex topics in their day-to-day practice by clarifying clinical interactions that are culturally unfamiliar to the students. Educators interested in developing cross-cultural curricula should refer to Table 5–1 for resources.

The CFI can be used as a tool to facilitate cross-cultural communication and negotiation in the patient-doctor relationship. Other tools that assist with these tasks include commonly taught frameworks such as ETHNIC (Levin et al. 2000) and BELIEF (Dobbie et al. 2003). The CFI has particular strengths over and above these frameworks in that it also addresses questions about cultural identity, the therapeutic relationship, and psychosocial stressors and cultural features of vulnerability and resilience (social supports).

To ensure uniform application of the CFI for medical students from all specialty interests, the core CFI questions can be integrated into the standard medical interviewing format. The inclusion of the CFI questions in the standard medical interview will help medical students obtain richer medical histories while also helping to ensure that the patient's cultural histories are sensitively obtained. Using this format, the core CFI can be introduced in general medical interviewing courses that are usually taught in the first year. Cultural competence workshops can then teach students to develop a framework for interpreting the cultural histories. Clinical clerkships can help students learn to apply these questions to real patient interviews and clinical assessments and in treatment planning. In Table 5–2, the authors of this chapter propose a new model, the CFI-Enhanced Medical Interview.

The final three questions (14–16) of the core CFI (see Appendix A in this handbook), modified for all specialty contexts, can be used to help medical students facilitate the process of shared decision making as they conclude the history-taking portion of the interview.

Sample Curriculum

At the University of California Davis (UCD) School of Medicine, medical students progress through a 4-year curriculum titled Teamwork for Professionalism, Ethics,

TABLE 5–1.   Resources for medical student education in cultural competence

Curriculum assessment

Tool for Assessing Cultural Competence Training (TACCT; Lie et al. 2008)

Curriculum design

Association of American Medical Colleges: Cultural Competence Education for Medical Students. Washington, DC, Association of American Medical Colleges, 2005

Expert Panel on Cultural Competence Education for Students in Medicine and Public Health: Cultural Competence Education for Students in Medicine and Public Health: Report of an Expert Panel. Washington, DC, Association of American Medical Colleges and Association of Schools of Public Health, 2012. Available at: https://www.mededportal.org/download/ 303534/data/culturalcompetencereport.pdf. Accessed June 15, 2014.

Curriculum implementation

MedEdPORTAL, www.mededportal.org

Note. TACCT provides validated recommendations for learning objectives organized across five domains of cultural competence for educators who wish to systematically assess and address gaps in their curriculum. Combined with actual learning modules, such as those found in MedEdPORTAL, on the American Association of Medical Colleges Web site, TACCT can be a powerful asset for curriculum development.

TABLE 5–2.   Proposed Cultural Formulation Interview (CFI)–Enhanced Medical Interview

Standard interview component	Resequenced core CFI questions[a]
Chief complaint	CFI question 1
History of present illness	CFI questions 2, 3, 4, 5, 6, 7, 11
Past medical/psychiatric history	CFI question 12
Social history	CFI questions 8, 9, 10, 13

Note. [a]Original numbering scheme retained for reference to core CFI.

and Cultural Competence Enrichment (Team PEACE). Students achieve cultural competence milestones over the 4 years through small-group exercises, standardized patient interviews, didactics, and clinical exposures that are embedded in various courses throughout their education (Table 5–3). Each milestone and its accompanying learning method build on the prior step, enhancing synergy and reinforcing cultural competence throughout all years of medical student education. These milestones are assessed at various intervals through observed standardized patient interviews, self-assessments, reflective writing, multiple-choice tests, and observation by faculty.

Although efforts to infuse the CFI into the Team PEACE curriculum are just beginning, training in CFI-enhanced medical interviewing will be introduced in the first-year interviewing course. In medical student year 1 (MS-1), the Team PEACE modules would address why these questions are asked; in MS-2 through MS-4, the modules would address how the information obtained from these questions can be used to render and deliver culturally appropriate assessments and treatment.

TABLE 5–3. Team PEACE cultural competence curriculum thread

School year	Learning milestones: medical students will be able to	Learning method
Mid MS-1	1. Describe culture and its components in broad and inclusive terms	SGDs with trigger videos
	2. Describe their own cultural background and belief systems	
	3. Appreciate the meaning of health and illness from different perspectives	
End MS-1	4. Describe health disparities and sociocultural, genetic, and epidemiologic factors that may contribute to these disparities	SGDs with trigger videos
	5. Describe the impact of language on health status and health care	Project Implicit Hidden Bias Tests (Project Implicit, https:// implicit.harvard.edu/ implicit/)
	6. Appreciate conscious and unconscious bias in themselves and its impact on health care delivery	
	7. Work collaboratively with peers across cultural groups	Large group didactic sessions
Mid MS-2	8. Describe and begin to implement approaches to understanding and working effectively with patients from culturally diverse backgrounds	SGDs Culturally diverse patient panel
End MS-2	9. Describe the components, challenges, and benefits of the effective use of a health care interpreter	Large group demonstration Small-group standardized patient scenarios
Mid MS-3	10. Develop rapport and effectively communicate with patients across various cultural groups	Clinical exposure and didactics
End MS-3	11. Demonstrate incorporation of cultural beliefs, practices, and supports into assessment and treatment planning	Clinical exposure and didactics
	12. Demonstrate effective use of a health care interpreter in actual clinical care	
End MS-4	13. Apply knowledge of health care disparities and sociocultural, genetic, and epidemiologic factors to care of patient populations across various cultural backgrounds	1-month clinical course chosen by MS-4 trainees

Note.   MS=medical school; SGDs=small-group discussions; Team PEACE=Teamwork for Professionalism, Ethics, and Cultural Competence Enrichment.

Adult Psychiatric Resident Education

Residency curricula in cultural competence emphasize training in multiple areas, including culture-general skills, such as how to conduct a cultural assessment with a patient from any culture; culture-specific knowledge, such as idioms of distress common in particular groups; and fostering attitudes that support culturally appropriate assessment and treatment. "Guidelines for Training in Cultural Psychiatry" (Kirmayer et al. 2012) is a comprehensive guide to curriculum design originating from the Canadian Psychiatric Association that predates the release of the CFI. Many of its major components can now be taught using the CFI. For example, the Canadian guidelines emphasize the importance of 1) awareness of the clinician's own identity and relationship to patients from diverse backgrounds (the subject of core CFI question 16); 2) knowledge of how cultural context and background influence help seeking, coping, adaptations to illness, treatment response, healing, recovery, and well-being (core CFI questions 11, 12, 14, and 15); and 3) skill building in cultural formulation and treatment negotiation (the CFI as a whole). Other topics included in the Canadian guidelines and other curricula are presented in Table 5–4.

The backbone of any cultural psychiatry curriculum is clinical experience with diverse patients and supervision by culturally trained faculty (American Psychiatric Association 2013b). Teaching methods for cultural competence in adult psychiatric residency programs rely on a variety of approaches, as noted by a qualitative study in which 20 cultural psychiatry instructors in adult residency programs across the United States were interviewed (Hansen et al. 2012). These approaches include lectures, reflective experiences, role-playing, field trips for observation, small-group discussions, ethnographic writing, films, culturally themed meals, ethnic group–based didactics, case formulation using the DSM-IV (American Psychiatric Association 1994) Outline for Cultural Formulation (OCF), and modeling interviewing techniques by faculty (American Psychiatric Association 2013b; Lim 2015). As a rule, the resident progresses through a series of stages: expanding cultural awareness (enhancing sensitivity, reducing bias), acquiring cultural knowledge, achieving cultural skills, and managing cultural encounters (Campinha-Bacote 1994). Experiencing increased awareness of blind spots, bias, and stereotyping improves openness toward cultural material and enhances understanding of differences. Small-group discussion after experiential exercises evoking bias and stereotyping can result in a powerful experience of self-reflection that facilitates changes in attitudes (Crenshaw et al. 2011; Guzder and Rousseau 2013). Teaching methods should be adapted to the specific needs of the residency program from the variety of modalities described above, and they should be aligned with proven teaching techniques, such as incorporating adult learning principles and including experiential exercises and small-group discussions. Moreover, the courses should include comprehensive evaluations with formative and summative feedback for trainees.

Many curricula in cultural psychiatry focus on specific topics, such as cultural minority groups, women, sexual orientation, elderly people, children, and religion and spirituality (Al-Mateen et al. 2011; American Psychiatric Association 2013b). These curricula usefully identify thematic areas for discussion, such as during seminars for residents and/or fellows. However, if this is the extent of the cultural curriculum, the topic-based approach runs the risk of replacing old stereotypes with new ones. A skills-based approach can avoid group-based teaching (e.g., the black patient, the female patient). The goal is to teach clinicians how to use their experience as normative data for the interpretation of the patient's illness experience (Aggarwal and Rohrbaugh 2011). The CFI as a whole offers an excellent new approach for fostering

TABLE 5–4. **Cultural curriculum recommendations for adult psychiatry residency programs**

Knowledge	Skills
Definition of culture, general concepts	Clinical interviewing with the CFI to elicit cultural concepts of distress
Stigma, stereotypes, and unconscious bias	
Health and mental health disparities	Ethnographic writing exercises
Structural systems and public health	Patient-centered care using the CFI
Ethnopsychopharmacology	Case formulation using the DSM-IV OCF
Berry et al. (1986) model of acculturation	Training in the use of interpreters at specialty clinics and use of cultural brokers
Religion, spirituality	
Sexual orientation (LGBTQ)	Identification and management of interethnic and intraethnic transference and counter-transference
Women's issues	
Cultural concepts of distress	
Attitude	**Institutional infrastructure**
Experiential learning	Grand rounds focused on culture
Movies and articles evoking stereotyping and bias	Lecture and discussion on how policies affect health and mental health and how to intervene
Videos of role-plays for self-assessment	Visits to local community
Exercises to instill cultural humility as a life-long process	Recruitment of diverse residents and faculty
	Cultural case conferences
Diversity training (cultural identity exploration)	Integration of cultural content across courses
	Minority fellowships for residents and junior faculty

Note. CFI=Cultural Formulation Interview; LGBTQ=lesbian-gay-bisexual-transgender-queer; OCF=Outline for Cultural Formulation.

skill development. The core CFI, the CFI–Informant Version, and the 12 supplementary modules can guide trainees in eliciting crucial information on the specific needs of the patient, by covering topics related to cultural identity, social networks, and certain social determinants of health. The 16 core CFI questions can be a basic tool to understand how health disparities affect individuals and perhaps to formulate ways to intervene. Introduction of the CFI–Informant Version and the 12 supplementary modules in advanced courses may foster deeper understanding of cultural issues and give meaning and support for the ongoing use of the CFI.

Programs will need to decide at which point in the training to introduce any of the components of the CFI. We recommend using the CFI early on after creating a culturally receptive environment through supportive discussions of bias and stereotyping, followed by self-reflection activities. The CFI should not be taught as a rigid set of questions; after clearly explaining the intent of each question, trainees should be encouraged to create their own versions of the CFI questions that they can use comfortably. Programs should consider creating or modifying intake forms to include cultural formulation questions and providing fields in the database to collect such information, as well as adding cultural formulation to the resident's evaluation form.

Other factors influencing the preparation of cultural curricula include the patient population being served, the availability of culturally competent faculty, the level of administration support, and the input of a core committee of instructors to ensure the curriculum's sustainability (Lewis-Fernández 2013). The importance of institutional support and the value of having a member of the residency training committee advocate for cultural education programs cannot be overemphasized (American Psychiatric Association 2013b). A major challenge to the implementation of cultural curricula is the recruitment of qualified supervisors with interest, experience, and knowledge in teaching cultural psychiatry. Departments of psychiatry should expand their efforts to recruit culturally trained faculty by utilizing resources such as graduates of the American Psychiatric Association/Substance Abuse and Mental Health Services Administration (APA/SAMHSA) Minority Fellowship and other training programs and by encouraging an interest in cultural psychiatry among their own residents and faculty. For example, the department could nominate a resident to be an APA/SAMHSA Minority Fellow to develop curricula for the program (Lim et al. 2008).

Obviously, the CFI alone will not be sufficient to build a curriculum. Other components, such as cultural grand rounds, CME programs, and case conferences, with oversight by a committee dedicated to the cultural curriculum, will need to be included. It is crucial that the medical school and residency program administration convey the importance of cultural competence by prioritizing it among competing centralized didactics.

Model Curricula in Cultural Psychiatry

In 2010, the American Association of Directors of Psychiatric Residency Training sponsored a national call for model curricula in cultural psychiatry aimed at adult psychiatric residency programs. Two model curricula were chosen, one from New York University (NYU), which follows a yearlong course format, and another from UCD, which has a longitudinal design, with seminars throughout all 4 years of residency training. The NYU course, offered during PGY-3, is called Culture and Psychiatry. Modules address three main goals: cultural competence, cultural humility, and cultural critiques. One module, for example, focuses on the patient-clinician interaction and includes the following subtopics: perceiving the other, perceiving the self, and working through cultural transference and countertransference (Hansen et al. 2010).

The UCD cultural psychiatry curriculum exposes trainees to an ethnically diverse faculty and population of patients (Lim et al. 2010) and is supported by department administration, which sustains the development of the longitudinal curriculum. A safe environment is developed to help trainees practice self-reflection and learn skills for clinical assessments using the OCF and CFI. The use of the CFI through a range of clinical tasks is encouraged, including psychiatric intakes, psychotherapy, and case presentations.

Other Examples of Adult Psychiatric Residency Curricula

Two other programs that deserve mention for their cultural curricula are those at the University of Toronto and Yale University. At the University of Toronto, an integrative curriculum has been developed that focuses on generic cultural competencies, including the application of the CFI and psychotherapeutic and pharmacological interventions with diverse cultural groups, as well as training in the use of interpreters and specific cultural competencies, such as eliciting cultural concepts of distress and illness explanatory models (Fung et al. 2008). The development process for the University of Toronto curriculum included a needs assessment and a survey of residents' interests, followed by the creation of a faculty working group, a standing steering committee, and a faculty retreat to discuss the proposed changes. The cultural psychiatric curriculum at Yale relies on residents as teachers, is incorporated into centralized didactics, and is overseen by a committee of residents and faculty. The focus is on person-centered care, health disparities, experiential learning, and videos of residents role-playing the OCF and CFI, followed by self-reflection (Díaz et al. 2015).

Continuing Medical Education for Practicing Clinicians

The U.S. Office of Minority Health has developed federal regulations requiring health care organizations to provide culturally and linguistically appropriate services (U.S. Department of Health and Human Services, Office of Minority Health 2013). These standards link systemic cultural competence to quality/performance improvement activities. Both live and Web-based CME courses have been developed to help providers comply with the standards. Several of these courses are described in the psychiatric literature, but so far, published reports have not included the CFI. For example, one live course based on the DSM-IV OCF focuses on cross-cultural diagnosis and treatment planning (Lim 2015); in 2014, the course incorporated the CFI for the first time along with the OCF. The Annual Summer Program in Cultural Psychiatry at McGill University (www.mcgill.ca/tcpsych) offers CME training in cultural competence that is grounded in the social sciences (see source reference included in American Psychiatric Association 2013b).

Web-based CME courses make it easier to reach busy clinicians and clinicians in isolated rural settings and to address time and economic constraints. Web-based resources have grown exponentially over the last two decades (Díaz et al. 2012; Quality Interactions 2014; U.S. Department of Health and Human Services, Office of Minority Health 2011), but it is unknown to what extent they have incorporated training in the CFI. Yale's CME course uses the OCF as a guide. Web sites and videos dedicated to cultural competence are available through the U.S. Office of Minority Health (U.S. Department of Health and Human Services, Office of Minority Health 2011); educational institutions such as the University of Pennsylvania, Drexel University, and the University of California, San Francisco; health insurance companies; and health care information providers such as Medscape and Quality Interactions (Quality Interactions 2014). These programs aim to develop knowledge and skills to enhance the cultural sensitivity of treatment providers, leading to greater self-reflection, critical thinking, and cultural humility in practitioners. CME Web sites also attempt to address a relatively neglected area: strategies to address health disparities (Like 2011).

In the future, CME courses can be developed based on the CFI, ranging from a single course focused on the core CFI to advanced courses that facilitate more comprehensive training based on the core CFI plus the supplementary modules. Expanding state medical boards' requirements for cultural competence training would likely help increase CME course attendance. Live or Web site training should include use of the CFI and should encourage participants to either videotape their patient encounters using the CFI or have a qualified proctor sit with the clinician during an interview in which the CFI is used.

Conclusion

The publication of the CFI in DSM-5 presents medical educators with the opportunity to teach medical students, psychiatric residents, and practicing psychiatrists how to collect clinical information in order to develop a cultural formulation. Learning how to use the CFI is a key skill that supplements any teaching regarding cultural concepts of distress, differing health beliefs and values, and treatment expectations. Medical students can learn to include the CFI questions in their routine interviews. Psychiatric residents can use the core CFI, the CFI-Informant Version, and the supplementary modules to create comprehensive cultural formulations. CME courses can demonstrate to practicing clinicians how the CFI can help them develop rapport and collaborate with patients to create a mutually acceptable, culturally appropriate treatment plan. Over time, the CFI will become a standard training intervention primarily aimed at skill building that will be incorporated into most training resources used to develop cultural competence, including those listed in Table 5–5.

KEY CLINICAL POINTS

- The Cultural Formulation Interview (CFI) can be used for teaching culturally appropriate assessment to medical students, psychiatry residents, and practicing clinicians through continuing education courses.

- Using the CFI, trainees may be able to learn how to better negotiate treatment plans with patients because of its patient-centered focus and attention to the patient's and social network's cultural conceptions of distress.

- Using the information elicited from the CFI, clinicians can enlist existing support systems, reduce the impact of stressors, and bridge the patient's and clinician's explanatory models to enhance adherence with treatment recommendations.

TABLE 5–5. Cultural competence training resources for educators

American Psychiatric Association: Resource Document on Cultural Psychiatry as a Specific Field of Study Relevant to the Assessment and Care of All Patients. Arlington, VA, American Psychiatric Association, 2013b. Available at: http://www.psychiatry.org/File%20Library/Learn/Archives/rd2013_CulturalPsychiatry.pdf. Accessed July 14, 2014.

Beamon CJ, Devisetty V, Forcina Hill JM, et al: A Guide to Incorporating Cultural Competency into Health Professionals' Education and Training. Washington, DC, National Health Law Program, 2006. Available at: http://njms.rutgers.edu/culweb/medical/documents/CulturalCompetencyGuide.pdf. Accessed June 15, 2014.

Betancourt JR, Green AR, Carrillo JE: Cultural Competence in Health Care: Emerging Frameworks and Practical Approaches. New York, The Commonwealth Fund, October 2002. Available at: http://www.commonwealthfund.org/usr_doc/betancourt_culturalcompetence_576.pdf. Accessed February 12, 2004.

California Endowment: A Manager's Guide to Cultural Competence Education for Health Care Professionals. Woodland Hills, CA, California Endowment, 2003. Available at: http://www.calendow.org/uploadedfiles/managers_guide_cultural_competence(1).pdf. Accessed February 12, 2004.

California Endowment: Principles and Recommended Standards for Cultural Competence Education of Health Care Professionals. Woodland Hills, CA, California Endowment, 2003. Available at: http://www.calendow.org/uploadedfiles/principles_standards_cultural_competence.pdf. Accessed February 12, 2004.

California Endowment: Resources in Cultural Competence Education for Health Care Professionals. Woodland Hills, CA, California Endowment, 2003. Available at: http://www.calendow.org/uploadedFiles/resources_in_cultural_competence.pdf. Accessed February 12, 2004.

Comas-Diaz: Multicultural Assessment. Washington, DC, American Psychological Association, 2012

Comas-Diaz L, Jacobsen FM: Ethnocultural transference and countertransference in the therapeutic dyad. Am J Orthopsychiatry 61:392–402, 1991

Group for the Advancement of Psychiatry: Cultural Assessment in Clinical Psychiatry. Washington, DC, American Psychiatric Publishing, 2002

Hays PA: Addressing Cultural Complexities in Practice: Assessment, Diagnosis, and Therapy, 2nd Edition. Washington, DC, American Psychological Association, 2008

Kirmayer LJ, Fung K, Rousseau C, et al: Guidelines for training in cultural psychiatry. Can J Psychiatry 57(insert):1–16, 2012

Lim RF: Clinical Manual of Cultural Psychiatry, 2nd Edition. Washington, DC, American Psychiatric Publishing, 2015

Lu FG: Annotated Bibliography on Cultural Psychiatry and Related Topics. Arlington, VA, National Alliance on Mental Illness, February 2005. Available at: http://www.nami.org/Content/ContentGroups/Multicultural_Support1/Fact_Sheets1/Dr_Lu_Cultural_Bibliography.pdf. Accessed February 19, 2008.

Tseng WS, Strelzer J: Culture and Psychotherapy. Washington, DC, American Psychiatric Publishing, 2001

Questions

For Educators

1. What are the best methods for teaching the CFI in undergraduate, graduate, and postgraduate medical education?

2. How do medical educators engage and encourage medical students, residents, and clinicians in practice to use the CFI?

3. How can educators teach trainees about stereotyping and bias toward ethnic minorities and discuss concepts such as racism with racially mixed or homogeneous audiences?

For Learners

1. How do clinicians best address the impact of cultural health beliefs and practices on patients' ways of understanding illness and expectations of care?

2. What are the best methods for teaching culturally appropriate assessment skills?

References

Accreditation Council of Graduate Medical Education, American Board of Psychiatry and Neurology: The Psychiatry Milestone Project, 2013. Available at: https://www.acgme.org/acgmeweb/Portals/0/PDFs/Milestones/PsychiatryMilestones.pdf. Accessed February 13, 2013.

Aggarwal NK, Rohrbaugh RM: Teaching cultural competency through an experiential seminar on anthropology and psychiatry. Acad Psychiatry 35(5):331–334, 2011 22007094

Al-Mateen CS, Mian A, Pumariega A, et al: Diversity and Cultural Competency Curriculum for Child and Adolescent Psychiatry Training. Washington, DC, American Academy of Child and Adolescent Psychiatry, 2011. Available at: http://www.aacap.org/aacap/Resources_for_Primary_Care/Diversity_and_Cultural_Competency_Curriculum/Home.aspx. Accessed March 2, 2014.

American Psychiatric Association: Diagnostic and Statistical Manual of Mental Disorders, 4th Edition. Washington, DC, American Psychiatric Association, 1994

American Psychiatric Association: Diagnostic and Statistical Manual of Mental Disorders, 5th Edition. Arlington, VA, American Psychiatric Association, 2013a

American Psychiatric Association: Resource Document on Cultural Psychiatry as a Specific Field of Study Relevant to the Assessment and Care of All Patients. Arlington, VA, American Psychiatric Association, 2013b. Available at: http://www.psychiatry.org/File%20Library/Learn/Archives/rd2013_CulturalPsychiatry.pdf. Accessed July 14, 2014.

Berry JW, Trimble JE, Olmedo EL: Assessment of acculturation, in Field Methods in Cross-Cultural Research, edited by Berry JW, Lonner WJ. Thousand Oaks, CA, Sage, 1986 pp 291–324

Betancourt JR: Cross-cultural medical education: conceptual approaches and frameworks for evaluation. Acad Med 78(6):560–569, 2003 12805034

Campinha-Bacote J: The Process of Cultural Competence in Health Care: A Culturally Competent Model of Care. Wyoming, OH, C.A.R.E. Associates, 1994

Crenshaw K, Shewchuk RM, Qu H, et al: What should we include in a cultural competence curriculum? An emerging formative evaluation process to foster curriculum development. Acad Med 86(3):333–341, 2011 21248602

Department of Public Health: Continuing Medical Education. 2013. Available at: http://www.ct.gov/dph/cwp/view.asp?a=3121&q=389490. Accessed February 12, 2014.

Díaz E, Armah T, Hersey D, et al: Enhancing Your Clinical Cultural Competence (psychiatric residency course). New Haven, CT, Yale University School of Medicine, 2012

Díaz E, Armah T, Linse C, et al: Novel brief cultural psychiatry training for residents. Acad Psychiatry Jan 31, 2015 25636254 [Epub ahead of print]

Dobbie AE, Medrano M, Tysinger J, et al: The BELIEF Instrument: a preclinical teaching tool to elicit patients' health beliefs. Fam Med 35(5):316–319, 2003 12772930

Fung K, Andermann L, Zaretsky A, et al: An integrative approach to cultural competence in the psychiatric curriculum. Acad Psychiatry 32(4):272–282, 2008 18695028

Guzder J, Rousseau C: A diversity of voices: the McGill 'Working with Culture' seminars. Cult Med Psychiatry 37(2):347–364, 2013 23549711

Hansen H, Trujillo M, Hopper K: Culture and Psychiatry: A Course for Third Year Psychiatry Residents. New York University, 2010. Available at: http://aadprt.org/secure/documents/model_curricula/cultural_psych_nyu_10.pdf. Accessed July 15, 2014.

Hansen H, Dugan T, Becker A, et al: Educating psychiatry residents about cultural aspects of care: a qualitative study of approaches used by U.S. expert faculty. Acad Psychiatry 37:412–416, 2012 24185288

Kai J, Spencer J, Wilkes M, et al: Learning to value ethnic diversity—what, why and how? Med Educ 33(8):616–623, 1999 10447850

Kirmayer LJ, Fung K, Rousseau C, et al: Guidelines for training in cultural psychiatry. Can J Psychiatry 57(insert):1–16, 2012

Levin SJ, Like RC, Gottlieb JE: ETHNIC: a framework for culturally competent ethical practice. Patient Care 34:188–189, 2000

Lewis-Fernández R: The use of the Cultural Formulation in training and practice. Paper presented at the annual meeting of the American Psychiatric Association, Washington, DC, May 2013

Lewis-Fernández R, Aggarwal NK, Bäärnhielm S, et al: Culture and psychiatric evaluation: operationalizing cultural formulation for DSM-5. Psychiatry 77(2):130–154, 2014 24865197

Liaison Committee on Medical Education: Functions and Structure of a Medical School: Standards for Accreditation of Medical Education Programs Leading to the M.D. Degree. Washington, DC, Liaison Committee on Medical Education, 2013. Available at: http://www.lcme.org/publications/functions2013june.pdf. Accessed March 6, 2014.

Lie DA, Boker J, Crandall S, et al: Revising the Tool for Assessing Cultural Competence Training (TACCT) for curriculum evaluation: findings derived from seven US schools and expert consensus. Med Educ Online 13:1–11, 2008 19756238

Like RC: Educating clinicians about cultural competence and disparities in health and health care. J Contin Educ Health Prof 31(3):196–206, 2011 21953661

Lim RF: Clinical Manual of Cultural Psychiatry, 2nd Edition. Washington, DC, American Psychiatric Publishing, 2015

Lim RF, Luo JS, Suo S, et al: Diversity initiatives in academic psychiatry: applying cultural competence. Acad Psychiatry 32(4):283–290, 2008 18695029

Lim RF, Koike AK, Gellerman DM, et al: A Four-Year Model Curriculum on Culture, Gender, LGBT, Religion, and Spirituality for General Psychiatry Residency Training Programs in the United States. Submitted to American Association for Directors of Psychiatric Residency Training, 2010. Available at: http://aadprt.org/secure/documents/model_curricula/Cultural_Competence_Curriculum.pdf. Accessed March 4, 2013.

Ling L, Derstine P, Cohen N: Implementing Milestones and Clinical Competency Committees. Accreditation Council for Graduate Medical Education webinar, April 24, 2013. Available at http://www.acgme.org/acgmeweb/Portals/0/PDFs/ACGMEMilestones-CCC-AssesmentWebinar.pdf. Accessed February 16, 2015.

National Consortium for Multicultural Education for Health Professionals: News and Events: Cultural Competency Legislation and Regulation 2009. Available at: http://culturalmeded.stanford.edu/news/laws.html. Accessed July 15, 2014.

Quality Interactions: Cultural Competency Solutions for Higher-Value Healthcare. Cambridge, MA, Quality Interactions, 2014. Available at: http://www.qualityinteractions.com/our-solutions/elearning/. Accessed June 14, 2014.

Reitmanova S: Cross-cultural undergraduate medical education in North America: theoretical concepts and educational approaches. Teach Learn Med 23(2):197–203, 2011 21516609

U.S. Department of Health and Human Services, Office of Minority Health: A Physician's Practical Guide to Culturally Competent Care (video series). Rockville, MD, U.S. Department of Health and Human Services, 2011. Available at: https://cccm.thinkculturalhealth.hhs.gov/videos/index.htm. Accessed March 6, 2014.

U.S. Department of Health and Human Services, Office of Minority Health: Think Cultural Health: CLAS and CLAS Standards. Rockville, MD, U.S. Department of Health and Human Services, 2013. Available at: https://www.thinkculturalhealth.hhs.gov/content/clas.asp. Accessed March 6, 2014.

CHAPTER 6

Conclusion

The Future of Cultural Formulation

Laurence J. Kirmayer, M.D.

The introduction of the Cultural Formulation Interview (CFI) in DSM-5 (American Psychiatric Association 2013) is a milestone in the development of cultural psychiatry and, more broadly, of person-centered mental health care. This volume provides detailed elaboration of the rationale, development, and application of the cultural formulation in diverse clinical settings. In this concluding chapter, I consider some directions for the future development of the CFI and of cultural formulation more generally, in terms of theory, research, and practice.

The Place of Culture in DSM

Recent decades have seen growing recognition in psychiatry of the importance of culture as the matrix within which people experience, express, and cope with mental health problems. The introduction of the Outline for Cultural Formulation (OCF) in DSM-IV (American Psychiatric Association 1994) was a major step in articulating what aspects of culture and context are relevant to everyday practice in the United States and other countries.

DSM-III-R (American Psychiatric Association 1987) had only a brief mention of culture in the introduction. The DSM-IV Work Group on Culture and Diagnosis, sponsored by the National Institute of Mental Health, made a concerted effort to elaborate cultural considerations for many of the disorders in the text (Mezzich et al. 1999). A large group of clinicians and researchers conducted systematic reviews of the literature on cultural variations in mental disorders and distilled these into lessons relevant for diagnostic assessment. However, the text was limited to comments on individual disorders, and no change in the overall structure of diagnostic categories was possible. Moreover, the basic concern of cultural psychiatry—understanding mental health problems in social context—was somewhat at odds with the aim of the nosology to describe problems in context-free, abstract, or general terms applicable in diverse settings (Thomas 2014). Some of the contrasts between DSM and a cultural-contextual approach are summarized in Table 6–1. These are not categorical differences but are, rather, shifts in emphasis, and ideally, the cultural perspective complements and expands the biomedical framework that is implicit in the structure and focus of DSM.

From the perspective of cultural psychiatry, the most significant innovation in DSM-IV was the OCF. Unfortunately, over the subsequent decades there was limited uptake and implementation of the DSM-IV OCF (Kirmayer et al. 2008). One reason for this limited use may have been the absence of any instruction within DSM-IV on how to collect the information needed to fill in the outline (Mezzich et al. 2009). The CFI in DSM-5 directly addresses this gap by giving clinicians a simple protocol to follow to collect basic information relevant to cultural formulation. The hope is that this will demystify the process of cultural assessment by providing a clear place to start and suggestions on how to pursue particular lines of inquiry with the supplementary modules. Further efforts to disseminate information on the CFI through workshops, publications (including this handbook), and video demonstrations make it likely that it will be better integrated into clinical training in the years to come.

The CFI is a work in progress. Although it is based on the knowledge of clinicians with long experience working in settings with high levels of cultural diversity in several countries, the hope is that it can continue to be refined and elaborated through research and clinical and training experiences (Lewis-Fernández et al. 2014). The American Psychiatric Association has made the CFI freely available online to encourage its wide distribution (www.psychiatry.org/practice/dsm/dsm5/online-assessment-measures). In effect, the CFI is a living document that will be modified with new knowledge. In particular, more needs to be known about how to adapt the core questions to different settings and types of patients, and there is much room to refine and add to the supplementary modules to clarify how experts pursue particular lines of inquiry to gain an understanding of patients' symptoms, concerns, and adaptation.

Dilemmas in the Design of the CFI

The development of the CFI involved several important trade-offs between the dynamic view of culture and context provided by anthropology and other social sciences and the practical demands and constraints of clinical work. Ethnographic research can provide extensive descriptions of individual lives and cultural communities that allow nuanced understanding of the complexities of illness experience, but this typically requires extended periods of time and access to individuals' lifeworlds through participant observation. Clinical work operates under intense constraints of time and resources and with an urgent mandate to come up with a clear assessment and intervention plan. Reflecting these constraints, the core CFI presents a limited set of questions that aim to elicit crucial elements of cultural context in the hopes that this will improve clinical care; however, it remains unclear how well any brief interview

TABLE 6–1. Contrasts between the DSM framing of disorders and a cultural perspective

Contrast category	DSM	Cultural perspective
Object of clinical attention	Discrete disorders	Predicaments
Medical semiotics	Symptoms viewed as indices of disorders	Symptoms viewed as acts of communication or behaviors embedded in cultural systems of meaning
Location of problem	Within patient	Within social situation or context
Locus of causal factors, sources of resilience	Individual	Family or social system
Interventions	Psychopharmacology, individual psychotherapy	Systemic individual, family, community, social network interventions
Outcomes	Symptom reduction	Recovery defined in terms of personal and communal values

such as the CFI can achieve an adequate level of understanding of particular patients, problems, or contexts.

Social science research also points out that the ways in which culture, race, and ethnicity are conceptualized in psychiatry reflect particular notions of identity. DSM is a U.S. publication, produced by the American Psychiatric Association, but it has global reach. Hence, examining some of the cultural assumptions built into DSM is important for its cultural adaptation and for understanding how the CFI can be maximally relevant in other countries or contexts. In U.S. psychiatry, *culture* has generally been taken to refer to ethnicity or racialized identities, which are often grouped together into five ethnoracial blocs: African American, American Indian and Alaska Native, Asian and Pacific Islander, Latino, and white (or Caucasian) (Good et al. 2011). These are extremely heterogeneous groups that reflect the history of U.S. migration and identity politics, organized by the imposition of labels in the U.S. Census. As such, these labels do not apply well in other countries and, in fact, fail to capture the diversity of identities important to people in the United States. Unfortunately, some approaches to cultural competence training tend to reify these categories by presenting capsule summaries or profiles of the blocs or other ethnoracial groups, hence minimizing internal variation or the complex ways in which individuals make use of cultural identities and resources.

The CFI makes an important break with this tradition of overgeneralizing or essentializing cultural identity by inquiring into identity on an individual basis. It thus encourages the clinician to think about identity as a personal project, in which the individual has at hand multiple potential sources of identity, which can be used in complex and idiosyncratic ways to construct a sense of self, belonging, and social positioning. The CFI allows for the possibility that facets of identity can be built around language, religion or spirituality, occupation, or indeed any aspect of family, group, or collective history. This open-ended approach should allow clinicians to work with the constantly changing forms of identity and community made possible by the Internet and globalization and fueled by culture change, conflict, and creative intermixing.

One dilemma that the CFI may not sufficiently address is that identity is a co-construction that emerges at the boundaries between different cultures, communities, and ways of being. Identity is always vis-à-vis another, so that how patients describe themselves and, more deeply, who they understand themselves to be depend on the context, including who is asking the questions, what setting they are in, and what larger social circumstances are in play. These larger circumstances may include relationships involving both local and transnational networks and events occurring both locally and in distant places that affect how individuals think and feel about identity and the kind of responses they expect to get from others. For example, when war is waged in one part of the world, people from groups involved in the conflict will experience intense pressures to affirm or disavow potential aspects of their identities, with consequences for how they narrate their identity. For the clinician to gain a more rounded picture of the range of identities relevant to patients' illness experience, it is useful to think of identity as socially situated and to ask about facets of identity that may be salient or in the foreground in specific contexts of home, school, workplace, or community, as well as in transnational networks maintained by travel and telecommunications (Doucerain et al. 2013).

Similar issues apply to every aspect of the CFI. The ways that people think about illness, adopt coping strategies, and seek help also depend on social contexts. The interaction of local and global processes is evident in illness experience and in psychosocial aspects of illness and healing. Patients may be influenced not only by their own cultural background but also by diverse perspectives within their families, among coworkers, and in local communities and global networks. There is a global circulation of information about mental health problems and treatments, both explicitly and indirectly through stories about media figures and others, that can exert strong effects on how individuals understand and approach their own difficulties. Some of these influences may occur outside of patients' awareness because they become part of taken-for-granted background knowledge. The CFI–Informant Version (and corresponding components of the CFI supplementary modules) can help clinicians understand some of this tacit social and cultural background. Community members, religious leaders, and others can provide more general information needed to make sense of the patient's predicament.

All of this diversity is part of the dynamic mix of culture. Appreciating these dynamics should encourage the clinician to think of culture not simply as traits shared by individuals with similar backgrounds but as complex histories and current contexts. Culture, then, is located not merely in the individual but also in the social world, and clinical assessment of culture is about this context as much as it is about the individual. Hence, the clinician needs to consider sources of information about current cultural frameworks beyond what the patient can explicitly describe.

Another related dilemma in the process of cultural assessment is that many aspects of culture reside in everyday practices, ways of looking at the world, and social arrangements that are taken for granted by participants. Hence, these aspects tend to be tacit or invisible and hard for the patient to articulate. It is not sufficient, therefore, for the clinician simply to ask the patient about his or her social context and experience. The clinician must know where to look for clinically relevant cultural issues: what aspects of life to inquire about, what language to use to elicit the patient's own understandings, and who else to speak with to gain some appreciation of contextual issues that are not part of the patient's current self-awareness even though they may be major social determinants of health and influences on his or her illness.

Implementing the CFI: Structure and Process

The CFI can contribute to a person-centered approach to psychiatry by emphasizing the patient's perspective. The core CFI begins with a question about the patient's reason for coming for help and makes that reason the center of the initial discussion before moving out to consider the wider context of illness. In effect, the CFI aims to elicit information that can complement the usual diagnostic formulation by assaying the social and cultural dimensions of illness experience, identity, coping, help seeking, and expectations for care. Ideally, the CFI would contribute to a comprehensive bio-psychosocial review of systems (Campbell and Rohrbaugh 2006; Harkness et al. 2014). Just as physicians learn to conduct a review of functional systems, organized in terms of underlying physiology, the CFI can be seen as a tool for conducting a psychosocial review of systems, which necessarily includes not only information on social determinants of health and illness in development and current life contexts but also patients' own narratives of identity, illness experience, values, and relationships, as well as the views of others in their social networks. The goal is to identify predisposing, precipitating, perpetuating, and protective factors, which may be at multiple systemic levels: individual, couple, family, community, health care system, and larger social networks (Weerasekera 1996).

The quality of information obtained by the CFI depends crucially on the clinician-patient relationship. Although use of the CFI can ultimately contribute to improving the relationship, the success of this process will reflect the extent to which the clinician is able to convey qualities of warmth, respect, competence, and concern. Beginning the interview with attention to the patient's presented complaints confirms the clinician's focus on the patient's concerns and on a line of inquiry that will lead to helpful interventions or recommendations. The various shifts of topic that occur in the CFI should occur in a natural way as the conversation unfolds but may require explicit discussion and justification with patients who do not see the connection between their presented complaints and the clinician's inquiries. This may be particularly the case when asking about cultural identity. For some patients, this line of questioning is welcome attention to a key aspect of their concerns, whereas for others it may be experienced as intrusive and threatening. Explaining the potential links between identity and health problems and solutions will suffice for most patients, but in some cases questions need to be deferred until further trust is built and the relationship strengthened.

Implementing the CFI requires attention to issues of cultural safety (Kirmayer 2012). People from groups that have experienced colonization, racism, discrimination, and marginalization by dominant groups in the society may approach institutions with caution or mistrust. Clinicians whom patients view as part of oppressive groups or institutions may have difficulty achieving the trust needed for effective assessment. Cultural safety requires thinking through some of these potential barriers to engagement in advance and taking steps to ensure that the institution, clinical setting, and conduct of health professionals convey respect for the history of structural violence and exclusion (Kirmayer 2011; Kirmayer et al. 2013).

The CFI can be an essential tool in culturally competent care. Skillful use of the CFI, however, requires broader cultural competence. Cultural competence begins with self-understanding. It goes on to include generic knowledge about how to explore culture (working with interpreters and culture brokers and elaborating questions to pursue particular lines of inquiry) and specific knowledge about the patient's culture, language, ethnicity, and religion. Competence at the level of the clinician must be complemented by competence at the level of the health care system, organization, or institution (see subchapter "Administrative Perspectives on the Implementation and Use of the Cultural Formulation Interview").

Working with interpreters, involving family and community, and taking the time needed to build trust and understand patients from different backgrounds all require additional time that must be factored into institutional practices and procedures, including resource allocation and reimbursement structures. The additional time that may be needed can pose a challenge in situations in which resources are limited or there are pressures for standardization of care, but it is important to recognize that providing equitable care requires addressing linguistic and cultural barriers to care by mobilizing appropriate resources.

From Interview to Formulation

The development of an interview to guide data collection is a first step in facilitating cultural formulation. The OCF provides a simple schema for recording the information under broad domains, but the DSM-5 process stopped short of developing a more structured template that could organize the data in ways that would facilitate access and help make links to specific clinical issues. The challenge that remains is providing guidance on how to integrate the data into a clinically useful formulation. Just as psychodynamic, behavioral, or systemic formulations depend on relevant knowledge and theoretical models (e.g., Chisolm and Lyketsos 2012; Hofmann 2014; Johnstone and Dallos 2013; Reilly and Newton 2011), so too does cultural formulation ultimately depend on evidence-based models and theory drawn from social science and cultural psychiatry (Hays 2008; Kirmayer et al. 2014a). Given the breadth of issues, there is no simple way to cover all of the potentially relevant links, which will differ by cultural context, type of disorder, and personal history. In this section, I draw from clinical experience in cultural psychiatry to outline the kinds of models and dimensions likely to be relevant and to suggest some potential organizing schemas.

Table 6–2 presents a list of common themes in cultural formulations conducted by the Cultural Consultation Service of the Jewish General Hospital in Montreal (Kirmayer et al. 2014a). To some extent, these themes reflect the particular patient population referred

---

TABLE 6–2. **Common themes in cultural formulations**

Family systems issues

  Family and couple conflicts

  Changes in configuration of extended family

  Intergenerational issues

  Family honor and obligations

Exposure to trauma and violence

  Impact of war, torture, and organized violence

  Domestic violence

  Effects of violence on child development

  Posttraumatic stress disorder, depression, and other sequelae

Migration issues

  Stresses and loss during migration trajectory

  Uncertainty of refugee or immigration status

  Family separation and reunification

  Homesickness and mourning for culture

Cultural identity, acculturation, and adjustment

  Shifting/hybrid cultural identity

  Adjusting to life in host country postmigration

  Changing gender roles

  Changing social roles and community relations

Cultural models of illness and healing

  Modes of symptom expression and idioms of distress

  Illness explanatory models and causal attributions

  Cultural influences on social determinants of health

  Treatment choice and expectations for care

Other social, economic, and structural issues

  Stereotyping, prejudice, racism, and discrimination

  Social isolation and marginalization

  Unemployment and underemployment

  Poverty and economic uncertainty

Source. Adapted from Kirmayer et al. 2014a, p. 38.

to this service (i.e., a high proportion of newcomers to Canada, with many refugees and asylum seekers, as well as many migrants from South Asia, Africa, and the Middle East). The themes also reflect the particular conceptual frameworks that consultants working for the Cultural Consultation Service bring to bear to make sense of the cases. Clinicians working with other populations and employing other conceptual frameworks will likely highlight somewhat different themes. In the end, the validity and clinical relevance of the theme must be judged by how much it resonates with patients' own understandings and, especially, how well it leads to effective clinical interventions.

Typically, a cultural formulation involves many themes that are intertwined. Some of these are related to how patients understand their problems, and they are crucial for effective clinical communication, engagement, and negotiation of treatment plans. Other themes point toward specific mechanisms or processes that may give rise to particular symptoms or forms of psychopathology and that can be targeted with specific interventions. Explaining the symptoms and course of psychopathology in terms of underlying mechanisms is a goal of psychiatric science, and the hope is that this will lead to more effective treatments. However, the assumption is often that the main mechanisms of psychopathology will be found in disturbed neurophysiology. Cultural psychiatry suggests that social factors can also be understood as causal explanations that have their own psychophysiological, sociophysiological, and psychosocial mechanisms. The study of these mechanisms can lead to new kinds of causal explanations, which contribute to a case formulation in terms of pathological processes (and sources of resilience and healing) that can guide clinical intervention.

This potential for cultural formulation including mechanisms is illustrated in Table 6–3, which identifies some processes that can be used to think about the interactions of culture with psychopathology and clinical presentations. This is necessarily an open-ended list with no simple structure yet apparent. Both theoretical and empirical work are needed to develop systematic frameworks to guide clinical thinking.

Integrating the information derived from the CFI into clinical case formulations requires attention to events and experiences in the patient's past (e.g., personal and family history), the current context (e.g., stressors and supports), and the values and expectations that guide future options (e.g., aspirations, norms, constraints). These can be thought of at an individual level, but some of the dimensions of culture affect a whole group, community, or population and exert their effects both directly on individuals and indirectly through effects on others or on social institutions and environments. These influences often are not discrete events but instead occur over extended periods of time, affecting developmental trajectories or the course of illness. Hence, a temporal perspective is required.

The cultural formulation can be integrated into the standard medical case history, with relevant aspects assigned to the history of present illness, personal and family history, and mental status examination. However, these may not provide sufficient reminders to the clinician to consider processes related to specific dimensions of culture and social context. The CFI and OCF provide broad categories, but the process of translating this information into a case formulation suggests additional components or dimensions. Table 6–4 suggests another way to organize cultural formulation in terms of a grid that considers factors that influence illness at different stages in its course or evolution: 1) the causes of illness; 2) the form of illness experience and symptomatology; 3) coping and help seeking; 4) treatment response; 5) adaptation, functional impairment, and recovery; and 6) the social responses to these outcomes, which may include stigmatization and marginalization or support and integration. Each of these stages in the evolution of illness can also be thought of in terms of a nested hierarchy of system levels: subpersonal processes of cognition and emotion, personal psychodynamics or self-systems, interpersonal, family, community (including institutional settings such as work, school, or the health care system itself), nation

---

TABLE 6–3. **Potential mechanisms in cultural formulation**

Social and cultural contributors to etiology
  Social determinants of health
  Differential exposure to stressors or other causal agents
Cultural issues that give rise to specific types of conflict
  Intrapsychic
  Interpersonal
  Between the family and the ethnic community (locally or transnationally)
  Between the person, family, or community and the larger society or its institutions
Problems directly related to migration, citizenship status, and acculturation
Problems related to family systems dynamics influenced by cultural variations in the composition and structure of the family, gender- and age-related roles and norms, developmental transitions, and cultural notions of honor

---

or society, transnational networks, and global systems. Each of these levels and stages is embedded in larger temporal processes that include collective histories that may antecede and frame patients' individual experiences; developmental trajectories; autobiographical narratives of the self that govern identity and life projects; current social contexts; and future aspirations. This third dimension of time can be included within the cells of the two-dimensional grid or added as specific description of relevant contexts and temporal trajectories (Table 6–5).

Evidence-Based Cultural Formulation

Cultural formulation should be evidence based, but developing the relevant evidence requires psychiatric research that addresses the diversity of populations, settings, and problems to identify specific aspects of culture and context that influence psychopathology, treatment, and recovery (Whitley et al. 2011). The ways in which knowledge of specific sociocultural processes can be integrated into cultural formulations can be illustrated with a few examples from the research literature.

In terms of causal processes, culturally mediated developmental experiences may increase vulnerability or resilience to specific types of mental health problems. Histories of colonization, ethnic conflict, slavery, and other events give rise to social structures of inequality and structural violence that powerfully affect individuals' mental health (Metzl and Hansen 2014). During development, individuals will have differential exposures to adverse life events and potential resources for resilience that will influence their developmental trajectories. The ways in which individuals come to frame their identities—which are partly a consequence of these collective histories and developmental experiences but which, at some point, involve a measure of choice and active self-fashioning—have implications for their positioning and subsequent vulnerability to illness. Cultural contexts also may give rise to specific social determinants of health, such as poverty and economic inequality, racism and discrimination, and social marginalization (Braveman et al. 2011). For example, there is much evi-

TABLE 6–4.   A grid for cultural formulation

Systemic level	Causal factors	Course of illness				
		Symptoms and signs of illness	Coping and help seeking	Treatment response	Functioning, adaptation, and recovery	Social response
Subpersonal						
Personal						
Interpersonal						
Family						
Community						
Society						
Transnational						
Global systems						

TABLE 6–5. Temporal Frames in Cultural Formulaton

Temporal frames	Examples
Collective social history	Colonization, slavery, collective violence
Developmental history	Child-rearing practices
Personal history	Identity, migration, trauma, acculturation
Current contexts	Structural violence, racism, discrimination
Future	Expectations and aspirations

dence for increased rates of psychosis among some populations that migrate to northern Europe from southern countries or former colonies (Cantor-Graae 2007). This increase does not seem to reflect elevated rates in countries of origin but is an effect that occurs over time in the new country, and the risk for psychosis is, in some instances, still greater for the second generation (Bourque et al. 2011). It is unclear precisely what social factors contribute to this increased risk, but exposure to structural violence, racism, and discrimination may play an important role. Additionally, the discrepancy between expectations and opportunities as a result of inequalities may be an important causal factor in feelings of demoralization or "social defeat" (Luhrmann 2007). Understanding patients' migration history and current exposures to discrimination (including subtle forms of microaggression and structural barriers to educational and economic advancement) therefore may be an important part of assessing risk and devising interventions that can reduce vulnerability and promote recovery and well-being (Sue et al. 2007). Attention to discrimination and structural processes of disadvantage has implications for public health interventions and social policy as well. There is evidence, for example, that neighborhood ethnic density may play a buffering role for some ethnocultural groups, reducing the stressful effects of being a discriminated-against minority (Bosqui et al. 2014). Considering the neighborhoods where patients live may thus be an important part of clinical assessment to identify both stressors and sources of resilience.

The experience and expression of mental health problems are shaped by symptom and illness schemas and explanations (Gone and Kirmayer 2010). Illness schemas can give rise to culture-specific symptoms and, when the attribution or interpretation results in emotional distress or stigmatization, may actually exacerbate symptoms and result in distress and disability (Kirmayer and Sartorius 2009). Such vicious circles mediated by culture-specific attributions have been well described for panic attacks (Hinton and Good 2009).

Explanatory models can also influence the diagnostic process and the course of illness. For example, there is evidence that paranoid thinking among patients from some ethnoracial minority groups may reflect consequences of endemic racism and discrimination (Whaley and Geller 2007). Experiences of racism and discrimination may contribute to symptom presentation, making patients with primary affective disorders appear to have psychotic symptoms. Knowledge of local cultural norms is needed to judge the level of paranoid ideation that indicates psychopathology (Chapman et al. 2014). Systematic evaluation of cultural norms and contexts of illness expression can improve the accuracy of diagnoses of psychosis (Adeponle et al. 2012a, 2014).

Cultural factors influence the ways in which patients and their families cope with illness and seek help. There is evidence that underutilization of mental health services among many groups may reflect negative perceptions of health care institutions based on collective histories, past experiences, or specific illness interpretations (Snowden and Yamada 2005).

Adaptation to illness, treatment response, and recovery are all shaped by cultural histories, contexts, and values. Evidence suggests that negative expressed emotion in families can exacerbate psychotic illness and increase relapse rates. Culturally based styles of emotional expression, as well as illness explanations, may mitigate negative expressed emotion in families, with effects on the course of illness (Aguilera et al. 2010; Karno et al. 1987). Recognizing such factors can allow the clinician to tailor psychoeducational and systemic interventions to improve outcome.

Current discussions of recovery highlight the diverse ways in which people may find meaning in their symptoms and suffering and the ways they may prioritize different domains of their life to judge whether or not interventions are helpful (Whitley and Drake 2010). The meanings of suffering, and the values, goals, and aspirations against which illness and recovery are assessed, vary with culture and social position (Adeponle et al. 2012b).

The examples discussed in this section are only meant to illustrate how the information collected through the CFI can be organized in clinically relevant formulations. Knowledge of specific processes, based on experience and research, can guide both the process of collecting information and the formulation to yield an expanded problem list, treatment plan, and strategies for interventions. The refinement of methods of cultural formulation requires further research on social and cultural processes in psychopathology (Alarcón et al. 2002). Research may lead to the recognition of new kinds of mechanisms of psychopathology and recovery, and this, in turn, can inform methods of clinical case formulation.

A Research Agenda for the CFI

There is a need for research on the CFI itself, to refine its components and to evaluate its effective implementation and impact on clinical outcomes. Although the CFI is based on a wealth of clinical experience in diverse settings, its contents and scope can be enlarged by research on the social and cultural determinants of health that identifies the kinds of social adversity and predicaments that give rise to or exacerbate specific types of mental health problems and the kinds of individual and collective resources and coping strategies that promote recovery. At the same time, the CFI provides a way to assess clinically relevant dimensions of history and context that can be integrated into research on other dimensions of mental health problems, such as helping to identify particular contexts or modes of gene-environment interaction that contribute to the epigenetic and behavioral processes that contribute to psychopathology.

There is also a need for research on the clinical process of cultural assessment itself. In particular, researchers need to examine how the CFI actually works in various contexts, in terms of both process (looking at interviews with various process-oriented methods, including conversation analysis) and outcomes (in terms of what kind of information the CFI collects that makes a difference to recovery). Both qualitative and quantitative studies of the interview process and the subsequent integration of cultural knowledge in diagnostic assessment and treatment planning are needed (e.g., Adeponle et al. 2014). Studies comparing the effects of reassessment of patients using the CFI with standard assessment can clarify the kinds of clinically relevant information a culturally oriented interview obtains (e.g., Bäärnhielm and Scarpinati Rosso 2009; Scarpinati Rosso and Bäärnhielm 2012).

Efforts were made to make the CFI as concise as possible. In actual practice, the length of the interview will depend on the patient's responses and the domains of clinical concern. However, this concision raises questions about how adequately a brief interview such as the CFI can elicit crucial clinical information, There is no single "gold standard" for cultural assessment against which the CFI can be compared, but comparisons with lengthier, more comprehensive assessments would be useful to determine whether there are certain types of information, patients, or contexts that require other interview strategies. Novel methods for eliciting cultural information can be explored as complements or alternatives to the CFI; these include the use of maps, time lines, and drawings (e.g., Saint Arnault and Shimabukuro 2012).

The structure of the CFI was designed to follow a typical sequence in clinical interviewing: beginning with questions about the patient's presented complaints and concerns and their meaning and interpretation; then moving to broader questions about psychosocial stresses and supports, issues of cultural identity, help seeking, and expectations for care; and finally posing questions about the clinician-patient relationship. This order may need to be modified in certain situations. For example, sometimes addressing identity issues at the outset can promote clinical trust and engagement, forestalling early breakdowns in communication. This consideration may be particularly important in settings where the safety or legitimacy of the clinician or the institutional setting has been called into question by patients' past histories of exposure to racism, discrimination, or other forms of structural violence.

Research on the interview process with the CFI would look at the microdynamics of the clinical interaction with and without the inclusion of an interpreter or culture broker. It could compare different interview formats, sequences, and contents to identify modifications that can improve the assessment process.

The use of the CFI can also make a difference to treatment teams and organizations. For example, discussing the results of culturally oriented interviews in multidisciplinary case conferences can influence the dynamics of the group by providing an explicit place for the perspectives of disciplines devoted to social-contextual understanding of mental health problems (Dinh et al. 2012). Making optimal use of the skills of diverse disciplines in cultural formulation may involve changes in the professional roles, modes of interaction, and organizational structure. Research on the organizational and systemic models of culturally responsive care will be important to guide effective implementation of the CFI.

Ultimately, research that shows how the CFI makes a difference to clinical outcomes is needed. These clinical impacts of the CFI that may be assessed in research studies include changes in diagnosis, recognition of other situational problems, increased treatment adherence, and improvements in the clinician-patient relationship. Each of these may have direct and indirect effects on clinical outcomes. Clearly, if a major diagnosis changes as a result of cultural formulation, the patient is likely to receive a new, more appropriate treatment, with corresponding improvement in outcome. Identifying additional problems, beyond diagnosis, that can be addressed through psychosocial or other interventions should also have measurable impacts that will interact with treatment for any psychiatric disorder. Improving clinical engagement and adherence will ensure that treatments are successfully delivered. Improving clinical communication should help patients better understand their problems and make more appropriate and effective use of mental health services. Studies of the effectiveness of the CFI, therefore, should consider these multiple levels of outcome.

Promoting Use of the CFI Through Training and Continuing Education

Clinical training aims to transmit the knowledge and skills needed to work in a wide variety of settings to address the range of problems presented by diverse patient populations. Learning to use the CFI should be a core clinical competency (Kirmayer et al. 2012). The CFI provides a way to explore the cultural context and meanings of illness experience and help seeking and therefore facilitates acquiring generic cultural competence.

In psychiatric training, practice in the use of the CFI (coupled with training in working with interpreters and culture brokers) can provide residents with basic skills to work in a wide variety of settings. Indeed, it is important to emphasize that the CFI can be used with any patient, and having trainees use it with patients from their own cultural background provides a good opportunity to help them become aware of their own cultural assumptions and the contexts in which they work, as well as the wide variations in experience within even familiar groups (Kirmayer et al. 2014b). This kind of pedagogical experience can help reduce the tendency to stereotype others and to encourage a more dynamic view of the interplay of individual agency with cultural resources and constraints. Intercultural work also requires a high tolerance for ambiguity and uncertainty, and training programs must provide safe spaces and role models for this work (Guzder and Rousseau 2013).

Accreditation standards for mental health training programs need to move beyond general criteria for cultural competence to include specific mention of the use of the CFI and related skills. New generations of clinicians will likely encounter the CFI as they become familiar with DSM-5, but particular efforts need to be made to reach earlier generations of clinicians currently in practice. Quality assurance and recertification standards that include cultural competence can make explicit note of skill in using the CFI as a criterion. To implement these standards, there is a need to develop further training materials, such as the videos that accompany this volume, as well as self-assessment tools that can be presented through continuing education workshops and online self-guided training and assessment.

Although developed as an interview protocol to explore cultural issues, the CFI operationalizes some key aspects of a patient-centered approach to health care (Mezzich et al. 2010) and therefore has implications beyond the challenge of addressing cultural diversity. The CFI also can be a useful tool in the training context, with relevance beyond psychiatry. Rooted as it is in the perspectives of medical anthropology, the CFI is useful for teaching patient-centered medicine at all levels of training (see Chapter 5, "Cultural Competence in Psychiatric Education Using the Cultural Formulation Interview"). Indeed, use of the CFI and similar interviews in primary care and internal medicine settings can help students and faculty grasp the elements of a person-centered approach to clinical assessment (Groleau et al. 2013). At the same time, the issues identified through the CFI provide an opportunity for trainees to learn more about specific social and cultural topics relevant to the care of particular kinds of patients and populations.

Conclusion

Culture is increasingly recognized as central to diagnostic assessment both to improve diagnostic accuracy and to deepen understanding of patients' problems in context. DSM-5 directly addresses several of the limitations of previous DSM editions. Concepts of culture have been refined based on current social science research. The OCF has been expanded to include a greater range of relevant cultural issues. Most significantly, DSM-5 includes the core CFI, the CFI–Informant Version, and the supplementary modules, which can guide clinical assessment of cultural dimensions. To become part of the tool kit of mental health practitioners, the CFI needs to be included in clinical training programs and incorporated into mental health services. Its increased use can contribute to improving mental health care for members of minority groups, migrants, and other communities likely to have distinctive illness experiences due to cultural differences. However, culture is important for everyone, and integrating the CFI into standard care can foster more patient-centered approaches that give due attention to each individual's unique history, lifeworld, and values that are rooted in particular social and cultural contexts. This attention to history and context is a matter not only of recognizing culture as a key dimension of identity but also as a path to more personalized care.

Culture is a moving target, undergoing constant transformation, and the ways in which identity is understood and clinically relevant aspects of social context are recognized today will likely change over time. Changing meanings of culture and social contexts will also give rise to new mechanisms of psychopathology or adaptation and corresponding new areas to explore in the CFI. For example, Internet use has created new forms of behavioral addiction or problematic use of media, and these will have neurobiological, psychological, social, and economic consequences for individuals— all of which may be relevant to cultural formulation that aims to clarify mechanisms, guide treatment planning, and predict outcome (Kirmayer et al. 2013).

Clearly, there is an ethical mandate to address culture when it constitutes a crucial element in delivering safe and effective care. Problems in communication due to cultural and linguistic differences can result in misunderstandings, inaccurate diagnostic assessments, inappropriate treatments, poor clinical engagement and adherence, and, ultimately, negative outcomes. Concerns about the time and effort involved in cultural formulation must be weighed against these potentially serious consequences of ignoring difference. Of course, there are limits to how well we as clinicians can know patients' experience, because of divergent life trajectories and situations. The ethical implications of the epistemic challenges and constraints of cultural assessment also point to a deeper problem of empathy at the limits of understanding (Kirmayer 2008). Recognizing the limits of understanding calls for cultural humility (Tervalon and Murray-García 1998). Indeed, the philosopher Emmanuel Levinas (Levinas 2003) argued that this situation is basic to the human condition—that is, each person is at once familiar and like us but also fundamentally different, strange and "other," and the recognition of otherness or alterity calls us to an ethical stance of respect, concern, and protectiveness toward the vulnerable other. This recognition that our understanding of the other is always limited and incomplete enjoins us to remain open to the other and to maintain a stance of collaborative inquiry in the clinical relationship. This ethics of inquiry grounded in respect and responsibility informs the guidelines for the CFI and can help the clinician tailor and adapt the interview process to meet the needs of each patient.

KEY CLINICAL POINTS

- Culture and context are relevant to every aspect of illness experience and health care for patients from every background.
- The Cultural Formulation Interview (CFI) addresses a key component of person-centered care by focusing attention on patients' experience as well as the social contexts of their illness.
- Further work is needed to systematize the process of translating the information collected through the CFI into a case formulation.
- Changes in organizational structure, training, and accreditation to ensure cultural safety and competence are needed to promote the use of the CFI.
- The meanings and mental health implications of cultural identity, knowledge, and practices need to be revisited as our local social worlds and global networks continue to evolve.

Questions

1. What are some of the differences between the DSM framing of disorders and a cultural perspective?

2. What trade-offs between practical and theoretical considerations were involved in the development of the CFI?

3. What are useful frameworks for organizing and recording the results of the CFI?

4. What kinds of research are needed for further development of the CFI?

5. How can the use of cultural formulation be promoted and institutionalized in psychiatric practice?

References

Adeponle AB, Thombs BD, Groleau D, et al: Using the cultural formulation to resolve uncertainty in diagnoses of psychosis among ethnoculturally diverse patients. Psychiatr Serv 63(2):147–153, 2012a 22302332

Adeponle AB, Whitley R, Kirmayer LJ: Cultural contexts and constructions of recovery, in Recovery of People With Mental Illness: Philosophical and Related Perspectives. Edited by Rudnick A. New York, Oxford University Press, 2012b pp. 109–132

Adeponle AB, Groleau D, Jarvis GE, et al: Clinician reasoning in the use of the cultural formulation to resolve uncertainty in the diagnosis of psychosis. Cult Med Psychiatry 2014 [Epub ahead of print]

Aguilera A, López SR, Breitborde NJ, et al: Expressed emotion and sociocultural moderation in the course of schizophrenia. J Abnorm Psychol 119(4):875–885, 2010 21090883

Alarcón RD, Bell CC, Kirmayer LJ, et al: Beyond the funhouse mirrors: research agenda on culture and psychiatric diagnosis, in A Research Agenda for DSM-V. Edited by Kupfer DJ, First MB, Regier DA. Washington, DC, American Psychiatric Publishing, 2002 pp 219–281

American Psychiatric Association: Diagnostic and Statistical Manual of Mental Disorders, 3rd Edition, Revised. Washington, DC, American Psychiatric Association, 1987

American Psychiatric Association: Diagnostic and Statistical Manual of Mental Disorders, 4th Edition. Washington, DC, American Psychiatric Association, 1994

American Psychiatric Association: Diagnostic and Statistical Manual of Mental Disorders, 5th Edition. Arlington, VA, American Psychiatric Association, 2013

Bäärnhielm S, Scarpinati Rosso M: The Cultural Formulation: a model to combine nosology and patients' life context in psychiatric diagnostic practice. Transcult Psychiatry 46(3):406–428, 2009 19837779

Bosqui TJ, Hoy K, Shannon C: A systematic review and meta-analysis of the ethnic density effect in psychotic disorders. Soc Psychiatry Psychiatr Epidemiol 49(4):519–529, 2014 24114240

Bourque F, van der Ven E, Malla A: A meta-analysis of the risk for psychotic disorders among first- and second-generation immigrants. Psychol Med 41(5):897–910, 2011 20663257

Braveman P, Egerter S, Williams DR: The social determinants of health: coming of age. Annu Rev Public Health 32:381–398, 2011 21091195

Campbell WH, Rohrbaugh RM: The Biopsychosocial Formulation Manual: A Guide for Mental Health Professionals. New York, Routledge, 2006

Cantor-Graae E: The contribution of social factors to the development of schizophrenia: a review of recent findings. Can J Psychiatry 52(5):277–286, 2007 17542378

Chapman LK, DeLapp R, Williams MT: Impact of race, ethnicity, and culture on the expression and assessment of psychopathology, in Adult Psychopathology and Diagnosis. Edited by Beidel D, Frueh BC, Hersen M. New York, John Wiley and Sons, 2014, pp 131–162

Chisolm MS, Lyketsos CG: Systematic Psychiatric Evaluation: A Step-by-Step Guide to Applying the Perspectives of Psychiatry. Baltimore, MD, Johns Hopkins University Press, 2012

Dinh NM, Groleau D, Kirmayer LJ, et al: Influence of the DSM-IV Outline for Cultural Formulation on multidisciplinary case conferences in mental health. Anthropol Med 19(3):261–276, 2012 22309357

Doucerain M, Dere J, Ryder AG: Travels in hyper-diversity: multiculturalism and the contextual assessment of acculturation. Int J Intercult Relat 37:686–699, 2013

Gone JP, Kirmayer LJ: On the wisdom of considering culture and context in psychopathology, in Contemporary Directions in Psychopathology: Scientific Foundations of the DSM-V and ICD-11. Edited by Millon T, Krueger RF, Simonsen E. New York, Guilford, 2010, pp 72–96

Good M-JD, Willen SS, Hannah SD, et al (eds): Shattering Culture: American Medicine Responds to Cultural Diversity. New York, Russell Sage Foundation, 2011

Groleau D, D'Souza NA, Bélanger E: Integrating the illness meaning and experience of patients: the McGill Illness Narrative Interview Schedule as a PCM clinical communication tool. Int J Pers Cent Med 3:140–146, 2013

Guzder J, Rousseau C: A diversity of voices: the McGill 'Working with Culture' seminars. Cult Med Psychiatry 37(2):347–364, 2013 23549711

Harkness AR, Reynolds SM, Lilienfeld SO: A review of systems for psychology and psychiatry: adaptive systems, Personality Psychopathology Five (PSY-5), and the DSM-5. J Pers Assess 96(2):121–139, 2014 23941204

Hays PA: Addressing Cultural Complexities in Practice: Assessment, Diagnosis, and Therapy, 2nd Edition. Washington, DC, American Psychological Association, 2008

Hinton DE, Good BJ (eds): Culture and Panic Disorder. Stanford, CA, Stanford University Press, 2009

Hofmann SG: Toward a cognitive-behavioral classification system for mental disorders. Behav Ther 45(4):576–587, 2014 24912469

Johnstone L, Dallos R: Formulation in Psychology and Psychotherapy: Making Sense of People's Problems, 2nd Edition. New York, Routledge, 2013

Karno M, Jenkins JH, de la Selva A, et al: Expressed emotion and schizophrenic outcome among Mexican-American families. J Nerv Ment Dis 175(3):143–151, 1987 3819710

Kirmayer LJ: Empathy and alterity in cultural psychiatry. Ethos 36:457–474, 2008

Kirmayer LJ: Multicultural medicine and the politics of recognition. J Med Philos 36(4):410–423, 2011 21804073

Kirmayer LJ: Rethinking cultural competence. Transcult Psychiatry 49(2):149–164, 2012 22508634

Kirmayer LJ, Sartorius N: Cultural models and somatic syndromes, in Somatic Presentations of Mental Disorders: Refining the Research Agenda for DSM-V. Edited by Dimsdale JE, Patel V, Xin Y, et al. Washington, DC, American Psychiatric Publishing, 2009, pp 23–46

Kirmayer LJ, Thombs BD, Jurcik T, et al: Use of an expanded version of the DSM-IV Outline for Cultural Formulation on a cultural consultation service. Psychiatr Serv 59(6):683–686, 2008 18511590

Kirmayer LJ, Fung K, Rousseau C, et al: Guidelines for training in cultural psychiatry. Can J Psychiatry 57(insert):1–16, 2012

Kirmayer LJ, Raikhel E, Rahimi S: Cultures of the Internet: identity, community and mental health. Transcult Psychiatry, 50(2):165–191 2013 23740931

Kirmayer LJ, Guzder J, Rousseau C (eds): Cultural Consultation: Encountering the Other in Mental Health Care. New York, Springer, 2014a

Kirmayer LJ, Rousseau C, Jarvis GE, et al: The cultural context of clinical assessment, in Psychiatry, 4th Edition. Edited by Tasman A, Maj M, First MB, et al. New York, Wiley, 2014b, pp 54–66

Levinas E: Humanism of the Other. Translated by Poller N. Chicago, University of Illinois Press, 2003

Lewis-Fernández R, Aggarwal NK, Bäärnhielm S, et al: Culture and psychiatric evaluation: operationalizing cultural formulation for DSM-5. Psychiatry 77(2):130–154, 2014 24865197

Luhrmann TM: Social defeat and the culture of chronicity: or, why schizophrenia does so well over there and so badly here. Cult Med Psychiatry 31(2):135–172, 2007 17534703

Metzl JM, Hansen H: Structural competency: theorizing a new medical engagement with stigma and inequality. Soc Sci Med 103:126–133, 2014 24507917

Mezzich JE, Kirmayer LJ, Kleinman A, et al: The place of culture in DSM-IV. J Nerv Ment Dis 187(8):457–464, 1999 10463062

Mezzich JE, Caracci G, Fabrega H Jr, et al: Cultural formulation guidelines. Transcult Psychiatry 46(3):383–405, 2009 19837778

Mezzich JE, Salloum IM, Cloninger CR, et al: Person-centred integrative diagnosis: conceptual bases and structural model. Can J Psychiatry 55(11):701–708, 2010 21070697

Reilly J, Newton R: Formulation: a proposal for a more structured, longitudinal approach. Australas Psychiatry 19(4):301–305, 2011 21879865

Saint Arnault D, Shimabukuro S: The Clinical Ethnographic Interview: a user-friendly guide to the cultural formulation of distress and help seeking. Transcult Psychiatry 49(2):302–322, 2012 22194348

Scarpinati Rosso M, Bäärnhielm S: Use of the Cultural Formulation in Stockholm: a qualitative study of mental illness experience among migrants. Transcult Psychiatry 49(2):283–301, 2012 22508638

Snowden LR, Yamada AM: Cultural differences in access to care. Annu Rev Clin Psychol 1:143–166, 2005 17716085

Sue DW, Capodilupo CM, Torino GC, et al: Racial microaggressions in everyday life: implications for clinical practice. Am Psychol 62(4):271–286, 2007 17516773

Tervalon M, Murray-García J: Cultural humility versus cultural competence: a critical distinction in defining physician training outcomes in multicultural education. J Health Care Poor Underserved 9(2):117–125, 1998 10073197

Thomas P: Psychiatry in Context: Experience, Meaning and Communities. Monmouth, UK, PCCS Books, 2014

Weerasekera P: Multiperspective case formulation: a step towards treatment integration. Malabar, FL, Krieger Publishing Company, 1996

Whaley AL, Geller PA: Toward a cognitive process model of ethnic/racial biases in clinical judgment. Rev Gen Psychol 11:75–96, 2007

Whitley R, Drake RE: Recovery: a dimensional approach. Psychiatr Serv 61(12):1248–1250, 2010 21123410

Whitley R, Rousseau C, Carpenter-Song E, et al: Evidence-based medicine: opportunities and challenges in a diverse society. Can J Psychiatry 56(9):514–522, 2011 21959026

Suggested Readings

Kirmayer LJ, Guzder J, Rousseau C: Conclusion: the future of cultural consultation, in Cultural Consultation: Encountering the Other in Mental Health Care. Edited by Kirmayer LJ, Rousseau C, Guzder J. New York, Springer, 2013, pp 335–351

Kirmayer LJ, Rousseau C, Jarvis GE, et al: The cultural context of clinical assessment, in Psychiatry, 4th Edition. Edited by Tasman A, Maj M, First MB, et al. New York, Wiley, 2014, pp 54–66

Metzl JM, Hansen H: Structural competency: theorizing a new medical engagement with stigma and inequality. Soc Sci Med 103:126–133, 2014 24507917

Multicultural Mental Health Resource Centre: Available at: http://www.mmhrc.ca. Accessed February 12, 2015.

Appendixes A–C

Cultural Formulation Interview–Core Version

Cultural Formulation Interview–Informant Version

Supplementary Modules

The APA is offering the Cultural Formulation Interview (including the Informant Version) and the Supplementary Modules to the core Cultural Formulation Interview for further research and clinical evaluation. They should be used in research and clinical settings as potentially useful tools to enhance clinical understanding and decision-making and not as the sole basis for making a clinical diagnosis. Additional information can be found in DSM-5 in the Section III chapter "Cultural Formulation." The APA requests that clinicians and researchers provide further data on the usefulness of these cultural formulation interviews at http://www.dsm5.org/Pages/Feedback-Form.aspx. To request permission for any other use beyond what is stipulated above, contact: http://www.appi.org/CustomerService/Pages/Permissions.aspx

Appendix A

Cultural Formulation Interview (CFI)–Core Version

The Cultural Formulation Interview (CFI) is a set of 16 questions that clinicians may use to obtain information during a mental health assessment about the impact of culture on key aspects of an individual's clinical presentation and care. In the CFI, *culture* refers to

- The values, orientations, knowledge, and practices that individuals derive from membership in diverse social groups (e.g., ethnic groups, faith communities, occupational groups, veterans groups).
- Aspects of an individual's background, developmental experiences, and current social contexts that may affect his or her perspective, such as geographical origin, migration, language, religion, sexual orientation, or race/ethnicity.
- The influence of family, friends, and other community members (the individual's *social network*) on the individual's illness experience.

The CFI is a brief semistructured interview for systematically assessing cultural factors in the clinical encounter that may be used with any individual. The CFI focuses on the individual's experience and the social contexts of the clinical problem. The CFI follows a person-centered approach to cultural assessment by eliciting information from the individual about his or her own views and those of others in his or her social network. This approach is designed to avoid stereotyping, in that each individual's cultural knowledge affects how he or she interprets illness experience and guides how he or she seeks help. Because the CFI concerns the individual's personal views, there are no right or wrong answers to these questions. The interview follows and is available online at www.psychiatry.org/practice/dsm/dsm5/online-assessment-measures.

The CFI is formatted as two text columns. The left-hand column contains the instructions for administering the CFI and describes the goals for each interview domain. The questions in the right-hand column illustrate how to explore these domains, but they are not meant to be exhaustive. Follow-up questions may be needed to clarify individuals' answers. Questions may be rephrased as needed. The CFI is intended as a guide to cultural assessment and should be used flexibly to maintain a natural flow of the interview and rapport with the individual.

The CFI is best used in conjunction with demographic information obtained prior to the interview in order to tailor the CFI questions to address the individual's background and current situation. Specific demographic domains to be explored with the CFI will vary across individuals and settings. A comprehensive assessment may include place of birth, age, gender, racial/ethnic origin, marital status, family composition, education, language fluencies, sexual orientation, religious or spiritual affiliation, occupation, employment, income, and migration history.

The CFI can be used in the initial assessment of individuals in all clinical settings, regardless of the cultural background of the individual or of the clinician. Individuals and clinicians who appear to share the same cultural background may nevertheless differ in ways that are relevant to care. The CFI may be used in its entirety, or components may be incorporated into a clinical evaluation as needed. The CFI may be especially helpful when there is

- Difficulty in diagnostic assessment owing to significant differences in the cultural, religious, or socioeconomic backgrounds of clinician and the individual.
- Uncertainty about the fit between culturally distinctive symptoms and diagnostic criteria.
- Difficulty in judging illness severity or impairment.
- Disagreement between the individual and clinician on the course of care.
- Limited engagement in and adherence to treatment by the individual.

The CFI emphasizes four domains of assessment: Cultural Definition of the Problem (questions 1–3); Cultural Perceptions of Cause, Context, and Support (questions 4–10); Cultural Factors Affecting Self-Coping and Past Help Seeking (questions 11–13); and Cultural Factors Affecting Current Help Seeking (questions 14–16). Both the person-centered process of conducting the CFI and the information it elicits are intended to enhance the cultural validity of diagnostic assessment, facilitate treatment planning, and promote the individual's engagement and satisfaction. To achieve these goals, the information obtained from the CFI should be integrated with all other available clinical material into a comprehensive clinical and contextual evaluation. An Informant version of the CFI can be used to collect collateral information on the CFI domains from family members or caregivers.

Supplementary modules have been developed that expand on each domain of the CFI and guide clinicians who wish to explore these domains in greater depth. Supplementary modules have also been developed for specific populations, such as children and adolescents, elderly individuals, and immigrants and refugees. These supplementary modules are referenced in the CFI under the pertinent subheadings and are available online at www.psychiatry.org/practice/dsm/dsm5/online-assessment-measures.

Supplementary modules used to expand each CFI subtopic are noted in parentheses.

GUIDE TO INTERVIEWER	**INSTRUCTIONS TO THE INTERVIEWER ARE ITALICIZED.**
The following questions aim to clarify key aspects of the presenting clinical problem from the point of view of the individual and other members of the individual's social network (i.e., family, friends, or others involved in current problem). This includes the problem's meaning, potential sources of help, and expectations for services.	*INTRODUCTION FOR THE INDIVIDUAL:* I would like to understand the problems that bring you here so that I can help you more effectively. I want to know about *your* experience and ideas. I will ask some questions about what is going on and how you are dealing with it. Please remember there are no right or wrong answers.

CULTURAL DEFINITION OF THE PROBLEM

CULTURAL DEFINITION OF THE PROBLEM

(Explanatory Model, Level of Functioning)

Elicit the individual's view of core problems and key concerns.	1. What brings you here today?
Focus on the individual's own way of understanding the problem.	*IF INDIVIDUAL GIVES FEW DETAILS OR ONLY MENTIONS SYMPTOMS OR A MEDICAL DIAGNOSIS, PROBE:*
Use the term, expression, or brief description elicited in question 1 to identify the problem in subsequent questions (e.g., "your conflict with your son").	People often understand their problems in their own way, which may be similar to or different from how doctors describe the problem. How would *you* describe your problem?
Ask how individual frames the problem for members of the social network.	2. Sometimes people have different ways of describing their problem to their family, friends, or others in their community. How would you describe your problem to them?
Focus on the aspects of the problem that matter most to the individual.	3. What troubles you most about your problem?

CULTURAL PERCEPTIONS OF CAUSE, CONTEXT, AND SUPPORT

CAUSES

(Explanatory Model, Social Network, Older Adults)

This question indicates the meaning of the condition for the individual, which may be relevant for clinical care.	4. Why do you think this is happening to you? What do you think are the causes of your [PROBLEM]?
Note that individuals may identify multiple causes, depending on the facet of the problem they are considering.	*PROMPT FURTHER IF REQUIRED:* Some people may explain their problem as the result of bad things that happen in their life, problems with others, a physical illness, a spiritual reason, or many other causes.
Focus on the views of members of the individual's social network. These may be diverse and vary from the individual's.	5. What do others in your family, your friends, or others in your community think is causing your [PROBLEM]?

GUIDE TO INTERVIEWER	**INSTRUCTIONS TO THE INTERVIEWER ARE ITALICIZED.**

STRESSORS AND SUPPORTS

(Social Network, Caregivers, Psychosocial Stressors, Religion and Spirituality, Immigrants and Refugees, Cultural Identity, Older Adults, Coping and Help Seeking)

Elicit information on the individual's life context, focusing on resources, social supports, and resilience. May also probe other supports (e.g., from co-workers, from participation in religion or spirituality).

6. Are there any kinds of support that make your [PROBLEM] better, such as support from family, friends, or others?

Focus on stressful aspects of the individual's environment. Can also probe, e.g., relationship problems, difficulties at work or school, or discrimination.

7. Are there any kinds of stresses that make your [PROBLEM] worse, such as difficulties with money, or family problems?

ROLE OF CULTURAL IDENTITY

(Cultural Identity, Psychosocial Stressors, Religion and Spirituality, Immigrants and Refugees, Older Adults, Children and Adolescents)

Sometimes, aspects of people's background or identity can make their [PROBLEM] better or worse. By **background** or **identity**, I mean, for example, the communities you belong to, the languages you speak, where you or your family are from, your race or ethnic background, your gender or sexual orientation, or your faith or religion.

Ask the individual to reflect on the most salient elements of his or her cultural identity. Use this information to tailor questions 9–10 as needed.

8. For you, what are the most important aspects of your background or identity?

Elicit aspects of identity that make the problem better or worse.

9. Are there any aspects of your background or identity that make a difference to your [PROBLEM]?

Probe as needed (e.g., clinical worsening as a result of discrimination due to migration status, race/ethnicity, or sexual orientation).

Probe as needed (e.g., migration-related problems; conflict across generations or due to gender roles).

10. Are there any aspects of your background or identity that are causing other concerns or difficulties for you?

CULTURAL FACTORS AFFECTING SELF-COPING AND PAST HELP SEEKING

SELF-COPING

(Coping and Help Seeking, Religion and Spirituality, Older Adults, Caregivers, Psychosocial Stressors)

Clarify self-coping for the problem.

11. Sometimes people have various ways of dealing with problems like [PROBLEM]. What have you done on your own to cope with your [PROBLEM]?

GUIDE TO INTERVIEWER	INSTRUCTIONS TO THE INTERVIEWER ARE *ITALICIZED.*

PAST HELP SEEKING

(Coping and Help Seeking, Religion and Spirituality, Older Adults, Caregivers, Psychosocial Stressors, Immigrants and Refugees, Social Network, Clinician-Patient Relationship)

Elicit various sources of help (e.g., medical care, mental health treatment, support groups, work-based counseling, folk healing, religious or spiritual counseling, other forms of traditional or alternative healing).

Probe as needed (e.g., "What other sources of help have you used?").

Clarify the individual's experience and regard for previous help.

12. Often, people look for help from many different sources, including different kinds of doctors, helpers, or healers. In the past, what kinds of treatment, help, advice, or healing have you sought for your [PROBLEM]?

PROBE IF DOES NOT DESCRIBE USE-FULNESS OF HELP RECEIVED:

What types of help or treatment were most useful? Not useful?

BARRIERS

(Coping and Help Seeking, Religion and Spirituality, Older Adults, Psychosocial Stressors, Immigrants and Refugees, Social Network, Clinician-Patient Relationship)

Clarify the role of social barriers to help seeking, access to care, and problems engaging in previous treatment.

Probe details as needed (e.g., "What got in the way?").

13. Has anything prevented you from getting the help you need?

PROBE AS NEEDED:

For example, money, work or family commitments, stigma or discrimination, or lack of services that understand your language or background?

CULTURAL FACTORS AFFECTING CURRENT HELP SEEKING

PREFERENCES

(Social Network, Caregivers, Religion and Spirituality, Older Adults, Coping and Help Seeking)

Clarify individual's current perceived needs and expectations of help, broadly defined.

Probe if individual lists only one source of help (e.g., "What other kinds of help would be useful to you at this time?").

Focus on the views of the social network regarding help seeking.

Now let's talk some more about the help you need.

14. What kinds of help do you think would be most useful to you at this time for your [PROBLEM]?

15. Are there other kinds of help that your family, friends, or other people have suggested would be helpful for you now?

CLINICIAN-PATIENT RELATIONSHIP

(Clinician-Patient Relationship, Older Adults)

Elicit possible concerns about the clinic or the clinician-patient relationship, including perceived racism, language barriers, or cultural differences that may undermine goodwill, communication, or care delivery.

Probe details as needed (e.g., "In what way?").

Address possible barriers to care or concerns about the clinic and the clinician-patient relationship raised previously.

Sometimes doctors and patients misunderstand each other because they come from different backgrounds or have different expectations.

16. Have you been concerned about this and is there anything that we can do to provide you with the care you need?

Appendix B

Cultural Formulation Interview (CFI)–Informant Version

The CFI–Informant Version collects collateral information from an informant who is knowledgeable about the clinical problems and life circumstances of the identified individual. This version can be used to supplement information obtained from the core CFI or can be used instead of the core CFI when the individual is unable to provide information—as might occur, for example, with children or adolescents, floridly psychotic individuals, or persons with cognitive impairment.

GUIDE TO INTERVIEWER	INSTRUCTIONS TO THE INTERVIEWER ARE ITALICIZED.
The following questions aim to clarify key aspects of the presenting clinical problem from the informant's point of view. This includes the problem's meaning, potential sources of help, and expectations for services.	*INTRODUCTION FOR THE INFORMANT:* I would like to understand the problems that bring your family member/friend here so that I can help you and him/her more effectively. I want to know about *your* experience and ideas. I will ask some questions about what is going on and how you and your family member/friend are dealing with it. There are no right or wrong answers.

RELATIONSHIP WITH THE PATIENT

Clarify the informant's relationship with the individual and/or the individual's family.	1. How would you describe your relationship to [INDIVIDUAL OR TO FAMILY]? *PROBE IF NOT CLEAR:* How often do you see [INDIVIDUAL]?

CULTURAL DEFINITION OF THE PROBLEM

Elicit the informant's view of core problems and key concerns.	2. What brings your family member/friend here today?
Focus on the informant's way of understanding the individual's problem.	*IF INFORMANT GIVES FEW DETAILS OR ONLY MENTIONS SYMPTOMS OR A MEDICAL DIAGNOSIS, PROBE:*
Use the term, expression, or brief description elicited in question 1 to identify the problem in subsequent questions (e.g., "her conflict with her son").	People often understand problems in their own way, which may be similar or different from how doctors describe the problem. How would *you* describe [INDIVIDUAL'S] problem?
Ask how informant frames the problem for members of the social network.	3. Sometimes people have different ways of describing the problem to family, friends, or others in their community. How would *you* describe [INDIVIDUAL'S] problem to them?
Focus on the aspects of the problem that matter most to the informant.	4. What troubles you most about [INDIVIDUAL'S] problem?

GUIDE TO INTERVIEWER	INSTRUCTIONS TO THE INTERVIEWER ARE *ITALICIZED.*

CULTURAL PERCEPTIONS OF CAUSE, CONTEXT, AND SUPPORT

CAUSES

This question indicates the meaning of the condition for the informant, which may be relevant for clinical care.

Note that informants may identify multiple causes depending on the facet of the problem they are considering.

5. Why do you think this is happening to [INDIVIDUAL]? What do you think are the causes of his/her [PROBLEM]?

    PROMPT FURTHER IF REQUIRED:

    Some people may explain the problem as the result of bad things that happen in their life, problems with others, a physical illness, a spiritual reason, or many other causes.

Focus on the views of members of the individual's social network. These may be diverse and vary from the informant's.

6. What do others in [INDIVIDUAL'S] family, his/her friends, or others in the community think is causing [INDIVIDUAL'S] [PROBLEM]?

STRESSORS AND SUPPORTS

Elicit information on the individual's life context, focusing on resources, social supports, and resilience. May also probe other supports (e.g., from co-workers, from participation in religion or spirituality).

7. Are there any kinds of supports that make his/her [PROBLEM] better, such as from family, friends, or others?

Focus on stressful aspects of the individual's environment. Can also probe, e.g., relationship problems, difficulties at work or school, or discrimination.

8. Are there any kinds of stresses that make his/her [PROBLEM] worse, such as difficulties with money, or family problems?

ROLE OF CULTURAL IDENTITY

Sometimes, aspects of people's background or identity can make the [PROBLEM] better or worse. By **background** or **identity**, I mean, for example, the communities you belong to, the languages you speak, where you or your family are from, your race or ethnic background, your gender or sexual orientation, and your faith or religion.

Ask the informant to reflect on the most salient elements of the individual's cultural identity. Use this information to tailor questions 10–11 as needed.

9. For you, what are the most important aspects of [INDIVIDUAL'S] background or identity?

Elicit aspects of identity that make the problem better or worse.

10. Are there any aspects of [INDIVIDUAL'S] background or identity that make a difference to his/her [PROBLEM]?

Probe as needed (e.g., clinical worsening as a result of discrimination due to migration status, race/ethnicity, or sexual orientation).

Probe as needed (e.g., migration-related problems; conflict across generations or due to gender roles).

11. Are there any aspects of [INDIVIDUAL'S] background or identity that are causing other concerns or difficulties for him/her?

| GUIDE TO INTERVIEWER | INSTRUCTIONS TO THE INTERVIEWER ARE *ITALICIZED.* |

CULTURAL FACTORS AFFECTING SELF-COPING AND PAST HELP SEEKING

SELF-COPING

Clarify individual's self-coping for the problem.

12. Sometimes people have various ways of dealing with problems like [PROBLEM]. What has [INDIVIDUAL] done on his/her own to cope with his/her [PROBLEM]?

PAST HELP SEEKING

Elicit various sources of help (e.g., medical care, mental health treatment, support groups, work-based counseling, folk healing, religious or spiritual counseling, other alternative healing).

Probe as needed (e.g., "What other sources of help has he/she used?").

Clarify the individual's experience and regard for previous help.

13. Often, people also look for help from many different sources, including different kinds of doctors, helpers, or healers. In the past, what kinds of treatment, help, advice, or healing has [INDIVIDUAL] sought for his/her [PROBLEM]?

PROBE IF DOES NOT DESCRIBE USE-FULNESS OF HELP RECEIVED:

What types of help or treatment were most useful? Not useful?

BARRIERS

Clarify the role of social barriers to help-seeking, access to care, and problems engaging in previous treatment.

Probe details as needed (e.g., "What got in the way?").

14. Has anything prevented [INDIVIDUAL] from getting the help he/she needs?

PROBE AS NEEDED:

For example, money, work or family commitments, stigma or discrimination, or lack of services that understand his/her language or background?

CULTURAL FACTORS AFFECTING CURRENT HELP SEEKING

PREFERENCES

Clarify individual's current perceived needs and expectations of help, broadly defined, from the point of view of the informant.

Probe if informant lists only one source of help (e.g., "What other kinds of help would be useful to [INDIVIDUAL] at this time?").

Focus on the views of the social network regarding help seeking.

Now let's talk about the help [INDIVIDUAL] needs.

15. What kinds of help would be most useful to him/her at this time for his/her [PROBLEM]?

16. Are there other kinds of help that [INDIVIDUAL'S] family, friends, or other people have suggested would be helpful for him/her now?

CLINICIAN-PATIENT RELATIONSHIP

Elicit possible concerns about the clinic or the clinician-patient relationship, including perceived racism, language barriers, or cultural differences that may undermine goodwill, communication, or care delivery.

Probe details as needed (e.g., "In what way?").

Address possible barriers to care or concerns about the clinic and the clinician-patient relationship raised previously.

Sometimes doctors and patients misunderstand each other because they come from different backgrounds or have different expectations.

17. Have you been concerned about this, and is there anything that we can do to provide [INDIVIDUAL] with the care he/she needs?

Appendix C
Supplementary Modules to the Core Cultural Formulation Interview (CFI)

Guidelines for Implementing the CFI Supplementary Modules

These modules supplement the core Cultural Formulation Interview and can help clinicians conduct a more comprehensive cultural assessment. The first eight supplementary modules explore the domains of the core CFI in greater depth. The next three modules focus on populations with specific needs, such as children and adolescents, older adults, and immigrants and refugees. The last module explores the experiences and views of individuals who perform caregiving functions, in order to clarify the nature and cultural context of caregiving and how they affect social support in the immediate environment of the individual receiving care. In addition to these supplementary modules, an Informant version of the core CFI collects collateral information on the CFI domains from family members or caregivers.

Clinicians may use these supplementary modules in two ways:

- As adjuncts to the core CFI for additional information about various aspects of illness affecting diverse populations. The core CFI refers to pertinent modules under each subheading to facilitate such use of the modules.

- As tools for in-depth cultural assessment independent of the core CFI. Clinicians may administer one, several, or all modules depending on what areas of an individual's problems they would like to elaborate.

Clinicians should note that a few questions in the modules duplicate questions in the core CFI (indicated by an asterisk [*]) or in other modules. This makes it possible to administer each module independently. Clinicians who use the modules as an adjunct to the core CFI or who administer the modules independently may skip redundant questions.

As with the core CFI, follow-up questions may be needed to clarify the individual's answers. Questions may be rephrased as needed. The modules are intended as a guide to cultural assessment and should be used flexibly to maintain a natural flow of the interview and rapport with the individual. In situations where the individual cannot answer these questions (e.g., due to cognitive impairment or severe psychosis) these questions can be administered to the identified caregiver. The caregiver's own perspective can also be ascertained using the module for caregivers.

In every module, instructions to the interviewer are in *italics*. The modules may be administered during the initial clinical evaluation, at a later point in care, or several times over the course of treatment. Multiple administrations may reveal additional information as rapport develops, especially when assessing the patient-clinician relationship.

Please refer to DSM-5 Section III, chapter "Cultural Formulation," sections "Outline for Cultural Formulation" and "Cultural Formulation Interview (CFI) for additional suggestions regarding this type of interview.

---

1. Explanatory Model

Related Core CFI Questions: 1, 2, 3, 4, 5 Some of the core CFI questions are repeated below and are marked with an asterisk (*). The CFI question that is repeated is indicated in brackets.

GUIDE TO INTERVIEWER: This module aims to clarify the individual's understanding of the problem based on his or her ideas about cause and mechanism (explanatory models) and past experiences of, or knowing someone with, a similar problem (illness prototypes). The individual may identify the problem as a symptom, a specific term or expression (e.g., "nerves," "being on edge"), a situation (e.g., loss of a job), or a relationship (e.g., conflict with others). In the examples below, the individual's own words should be used to replace "[PROBLEM]". If there are multiple problems, each relevant problem can be explored. The following questions may be used to elicit the individual's understanding and experience of that problem or predicament.

INTRODUCTION FOR THE INDIVIDUAL BEING INTERVIEWED: I would like to understand the problems that bring you here so that I can help you more effectively. I will be asking you some questions to learn more about your own ideas about the causes of your problems and the way they affect your daily life.

General understanding of the problem
1. *Can you tell me more about how you understand your [PROBLEM]? [RELATED TO CFI Q#1-2.]
2. What did you know about your [PROBLEM] before it affected you?

Illness prototypes
3. Had you ever had anything like your [PROBLEM] before? Please tell me about that.
4. Do you know anyone else, or heard of anyone else, with this [PROBLEM]? If so, please describe that person's [PROBLEM] and how it affected that person. Do you think this will happen to you too?
5. Have you seen on television, heard on the radio, read in a magazine, or found on the internet anything about your [PROBLEM]? Please tell me about it.

Causal explanations
6. *Can you tell me what you think caused your [PROBLEM]? (*PROBE AS NEEDED*: Is there more than one cause that may explain it?] [RELATED TO CFI Q#4.)
7. Have your ideas about the cause of the [PROBLEM] changed? How? What changed your ideas about the cause?
8. *What do people in your family, friends, or others in your community think caused the [PROBLEM]? (*PROBE AS NEEDED*: Are their ideas about it different from yours? How so?) [RELATED TO CFI Q#5.]
9. How do you think your [PROBLEM] affects your body? Your mind? Your spiritual wellbeing?

Course of illness
10. What usually happens to people who have this [PROBLEM]? In your own case, what do you think is likely to happen?
11. Do you consider your [PROBLEM] to be serious? Why? What is the worst that could happen?
12. How concerned are other people in your family, friends or community about your having this [PROBLEM]? Please tell me about that.

Help seeking and treatment expectations
13. What do you think is the best way to deal with this kind of problem?
14. What do your family, friends, or others in your community think is the best way of dealing with this kind of problem?

---

2. Level of Functioning

Related Core CFI Question: 3

GUIDE TO INTERVIEWER: The following questions aim to clarify the individual's level of functioning in relation to his or her own priorities and those of the cultural reference group. The interview begins with a general question about everyday activities that are important for the individual. Questions follow about domains important for positive health (social relations, work/school, economic viability, and resilience). Questions should be kept relatively broad and open to elicit the individual's own priorities and perspective. For a more detailed evaluation of specific domains of functioning, a standard instrument such as the WHO-DAS II may be used together with this interview.

INTRODUCTION FOR THE INDIVIDUAL BEING INTERVIEWED: I would like to know about the daily activities that are most important to you. I would like to better understand how your [PROBLEM] has affected your ability to perform these activities, and how your family and other people around you have reacted to this.

1. How has your [PROBLEM] affected your ability to do the things you need to do each day, that is, your daily activities and responsibilities?
2. How has your [PROBLEM] affected your ability to interact with your family and other people in your life?
3. How has your [PROBLEM] affected your ability to work?
4. How has your [PROBLEM] affected your financial situation?
5. How has your [PROBLEM] affected your ability to take part in community and social activities?
6. How has your [PROBLEM] affected your ability to enjoy everyday life?
7. Which of these concerns are most troubling to you?
8. Which of these concerns are most troubling to your family and to other people in your life?

3. Social Network

Related Core CFI Questions: 5, 6, 12, 15

GUIDE TO INTERVIEWER: *The following questions identify the influences of the informal social network on the individual's problem.* **Informal social network** *refers to family, friends and other social contacts through work, places of prayer/worship or other activities and affiliations. Question #1 identifies important people in the individual's social network, and the clinician should tailor subsequent questions accordingly. These questions aim to elicit the social network's response, the individual's interpretation of how this would impact on the problem, and the individual's preferences for involving members of the social network in care.*

INTRODUCTION FOR THE INDIVIDUAL BEING INTERVIEWED: I would like to know more about how your family, friends, colleagues, co-workers, and other important people in your life have had an impact on your [PROBLEM].

Composition of the individual's social network
1. Who are the most important people in your life at present?
2. Is there anyone in particular whom you trust and can talk with about your [PROBLEM]? Who? Anyone else?

Social network understanding of problem
3. Which of your family members, friends, or other important people in your life know about your [PROBLEM]?
4. What ideas do your family and friends have about the nature of your [PROBLEM]? How do they understand your [PROBLEM]?
5. Are there people who do not know about your [PROBLEM]? Why do they not know about your [PROBLEM]?

Social network response to problem
6. What advice have family members and friends given you about your [PROBLEM]?
7. Do your family, friends, and other people in your life treat you differently because of your [PROBLEM]? How do they treat you differently? Why do they treat you differently?
8. (IF HAS NOT TOLD FAMILY OR FRIENDS ABOUT PROBLEM): Can you tell me more about why you have chosen not to tell family or friends about the [PROBLEM]? How do you think they would respond if they knew about your [PROBLEM]?

Social network as a stress/buffer
9. What have your family, friends, and other people in your life done to make your [PROBLEM] better or easier for you to deal with? (*IF UNCLEAR:* How has that made your [PROBLEM] better?)
10. What kinds of help or support were you expecting from family or friends?
11. What have your family, friends, and other people in your life done to make your [PROBLEM] worse or harder for you to deal with? (*IF UNCLEAR:* How has that made your [PROBLEM] worse?)

Social network in treatment
12. Have any family members or friends helped you get treatment for your [PROBLEM]?
13. What would your family and friends think about your coming here to receive treatment?
14. Would you like your family, friends, or others to be part of your treatment? If so, who would you like to be involved and how?
15. How would involving family or friends make a difference in your treatment?

4. Psychosocial Stressors

Related Core CFI Questions: 7, 9, 10, 12

GUIDE TO INTERVIEWER: *The aim of these questions is to further clarify the stressors that have aggravated the problem or otherwise affected the health of the individual. (Stressors that initially caused the problem are covered in the module on Explanatory Models.) In the examples below, the individual's own words should be used to replace "[STRESSORS]". If there are multiple stressors, each relevant stressor can be explored.*

INTRODUCTION FOR THE INDIVIDUAL BEING INTERVIEWED: You have told me about some things that make your [PROBLEM] worse. I would like to learn more about that.

1. Are there things going on that have made your [PROBLEM] worse, for example, difficulties with family, work, money, or something else? Tell me more about that.
2. How are the people around you affected by these [STRESSORS]?
3. How do you cope with these [STRESSORS]?
4. What have other people suggested about coping with these [STRESSORS]?
5. What else could be done about these [STRESSORS]?

GUIDE TO INTERVIEWER: *Patients may be reluctant to discuss areas of their life they consider sensitive, which may vary across cultural groups. Asking specific questions may help the patient discuss these stressors. Insert questions about relevant stressors here. For example:*

6. Have you experienced discrimination or been treated badly as a result of your background or identity? By background or identity I mean, for example, the communities you belong to, the languages you speak, where you or your family are from, your racial or ethnic background, your gender or sexual orientation, and your faith or religion. Have these experiences had an impact on [STRESSORS] or your [PROBLEM]?

---

5. Spirituality, Religion, and Moral Traditions

Related Core CFI Questions: 6, 7, 8, 9, 10, 11, 12, 14, 15

GUIDE TO INTERVIEWER: *The following questions aim to clarify the influence of spirituality, religion, and other moral or philosophical traditions on the individual's problems and related stresses. People may have multiple spiritual, moral, and religious affiliations or practices. If the individual reports having specific beliefs or practices, inquire about the level of involvement in that tradition and its impact on coping with the clinical problem. In the examples below, the individual's own words should be used to replace "[NAME(S) OF SPIRITUAL, RELIGIOUS OR MORAL TRADITION(S)]". If the individual identifies more than one tradition, each can be explored. If the individual does not describe a specific tradition, use the phrase "spirituality, religion or other moral traditions" instead of the specific name of a tradition (e.g., Q5: "What role do spirituality, religion or other moral traditions play in your everyday life?").*

INTRODUCTION FOR THE INDIVIDUAL BEING INTERVIEWED: To help you more effectively, I would like to ask you some questions about the role that spirituality, religion or other moral traditions play in your life and how they may have influenced your dealing with the problems that bring you here.

Spiritual, religious, and moral identity
1. Do you identify with any particular spiritual, religious or moral tradition? Can you tell me more about that?
2. Do you belong to a congregation or community associated with that tradition?
3. What are the spiritual, religious or moral tradition backgrounds of your family members?
4. Sometimes people participate in several traditions. Are there any other spiritual, religious or moral traditions that you identify with or take part in?

Role of spirituality, religion, and moral traditions
5. What role does [NAME(S) OF SPIRITUAL, RELIGIOUS OR MORAL TRADITION(S)] play in your everyday life?
6. What role does [NAME(S) OF SPIRITUAL, RELIGIOUS OR MORAL TRADITION(S)] play in your family, for example, family celebrations or choices in marriage or schooling?
7. What activities related to [NAME(S) OF SPIRITUAL, RELIGIOUS OR MORAL TRADITION(S)] do you carry out in the home, for example, prayers, meditation, or special dietary laws? How often do you carry out these activities? How important are these activities in your life?
8. What activities do you engage in outside the home related to [NAME(S) OF SPIRITUAL, RELIGIOUS OR MORAL TRADITION(S)], for example, attending ceremonies or participating in a [CHURCH, TEMPLE OR MOSQUE]? How often do you attend? How important are these activities in your life?

Relationship to the [PROBLEM]
9. How has [NAME(S) OF SPIRITUAL, RELIGIOUS OR MORAL TRADITION(S)] helped you cope with your [PROBLEM]?
10. Have you talked to a leader, teacher or others in your [NAME(S) OF SPIRITUAL, RELIGIOUS OR MORAL TRADITION(S)] community, about your [PROBLEM]? How have you found that helpful?
11. Have you found reading or studying [BOOK(S) OF SPIRITUAL, RELIGIOUS OR MORAL TRADITION(S), (E.G. BIBLE, KORAN)], or listening to programs related to [NAME(S) OF SPIRITUAL, RELIGIOUS OR MORAL TRADITION(S)] on TV, radio, the Internet or other media [e.g., DVD, tape] to be helpful? In what way?
12. Have you found any practices related to [NAME(S) OF SPIRITUAL, RELIGIOUS OR MORAL TRADITION(S)], like prayer, meditation, rituals, or pilgrimages to be helpful to you in dealing with [PROBLEM]? In what way?

Potential stresses or conflicts related to spirituality, religion, and moral traditions
13. Have any issues related to [NAME(S) OF SPIRITUAL, RELIGIOUS OR MORAL TRADITION(S)] contributed to [PROBLEM]?
14. Have you experienced any personal challenges or distress in relation to your [NAME(S) OF SPIRITUAL, RELIGIOUS OR MORAL TRADITION(S)] identity or practices?
15. Have you experienced any discrimination due to your [NAME(S) OF SPIRITUAL, RELIGIOUS OR MORAL TRADITION(S)] identity or practices?
16. Have you been in conflict with others over spiritual, religious or moral issues?

6. Cultural Identity

Related Core CFI Questions: 6, 7, 8, 9, 10 Some of the core CFI questions are repeated below and are marked with an asterisk (*). The CFI question that is repeated is indicated in brackets.

GUIDE TO INTERVIEWER: *This module aims to further clarify the individual's cultural identity and how this has influenced the individual's health and well being. The following questions explore the individual's cultural identity and how this may have shaped his or her current problem. We use the word* **culture** *broadly to refer to all the ways the individual understands his or her identity and experience in terms of groups, communities or other collectivities, including national or geographic origin, ethnic community, racialized categories, gender, sexual orientation, social class, religion/spirituality, and language.*

INTRODUCTION FOR THE INDIVIDUAL BEING INTERVIEWED: Sometimes peoples' background or identity influences their experience of illness and the type of care they receive. In order to better help you, I would like to understand your own background or identity. By background or identity I mean, for example, the communities you belong to, the languages you speak, where you or your family are from, your racial or ethnic background, your gender or sexual orientation, and your faith or religion.

National, Ethnic, Racial Background
1. Where were you born?
2. Where were your parents and grandparents born?
3. How would you describe your family's national, ethnic, and/or racial background?
4. In terms of your background, how do you usually describe yourself to people outside your community? Sometimes people describe themselves somewhat differently to members of their own community. How do you describe yourself to them?
5. Which part of your background do you feel closest to? Sometimes this varies, depending on what aspect of your life we are talking about. What about at home? Or at work? Or with friends?
6. Do you experience any difficulties related to your background, such as discrimination, stereotyping, or being misunderstood?
7. *Is there anything about your background that might impact on your [PROBLEM] or impact on your health or health care more generally? [RELATED TO CFI Q#9.]

Language
8. What languages do you speak fluently?
9. What languages did you speak growing up?
10. What languages are spoken at home? Which of these do you speak?
11. What languages do you use at work or school?
12. What language would you prefer to use in getting health care?
13. What languages do you read? Write?

Migration
GUIDE TO INTERVIEWER: *If the individual was born in another country, ask questions 1-7. [For refugees, refer to the module on Immigrants and Refugees to obtain more detailed migration history.]*

14. When did you come to this country?
15. What made you decide to leave your country of origin?
16. How has your life changed since coming here?
17. What do you miss about the place or community you came from?
18. What are your concerns for your own and your family's future here?
19. What is your current status in this country (e.g., refugee claimant, citizen, student visa, work permit)? *Be aware this may be a sensitive or confidential issue for the individual, if they have precarious status.*
20. How has migration influenced your health or that of your family?
21. Is there anything about your migration experience or current status in this country that has made a difference to your [PROBLEM]?
22. Is there anything about your migration experience or current status that might influence your ability to get the right kind of help for your [PROBLEM]?

Spirituality, Religion, and Moral Traditions

23. Do you identify with any particular religious, moral or spiritual tradition?

GUIDE TO INTERVIEWER: *In the next question, the individual's own words should be used to replace "[NAME(S) OF SPIRITUAL, RELIGIOUS OR MORAL TRADITION(S)]".*

24. What role does [NAME(S) OF SPIRITUAL, RELIGIOUS OR MORAL TRADITION(S)] play in your everyday life?
25. Do your family members share your spiritual, religious or moral traditions? Can you tell me more about that?

Gender Identity

INTRODUCTION FOR THE INDIVIDUAL BEING INTERVIEWED: Some individuals feel that their gender [e.g. the social roles and expectations they have related to being male, female, transgender, genderqueer, or intersex] influences their health and the kind of health care they need.

GUIDE TO INTERVIEWER: *In the examples below, the individual's own words should be used to replace "[GENDER]". The interviewer may need to exemplify or explain the term 'GENDER" with relevant wording (e.g., "being a man," "being a transgender woman").*

26. Do you feel that your [GENDER] has influenced <u>your [PROBLEM] or your health</u> more generally?
27. Do you feel that your [GENDER] has influenced <u>your ability to get the kind of health care</u> you need?
28. Do you feel that health care providers have certain assumptions or attitudes about you or your [PROBLEM] because of your [GENDER]?

Sexual Orientation Identity

INTRODUCTION FOR THE INDIVIDUAL BEING INTERVIEWED: Sexual orientation may also be important to individuals and their comfort in seeking health care. I would like to ask you some questions about your sexual orientation. Are you comfortable answering questions about your sexual orientation?

29. How would you describe your sexual orientation (e.g., heterosexual, gay, lesbian, bisexual, queer, pansexual, asexual)?
30. Do you feel that your sexual orientation has influenced <u>your [PROBLEM] or your health</u> more generally?
31. Do you feel that your sexual orientation influences <u>your ability to get the kind of health care</u> you need for your [PROBLEM]?
32. Do you feel that health care providers have assumptions or attitudes about you or your [PROBLEM] that are related to your sexual orientation?

Summary

33. You have told me about different aspects of your background and identity and how this has influenced your health and well being. Are there other aspects of your identity I should know about to better understand your health care needs?
34. What are the most important aspects of your background or identity in relation to [PROBLEM]?

7. Coping and Help-Seeking

Related Core CFI Questions: 6, 11, 12, 14, 15 Some of the core CFI questions are repeated below and are marked with an asterisk (*). The CFI question that is repeated is indicated in brackets.

GUIDE TO INTERVIEWER: This module aims to clarify the individual's ways of coping with the current problem. The individual may have identified the problem as a symptom or mentioned a term or expression (e.g., "nerves," "being on edge," spirit possession), or a situation (e.g., loss of a job), or a relationship (e.g., conflict with others). In the examples below, the individual's own words should be used to replace "[PROBLEM]". If there are multiple problems, each relevant problem can be explored. The following questions may be used to learn more about the individual's understanding and experiencing of that problem.

INTRODUCTION FOR THE INDIVIDUAL BEING INTERVIEWED: I would like to understand the problems that bring you here so that I can help you more effectively. I will be asking you questions about how you have tried to cope with your problems and get help for them.

Self-coping
1. *Can you tell me more about how you are trying to cope with [PROBLEM] <u>at this time</u>? Has that way of coping with it been helpful? If so, how? [RELATED TO CFI Q#11.]
2. *Can you tell me more about how you tried to cope with the [PROBLEM] or with similar problems <u>in the past</u>? Was that way of coping with it helpful? If so, how? [RELATED TO CFI Q#11.]
3. Have you sought help for your [PROBLEM] on the internet, by reading books, by viewing television shows, or by listening to audiotapes, videos or other sources? If so, which of these? What did you learn? Was it helpful?
4. Do you engage <u>by yourself</u> in practices related to a spiritual, religious or moral tradition to help you cope with your [PROBLEM]? For example, prayer, meditation, or other practices that you carry out by yourself?
5. Have you sought help for your [PROBLEM] from natural remedies or medications that you take without a doctor's prescription, such as over-the-counter medicines? If so, which natural remedies or medications? Were they helpful?

Social network
6. *Have you told a <u>family member</u> about your [PROBLEM]? Have family members helped you cope with the [PROBLEM]? If so, how? What did they suggest you do to cope with the [PROBLEM]? Was it helpful? [RELATED TO CFI Q#15.]
7. *Have you told a <u>friend or co-worker</u> about your [PROBLEM]? Have friends or co-workers helped you cope with the [PROBLEM]? If so, how? What did they suggest you do to cope with the [PROBLEM]? Was it helpful? [RELATED TO CFI Q#15.]

Help- and treatment-seeking beyond social network
8. Are you involved in activities <u>that involve other people</u> related to a spiritual, religious or moral tradition? For example, do you go to worship or religious gatherings, speak with other people in your religious group or speak with the religious or spiritual leader? Have any of these been helpful in coping with [PROBLEM]? In what way?
9. Have you ever tried to get help for your [PROBLEM] from your <u>general doctor</u>? If so, who and when? What treatment did they give? Was it helpful?
10. Have you ever tried to get help for your [PROBLEM] from a <u>mental health clinician</u>, such as a counselor, psychologist, social worker, psychiatrist, or other professional? If so, who and when? What treatment did they give? Was it helpful?
11. Have you sought help from <u>any other kind of helper</u> to cope with your [PROBLEM] other than going to the doctor, for example, a chiropractor, acupuncturist, homeopath, or other kind of healer? What kind of treatment did they recommend to resolve the problem? Was it helpful?

Current treatment episode
12. What were the circumstances that led to your coming here for treatment for your [PROBLEM]? Did anyone suggest you come here for treatment? If so, who, and why did he or she suggest you come here?
13. What help are you hoping to get here [at this clinic] for your [PROBLEM]?

8. Patient–Clinician Relationship

Related Core CFI Question: 16 Some of the core CFI questions are repeated below and are marked with an asterisk (*). The CFI question that is repeated is indicated in brackets.

GUIDE TO INTERVIEWER: *The following questions address the role of culture in the patient–clinician relationship with respect to the individual's presenting concerns and to the clinician's evaluation of the individual's problem. We use the word* **culture** *broadly to refer to all the ways the individual understands his or her identity and experience in terms of groups, communities or other collectivities, including national or geographic origin, ethnic community, racialized categories, gender, sexual orientation, social class, religion/spirituality, and language.*

The first set of questions evaluates four domains in the clinician-patient relationship from the point of view of the patient: experiences, expectations, communication, and possibility of collaboration with the clinician. The second set of questions is directed to the clinician to guide reflection on the role of cultural factors in the clinical relationship, the assessment, and treatment planning.

INTRODUCTION FOR THE PATIENT: I would like to learn about how it has been for you to talk with me and other clinicians about your [PROBLEM] and your health more generally. I will ask some questions about your views, concerns, and expectations.

QUESTIONS FOR THE PATIENT:

1. What kind of experiences have you had with clinicians in the past? What was most helpful to you?
2. Have you had difficulties with clinicians in the past? What did you find difficult or unhelpful?
3. Now let's talk about the help that you would like to get here. Some people prefer clinicians of a similar background (for example, age, race, religion, or some other characteristic) because they think it may be easier to understand each other. Do you have any preference or ideas about what kind of clinician might understand you best?
4. *Sometimes differences among patients and clinicians make it difficult for them to understand each other. Do you have any concerns about this? If so, in what way? [RELATED TO CFI Q#16.]

GUIDE TO INTERVIEWER: *Question #5 addresses the patient-clinician relationship moving forward in treatment. It elicits the patient's expectations of the clinician and may be used to start a discussion on how the two of them can collaborate in the individual's care.*

5. What patients expect from their clinicians is important. As we move forward in your care, how can we best work together?

QUESTIONS FOR THE CLINICIAN AFTER THE INTERVIEW:

1. How did you feel about your relationship with the patient? Did cultural similarities and differences influence your relationship? In what way?
2. What was the quality of communication with the patient? Did cultural similarities and differences influence your communication? In what way?
3. If you used an interpreter, how did the presence of an interpreter or his/her way of interpreting influence your relationship or your communication with the patient and the information you received?
4. How do the patient's cultural background or identity, life situation, and/or social context influence your understanding of his/her problem and your diagnostic assessment?
5. How do the patient's cultural background or identity, life situation, and/or social context influence your treatment plan or recommendations?
6. Did the clinical encounter confirm or call into question any of your prior ideas about the cultural background or identity of the patient? If so, in what way?
7. Are there aspects of your own identity that may influence your attitudes toward this patient?

9. School-Age Children and Adolescents

Related Core CFI Questions: 8, 9, 10

GUIDE TO INTERVIEWER: This supplement is directed to adolescents and mature school-age children. It should be used in conjunction with standard child mental health assessments that evaluate family relations (including intergenerational issues), peer relations, and the school environment. The aim of these questions is to identify, from the perspective of the child/youth, the role of age-related cultural expectations, the possible cultural divergences between school, home, and the peer group, and whether these issues impact on the situation or problem that brought the youth for care. The questions indirectly explore cultural challenges, stressors and resilience, and issues of cultural hybridity, mixed ethnicity or multiple ethnic identifications. Peer group belonging is important to children and adolescents, and questions exploring ethnicity, religious identity, racism or gender difference should be included following the child's lead. Some children may not be able to answer all questions; clinicians should select and adapt questions to ensure they are developmentally appropriate for the individual. Children should not be used as informants to provide socio-demographic information on the family or an explicit analysis of the cultural dimensions of their problems. An Addendum lists cultural aspects of development and parenting that can be evaluated during parents' interviews.

INTRODUCTION FOR THE CHILD/YOUTH: We have talked about the concerns of your family. Now I would like to know more about how you feel about being ___ years old.

Feelings of age appropriateness in different settings
1. Do you feel you are like other children/youth your age? In what way?
2. Do you sometimes feel different from other children/youth your age? In what way?
3. *IF THE CHILD/YOUTH ACKNOWLEDGES SOMETIMES FEELING DIFFERENT:* Does this feeling of being different happen more at home, at school, at work, and/or some other place?
4. Do you feel your family is different from other families?
5. Do you use different languages? With whom and when?
6. Does your name have any special meaning for you? Your family? Your community?
7. Is there something special about you that you like or that you are proud of?

Age-related stressors and supports
8. What <u>do</u> you like about being a child/youth at home? At school? With friends?
9. What <u>don't</u> you like about being a child/youth at home? At school? With friends?
10. Who is there to support you when you feel you need it? At home? At school? Among your friends?

Age-related expectations
GUIDE TO INTERVIEWER: Concepts of childhood and age-appropriate behavior vary significantly across cultures. The aim of these questions is to elicit the normative frame(s) of the child /family and how this may be different from other cultural environments.

11. What do your <u>parents or grandparents</u> expect from a child/youth your age? (*CLARIFY:* For example, chores, schoolwork, play, religious observance.)
12. What do your <u>school teachers</u> expect from a child/youth your age?
13. *IF INDIVIDUAL HAS SIBLINGS:* What do your <u>siblings</u> expect from a child/youth your age? (*CLARIFY:* For example, babysitting, help with homework, dating, dress.)
14. What do other <u>children/youth your age</u> expect from a child/youth your age?

Transition to adulthood/maturity (FOR ADOLESCENTS ONLY)
15. Are there any important celebrations or events in your community to recognize reaching a certain age or growing up?
16. When is a youth considered ready to become an adult <u>in your family or community</u>?
17. When is a youth considered ready to become an adult <u>according to your school teachers</u>?
18. What is good or difficult about becoming a young woman or a young man in your family? In your school? In your community?
19. How do you feel about "growing up" or becoming an adult?
20. In what ways are your life and responsibilities different from the life and responsibilities of your parents?

ADDENDUM FOR PARENTS' INTERVIEW
GUIDE TO INTERVIEWER: Information on cultural influences on development and parenting is best obtained by interviewing the child's parents or caretakers. In addition to issues directly related to presenting problems, it is useful to inquire about:

- The child's particular place in the family (e.g., oldest boy, only girl)
- The process of naming the child (Who chose the name? Does it have special meaning? Who else is called like this?)
- Developmental milestones in the culture of origin of the mother (and father): expected age for weaning, walking, toilet training, speaking. Vision of normal autonomy/dependency, appropriate disciplining and so on
- Perceptions of age-appropriate behaviors (e.g., age for staying home alone, participation in chores, religious observance, play)
- Child-adult relations (e.g., expression of respect, eye contact, physical contact)
- Gender relations (expectations around appropriate girl-boy behavior, dress code)
- Languages spoken at home, in daycare, at school
- The importance of religion, spirituality, and community in family life and related expectations for the child.

10. Older Adults

Related Core CFI Questions: 5, 6, 7, 8, 9, 10, 12, 13, 15, 16

GUIDE TO INTERVIEWER: *The following questions are directed to older adults. The goal of these questions is to identify the role of cultural conceptions of aging and age-related transitions on the illness episode.*

INTRODUCTION FOR THE INDIVIDUAL BEING INTERVIEWED: I would like to ask some questions to better understand your problem and how we can help you with it, taking into account your age and specific experiences.

Conceptions of aging and cultural identity
1. How would you describe a person of your age?
2. How does your experience of aging compare to that of your friends and relatives who are of a similar age?
3. Is there anything about being your age that helps you cope with your current life situation?

Conceptions of aging in relationship to illness attributions and coping
4. How does being older influence your [PROBLEM]? Would it have affected you differently when you were younger?
5. Are there ways that being older influences how you deal with your [PROBLEM]? Would you have dealt with it differently when you were younger?

Influence of comorbid medical problems and treatments on illness
6. Have you had health problems due to your age?
7. How have your health conditions or the treatments for your health conditions affected <u>your [PROBLEM]</u>?
8. Are there any ways that your health conditions or treatments influence how you <u>deal with</u> your [PROBLEM]?
9. Are there things that are important to you that you are unable to do because of your health or age?

Quality and nature of social supports and caregiving
10. Who do you rely on for help or support in your daily life in general? Has this changed now that you are going through [PROBLEM]?
11. How has [PROBLEM] affected your relationships with family and friends?
12. Are you receiving the amount and kind of support you expected?
13. Do the people you rely on share your view of your [PROBLEM]?

Additional age-related transitions
14. Are there other changes you are going through related to aging that are important for us to know about in order to help you with your [PROBLEM]?

Positive and negative attitudes towards aging and clinician-patient relationship
15. How has your age affected how health providers treat you?
16. Have any people, including health care providers, discriminated against you or treated you poorly because of your age? Can you tell me more about that? How has this experience affected your [PROBLEM] or how you deal with it?
17. *[IF THERE IS A SIGNIFICANT AGE DIFFERENCE BETWEEN PROVIDER AND PATIENT:]* Do you think that the difference in our ages will influence our work in any way? If so, how?

11. Immigrants and Refugees

Related Core CFI Questions: 7, 8, 9, 10, 13

GUIDE TO INTERVIEWER: The following questions aim to collect information from refugees and immigrants about their experiences of migration and resettlement. Many refugees have experienced stressful interviews with officials or health professionals in their home country, during the migration process (which may involve prolonged stays in refugee camps or other precarious situations), and in the receiving country, so it may take longer than usual for the interviewee to feel comfortable with and trust the interview process. When patient and clinician do not share a high level of fluency in a common language, accurate language translation is essential.

INTRODUCTION FOR THE INDIVIDUAL BEING INTERVIEWED: Leaving one's country of origin and resettling elsewhere can have a great impact on people's lives and health. To better understand your situation, I would like to ask you some questions related to your journey here from your country of origin.

Background information
1. What is your country of origin?
2. How long have you been living here in _____ (HOST COUNTRY)?
3. When and with whom did you leave _____ (COUNTRY OF ORIGIN)?
4. Why did you leave _____ (COUNTRY OF ORIGIN)?

Pre-migration difficulties
5. Prior to arriving in _____ (HOST COUNTRY), were there any challenges in your country of origin that you or your family found especially difficult?
6. Some people experience hardship, persecution, or even violence before leaving their country of origin. Has this been the case for you or members of your family? Can you tell me something about your experiences?

Migration-related losses and challenges
7. Of the persons important/close to you, who stayed behind?
8. Often people leaving a country experience losses. Did you or any of your family members experience losses upon leaving the country? If so, what are they?
9. Were there any challenges on your journey to _____ (HOST COUNTRY) that you or your family found especially difficult?
10. Do you or your family miss anything about your way of life in (COUNTRY OF ORIGIN)?

Ongoing relationship with country of origin
11. Do you have concerns about relatives that remain in (COUNTRY OF ORIGIN)?
12. Do relatives in (COUNTRY OF ORIGIN) have any expectations of you?

Resettlement and new life
13. Have you or your family experienced any difficulties related to your visa, citizenship, or refugee status here in _____ (HOST COUNTRY)?
14. Are there any (other) challenges or problems you or others in your family are facing related to your resettlement here?
15. Has coming to (HOST COUNTRY) resulted in something positive for you or your family? Can you tell me more about that?

Relationship with problem
16. Is there anything about your migration experience or current status in this country that has made a difference to your [PROBLEM]?
17. Is there anything about your migration experience or current status that might make it easier or harder to get help for your [PROBLEM]?

Future expectations
18. What hopes and plans do you have for you and your family in the coming years?

_____

12. Caregivers

Related Core CFI Questions: 6, 12, 14

GUIDE TO INTERVIEWER: *This module is designed to be administered to individuals who provide caregiving for the individual being assessed with the CFI. This module aims to explore the nature and cultural context of caregiving, and the social support and stresses in the immediate environment of the individual receiving care, from the perspective of the caregiver.*

INTRODUCTION FOR THE CAREGIVER: People like yourself who take care of the needs of patients are very important participants in the treatment process. I would like to understand your relationship with [INDIVIDUAL RECEIVING CARE] and how you help him/her with his/her problems and concerns. By *help,* I mean support in the home, community, or clinic. Knowing more about that will help us plan his/her care more effectively.

Nature of relationship
1. How long have you been taking care of [INDIVIDUAL RECEIVING CARE]? How did this role for you start?
2. How are you connected to [INDIVIDUAL RECEIVING CARE]?

Caregiving activities and cultural perceptions of caregiving
3. How do you help him/her with the [PROBLEM] or with day-to-day activities?
4. What is most rewarding about helping him/her?
5. What is most challenging about helping him/her?
6. How, if at all, has his/her [PROBLEM] changed your relationship?

Sometimes caregivers like yourself are influenced in doing what they do by cultural traditions of helping others, such as beliefs and practices in your family or community. By cultural traditions I mean, for example, what is done in the communities you belong to, where you or your family are from, or among people who speak your language or who share your race or ethnic background, your gender or sexual orientation, or your faith or religion.

7. Are there any cultural traditions that influence how you approach helping [INDIVIDUAL RECEIVING CARE]?
8. Is the amount or kind of help you are giving him/her different in any way from what would be expected in the community that you come from or the one he/she comes from? Is it different from what society in general would expect?

Social context of caregiving
9. *[IF CAREGIVER IS A FAMILY MEMBER:]* How do you, as a family, cope with this [PROBLEM]?
10. Are there others, such as family members, friends, or neighbors, who also help him/her with the [PROBLEM]? If so, what do they do?
11. How do you feel about how much or how little others are helping with his/her [PROBLEM]?

Clinical support for caregiving
12. How do you see yourself helping to provide care to [INDIVIDUAL RECEIVING CARE] now and in the future?
13. *[IF UNCLEAR:]* How do you see yourself helping with the care that he/she receives in this clinic?
14. How can we make it easier for you to be able to help [INDIVIDUAL RECEIVING CARE] with the [PROBLEM]?

INDEX

Page numbers printed in **boldface** refer to tables or figures.